# Handbook of Therapeutic

The *Handbook of Therapeutic Storytelling* enables people in the healing professions to utilise storytelling, pictures and metaphors as interventions to help their patients.

Communicating in parallel worlds and using simple images and solutions can help to generate positive attitudes, which can then be nurtured and enhanced to great effect. Following an "Introduction" to the therapeutic use of stories, which closes with helpful "Instructions for use", the book is divided into two parts, both of which contain a series of easily accessible chapters. Part One includes stories with specific therapeutic applications linked to symptoms and situations. Part Two explains and investigates methods and offers a wide range of tools; these include trance inductions, adaptation hints, reframing, the use of metaphor and intervention techniques, how stories can be structured, and how to invent your own. The book also contains a detailed reference section with cross-referenced keywords to help you find the story or tool that you need.

With clear guidance on how stories can be applied to encourage positive change in people, groups and organisations, the *Handbook of Therapeutic Storytelling* is an essential resource for psychotherapists and other professions of health and social care in a range of different settings, as well as coaches, supervisors and management professionals.

**Stefan Hammel** is a child and family therapist, a hypnotherapist and a chaplain in a psychiatric and a general hospital in Kaiserslautern, Germany. He studied Theology in Aberdeen (Scotland), Leipzig and Heidelberg (Germany), and has trained in Systemic Therapy and Child Hypnotherapy. He is a member of the German Milton Erickson Society for Clinical Hypnosis and has led seminars in the UK, France, USA, South Africa and other countries. For further information on the author and a blog with therapeutic stories in English, French and Spanish, see: www.stefanhammel.com

# Handbook of Therapeutic Storytelling

Stories and Metaphors in
Psychotherapy, Child and Family
Therapy, Medical Treatment,
Coaching and Supervision

Stefan Hammel

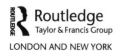
Routledge
Taylor & Francis Group

LONDON AND NEW YORK

First published in English 2019
by Routledge
2 Park Square, Milton Park, Abingdon, Oxon OX14 4RN

and by Routledge
711 Third Avenue, New York, NY 10017

*Routledge is an imprint of the Taylor & Francis Group, an informa business*

© 2019 Stefan Hammel

English translation by Joanne Reynolds

The right of Stefan Hammel to be identified as author of this work has been asserted by him in accordance with sections 77 and 78 of the Copyright, Designs and Patents Act 1988.

*British Library Cataloguing in Publication Data*
A catalogue record for this book is available from the British Library

*Library of Congress Cataloging in Publication Data*
Names: Hammel, Stefan, author.
Title: Handbook of therapeutic storytelling : stories and metaphors in psychotherapy, child and family therapy, medical treatment, coaching and supervision / Stefan Hammel ; English translation by Joanne Reynolds.
Other titles: Handbuch des therapeutischen Erzèahlens. English
Description: Milton Park, Abingdon, Oxon ; New York, NY : Routledge, 2018. | Includes bibliographical references and index.
Identifiers: LCCN 2018013420 (print) | LCCN 2018013628 (ebook) | ISBN 9780429461606 (Master e-book) | ISBN 9781138617513 (hbk) | ISBN 9781782205562 (pbk) | ISBN 9780429461606 (ebk)
Subjects: LCSH: Narrative therapy—Handbooks, manuals, etc. | Storytelling—Psychological aspects—Handbooks, manuals, etc. | Metaphor—Therapeutic use—Handbooks, manuals, etc. | Psychotherapist and patient—Handbooks, manual, etc.
Classification: LCC RC489.S74 (ebook) | LCC RC489.S74 H353 2018 (print) | DDC 616.89/165—dc23
LC record available at https://lccn.loc.gov/2018013420

ISBN: 978-1-138-61751-3 (hbk)
ISBN: 978-1-78220-556-2 (pbk)
ISBN: 978-0-429-46160-6 (ebk)

Typeset in Times New Roman
by Out of House Publishing

Printed and bound by CPI Group (UK) Ltd, Croydon, CR0 4YY

# Contents

*Foreword*                                                                viii

## Introduction                                                              I

1   The potential of stories                                                 3
    *Approach 3*
    *Tradition 4*
    *Application 5*
    *Benefits 7*
    *Trance, rapport and suggestions 8*
    *The world of dreams 11*
    *Structure versus substance 13*
    *Therapeutic principles 14*
    *Philosophical position 17*
    *Instructions for use 19*

## PART ONE
## The stories                                                             21

2   Promoting understanding                                                 23
    *Assigning meaning 23*
    *Perception and interpretation 25*
    *Understanding and misunderstanding 29*

3   Promoting health                                                        32
    *Heart, circulation, bleeding and blood flow 32*
    *Infections, allergies, autoimmune diseases 37*
    *Skin and hair 46*
    *Muscular tension and relaxation 49*

*Bodily sensations and the perception of pain  52*
*Sense of sight  60*
*Sense of hearing  62*
*Sense of balance  64*
*Speech  66*
*Memory and access to skills  69*
*Excretion  79*
*Sleep  82*
*Sexuality  88*
*Eating behaviours and addiction  90*

4   Promoting wellbeing                                          98
*Resource orientation and positive thinking  98*
*Attack and defence  102*
*Anxiety  113*
*Compulsion  118*
*Depression  122*
*Mania  128*
*Dream world, delusion and hallucination  130*
*Suicidal tendencies  138*
*Loss and farewell  141*

5   Promoting successful relationships                          148
*Romantic relationships  148*
*Family  155*
*Parenting and detachment from the parental home  162*
*Middle-aged and elderly people  169*
*Friends  171*

6   Promoting development                                       175
*Development and maturity  175*
*Learning  180*
*Wishes, will and vision  183*
*Economy, order, efficiency and quality  188*

**PART TWO**
**The methods**                                                 **201**

7   Identifying therapeutic stories                             203
*Using intuition  203*

*Using written sources  204*
*Using oral sources  205*
*Using one's own life as a source  205*
*Using films and other media as sources  206*
*Using other sources of communication  207*

8  Developing therapeutic stories through dialogue          209
*Developing stories through systemic questions  209*
*Changing problem metaphors into solution metaphors  210*
*Developing stories together with children  215*

9  Inventing therapeutic stories          217
*Types of therapeutic stories  217*
*Basic forms of suggestion  221*
*Basic therapeutic storytelling interventions  226*
*Storytelling structures  247*
*Genres  257*

10  Telling therapeutic stories          265
*Before storytelling  265*
*Starting storytelling  266*
*Trusting the power of stories  267*
*Trances and trance phenomena  269*
*Therapeutic interventions in detail  274*
*Stringing together and interweaving stories  281*
*After storytelling  282*

11  Experiencing therapeutic stories without words          284
*Painted and sculpted stories  284*
*Pantomime stories  287*
*Concrete stories and lived stories  287*

12  Appendix          289
*List of stories  289*

*Literature*          295
*Index*          299

# Foreword

When my sister and I visited our grandparents as children, we had the habit of crawling into their bed when we woke up between five and six each morning, and pressing the "story switch" – the button on my grandfather's pyjamas. He would then tell us many different kinds of stories, including stories he had heard, stories he had read, stories he had experienced himself and stories he had invented. There was one particular story I wanted to hear over and over again – the Parable of the Lost Sheep, from the Gospel of Luke (Luke 15:3–7). My grandfather must have wondered why I wanted to hear this story so often, but nevertheless he told it to me again and again. This was my story, and I needed to hear it. Two key passages appeared in each of my grandfather's retellings of this story; the first told how the shepherd heard the sheep's cry for the first time after having searched and called for so long, and then how the shepherd called and the sheep bleated in turn until the shepherd finally found the sheep, and the second told how the shepherd found the sheep stuck fast in a thornbush, unable to move forwards or backwards, and how he carefully freed the animal…

This story formed a constant backdrop to my childhood, and when I grew up it was this story that first brought home to me the therapeutic power of stories – a power that most people today probably still underestimate. This two-thousand-year-old story was written down because it helped the people who heard it, and it still influences people's thinking and experiences today.

Stories create reality. The aim of this handbook is to harness the transformative power of stories and to turn therapy into a living language.

My thanks go to all those who have interwoven their own stories with the story of this book. You know who you are.

# Introduction

# Chapter 1

# The potential of stories

## Approach

"Why shouldn't it work?" This was the motto I followed when I began to tell stories to my body – to my skin cells, to my immune system and even to the hay fever which made me so miserable. I used metaphors in these stories to explain what I wanted my body to do. I heaped praise on my body's immune system at the same time as negotiating with it. After just a short time my allergic reactions diminished in intensity, and eventually they disappeared altogether. I told one of my friends, a doctor from Mainz, about the success of my healing method. She laughed. "It's probably just that there's no pollen around at the moment! Pollen levels vary from year to year, so getting rid of hay fever is a long-term endeavour." The following day my hay fever had returned. How annoying! "Dear hay fever," I said. "Go to my colleague in Mainz – maybe she can find some use for you. I don't need you any more." The symptoms disappeared within seconds. This approach has provoked criticism from some, but the colleague claims that the hay fever never arrived...

Messages of this kind are highly effective, whether they are directed at ourselves or at others, and whether they are used deliberately or unintentionally. It is admittedly the case that the unconscious mind fails to implement a great deal of what it hears, but this is because the flood of suggestive statements that washes over us on a daily basis is categorised by the unconscious mind on the basis of certain criteria. This makes it possible for the unconscious mind to distinguish between important and irrelevant instructions, and to implement some while largely ignoring others.

In the case described above, a message from an expert ("You haven't really cured your hay fever!") was apparently implemented as a priority, and indeed messages of this kind are perceived very differently depending on whether they originate from a doctor or an amateur in the field. A further criterion that determines whether or not a message of this kind is implemented is the level of acceptance or resistance it induces in the recipient. Offering advice to someone in the depths of frustration is likely to frustrate him even more, yet there is a much greater chance that the same person will accept the very same suggestion if it is contained in a story about someone for whom happiness was an elusive goal until he had sought it for so long and experienced so much that happiness finally found him.

Stories tend to avoid the "yes but" structure of counselling conversations that operate on a cognitive level, since it is a great deal harder to respond to a story with the words, "I've already tried that!" than to a piece of advice or a potential solution. Suggestive stories circumvent conscious thinking, which has a tendency to be paralysed by the familiar and the feared, and instead address the problem-solving capacities of the unconscious mind, thereby introducing a lightness into counseling, which is often missing from cognitively focused conversations. The task of searching for a solution is assigned to the unconscious mind rather than rational thought, since the former is much more likely to succeed in finding one. This opens up the way for humour, curiosity and optimism during counselling sessions, for the simple reason that the client's attention is focused on something much more pleasant than the burden of his or her unsolved problems. The curious thing is that these problems are in fact often solved imperceptibly and in passing while the client listens to the stories; this is revealed by the client's relieved comments after the therapy session, by immediate bodily reactions (such as his breath, voice, face and movements showing signs of relief), by the frequent absence of further questions on how to solve the "real" problem, and most importantly by rapid changes in patterns of thinking and behaviour in the aftermath of the counselling session.

The above makes it clear that the messages contained in therapeutic stories are often open in substantive terms, and that instead of offering a clearly defined answer they suggest to the listener an avenue for future exploration or a searching attitude which may lead to various solutions. For example, concrete suggestions are framed as stories about situations that other people have experienced, so that the listener can examine their usefulness as a model for his or her own experiments. It is a fundamental tenet of counselling that the client himself or herself should identify these solutions wherever possible, and that no limits should be placed on their potential scope.

## Tradition

The working method described here is rooted *inter alia* in findings from systemic therapy. I base my approach on the Heidelberg School, the work of the Milan Group centred around Mara Selvini Palazzoli and that of the communication theorist Paul Watzlawick.

The methods developed by the American psychiatrist Milton Erickson, who is regarded as a pioneer of modern hypnotherapy, have had a particularly strong influence on my work. Somewhat astonishingly, during the latter part of his life Erickson rarely used formal hypnosis strategies, preferring to tell or act out stories for his clients and the students who attended his seminars.

The approach described here has also been influenced by the Judeo-Christian and Ancient Oriental traditions of storytelling. The writings of the Old Testament prophets, the parables of Jesus and the stories of the rabbis deal with spiritual, pedagogical and social therapy problems while simultaneously entertaining listeners. Throughout all of Christian, Jewish and Muslim history, metaphors have been deliberately used as effective prompts for problem solving.

With the exception of the stories told by clients about their biographical experiences, storytelling seemed for some time to have vanished almost entirely from the arsenal of therapeutic strategies, a fact which is all the more surprising because storytelling techniques have proven their worth through the millennia and across cultural boundaries. Back in the days before therapists, wisdom was dispensed to those seeking advice by sages (rabbis, prophets, priests, hermits, mullahs, gurus, Zen masters, healers, seers, teachers, philosophers, medicine men, shamans and druids, at different times and in different cultures); in many cases this task is now performed by therapists, social workers, doctors and alternative practitioners.

"No vice is so bad as advice," said Marie Dressler, and many counsellors of bygone ages took heed of this warning and refused to provide clear answers, preferring counter-questions, enigmatic riddles or stories. For example, someone is said to have once asked a Jewish scholar, "Why do you answer every question with a counterquestion?" whereupon the scholar replied, "Why not?" (Bonder, 1999: 15) A young monk asked, "What is the secret of enlightenment?" His teacher answered, "Eat when you are hungry and sleep when you are tired" (cf. Kopp, 1971: 77). Someone who had heard that one should love one's neighbours asked Jesus, "Who is my neighbour?" and Jesus answered, "A man was going down from Jerusalem to Jericho, when he was attacked by robbers. They stripped him of his clothes, beat him and went away, leaving him half dead…" And he told how two men of good standing walked past the injured man, but a Samaritan (despised by the Jews) stopped to look after the man, bandage his wounds and take him to a safe place (Luke 10:25).

Stories of this kind have been passed down over the centuries by the prophets of the Old Testament, the Jewish rabbis and the wise men of the Ancient Orient and of antique Greece; both the traditional fairy tales and aphorisms of the East and the corresponding Western traditions use invented stories to solve real problems. Stories are therapeutic remedies that complement psychotherapeutic and medical approaches and sometimes provide the missing piece of the treatment puzzle, yet the art of using stories for therapeutic and medical purposes has in many respects been lost and needs to be rediscovered.

## Application

The potential applications of therapeutic stories are as diverse as they are varied; in the field of hypnotherapy, for example, they can be used to reduce pain, stop bleeding, cure neurodermatitis and warts, overcome autoimmune diseases, eliminate tinnitus, regulate blood pressure and treat innumerable other disorders. Stories can provide relief for patients suffering from anxiety, compulsive behaviours, tics and stammering. Stories based around metaphors can be helpful in the context of addiction or couples therapy, or during counselling sessions with young people on the brink of adulthood. They can be interspersed into the conversation during coaching sessions or team meetings, and – last but not least – can also be used by trainers and supervisors to illustrate attitudes and techniques and to generate creative new ideas. Many interventions can be used in pedagogical practice with children or with adults, for pastoral care and for self-coaching.

A brief word should be said about the use of stories in medical and nursing fields; when a patient suffers from a somatic disorder, it is sometimes the case that the body does not heal itself to the best of its abilities, for example owing to beliefs which interfere with healing, poor priority setting (i.e. the non-optimum distribution of attention, energy and other resources) or a continual failure to be fully aware of the self-healing options available. Mental training and psychotherapeutic methods to optimise self-healing opportunities can complement the conventional medical remedies used for healing in such cases.

A colleague voiced his concern that the handbook might encourage people to think that a three-line story could be used to solve problems which present an almost insurmountable challenge for conventional medicine or which would require 300 hours or so of traditional psychotherapy. A differentiated approach must be taken to the potential of therapeutic storytelling; such effects can unquestionably be achieved for certain problems, but this will generally require the use of an interconnected web of stories and several hours of work by the therapist and the client. However, sometimes disorders that have been causing severe suffering to clients for a long time can be solved in a short time. Several sections of the handbook document complete short courses of therapy as they have taken place. For example, the three stories "The Persecuted I", "The Persecuted II" and "Celibacy" give witness of a four-hour course of therapy. "Zero-Problem Therapy" and "When Someone Says 'Stefan Hammel'" show a therapy that has taken place in two hours, just as are the stories "Anna's Submarine" and "Mrs Brain", or the story "The Bladder Alarm Clock".

In my experience, the targeted use of stories is just as effective as work with formal hypnosis techniques, and the majority of therapies last between two and eight hours in both cases. A likely reason for this is that both procedures are essentially similar in that they involve the combined use of trance, rapport and suggestions. One key difference is that the trances induced informally during storytelling would not be regarded by most people as "hypnosis", making it possible to use these methods with people who are sceptical about hypnosis and other common psychotherapy procedures. It is important to view suggestive procedures and storytelling interventions of any kind as a complement to other forms of treatment rather than as an alternative, and to combine the two.

The underlying context to these stories is the idea of short therapy courses, which are based on hypno-systemic principles and aimed at modifying the interconnected web of effects that lies at the root of the relevant symptoms and problems. This is achieved by means of paradigms, with the assumption that the unconscious mind will retain what is useful and reproduce it in adjacent areas of life. In my experience, most courses of therapy based on paradigmatic work of this kind last ten hours or less. Right from the very start the therapy is aimed at achieving as much change as possible in as safe and sustainable a way as possible, with a view to reducing suffering, increasing happiness and helping the client to tolerate any unavoidable stresses. The first task that must be tackled during such a course of therapy is to clarify the purpose and task of the therapeutic work and to discuss the biographical and current background to the problem being discussed. On the basis of this discussion, the therapist then works together with the client to develop an interconnected web of interventions that move the client closer to the overall objective. The therapist investigates whether achievement of the task might be associated with any undesirable side effects and how these might be avoided, and has the right to reject any goals that he or she believes would be harmful for his or her client, unethical or unachievable. The therapist must maintain a positive attitude towards the interventions while at the same time carefully and continually monitoring the quality of the outcomes that have been achieved.

## Benefits

Storytelling makes it possible to overcome obstacles. The sense of paralysis and entanglement experienced in connection with problems often infiltrates any conversation about them. The storytelling approach involves discussing a representative story rather than problems and traumatic experiences, facilitating a stress-free conversation which is more conducive to the identification of solutions. Conversations about stories that stand in for the real situation inject a sense of lightness and humour into therapy sessions, and discussions about metaphors, paradigmatic stories and solutions in non-problematic areas inspire creativity in both parties to the discussion. It is often possible to avoid mentioning the real problem for a significant length of time, sometimes only discussing it again at the end of the course of therapy when effective solutions have already been found, or even consigning it to the past in silence because it has been resolved. Many clients choose to end a course of therapy shortly after discussing a problem on a metaphorical level; they are satisfied with the outcome, but are unable to explain exactly how their problem was solved.

It goes without saying that a narrative approach of this kind is more pleasant for clients, who often enjoy the therapy sessions and look forward to the next one. This is of particular relevance to therapeutic outcomes in the case of children and young people who are brought to therapy by their parents.

If we assume that storytelling differs in some way from what other counsellors before us have offered to clients, the facts are on our side from the outset; anyone who does things differently to his predecessors will achieve different results.

Empathic therapists often identify with their clients' experiences of powerlessness, fear, anger and emptiness, and find internal resonance with these experiences. This not only undermines the therapeutic process, but also entails the risk of emotional burnout for the counsellor as a result of long-term identification with these stressful experiences. The use of stories can be an effective way for a therapist to avoid burn-out, since they make it possible to concentrate more on subjects that avoid compromising (and even strengthen) the therapist's emotional balance, and to focus comparatively less on the client's suffering. Therapists who have used storytelling during a therapy session frequently feel energised and motivated afterwards, and often find that they have solved problems of their own while working with the client, without even noticing it.

## Trance, rapport and suggestions

The interventions described in this handbook stem from the efforts I have undertaken to optimise my therapeutic work. Ways of achieving the same outcomes as hypnotherapy without formal hypnosis are of particular interest to me; after all, trance, rapport and suggestions are ubiquitous everyday phenomena rather than merely characteristics of hypnotic work, and the effects of hypnotherapy should therefore be achievable without the ritual of induced hypnosis. The stories in this handbook incorporate methods developed in the field of hypnotherapy into a wide range of therapeutic situations without the use of hypnosis, and most can be used by hypnotherapists in modified form as trance stories in hypnotic settings.

When talking about the transfer of hypnotherapeutic findings into non-hypnotic therapy, it is useful to remember the role played by the fundamentals of hypnosis – trance, rapport and suggestive communication – in normal therapeutic dialogue.

I understand the term "trance" to mean physical and mental states that are characterised by the focusing of attention on a small number of sources of stimuli along with the dissociation of most others, and in particular by the focusing of attention inwards, which is towards remembered perceptions or perceptions constructed by the imagination. People experience trances on a daily basis when driving their car, playing, working, watching television or listening to or watching something with intense concentration, and trances also occur quite naturally during therapy, in various forms and intensities. There are in fact many possible states in which an individual's levels of alertness and attention differ from those which are regarded as normal for individuals or society as a whole, and "trance" is therefore a comparative term rather than one which is rigidly defined. In methodological terms, the trances that are most relevant to therapy are relaxation trances, which are characterised by an increased willingness and ability to learn, reduced physical and mental stress (regardless of the form taken by this stress), lowered inhibitions and more intense imagined experiences (daydreams). Storytelling is particularly suitable for inducing trances because it requires the listener to focus on the content of the story and internal images; this in turn makes it clear that trance is a ubiquitous feature of any therapy, and does not appear only as a result of formal hypnosis.

I use the term "rapport" to refer to a state of consonance in which two parties identify intensely with each other to the extent that the personal realities of the individuals merge in some sense and are experienced as a shared reality. Rapport means being on the same wavelength, in both verbal and non-verbal terms. Rapport behaviours include unconscious behaviours such as symmetrical body positions, simultaneous and similar movements, synchronised breathing, copying a counterpart's behaviour (infectious yawning), adopting a counterpart's vocabulary, accent and speech patterns and similar phenomena. From the viewpoint of behavioural biology, the purpose of rapport is to synchronise the behaviour of all pack members with each other and if necessary with a lead animal (for the purpose of attacking or fleeing together), to coordinate mating behaviour and to align the behaviour of inexperienced young animals with that of the experienced mother or parent animals. Storytelling creates a shared experience merging the identities of the storyteller and the listener, and rapport is particularly strengthened by stories that express conformity or which are experienced together on an emotional level. The involuntary mutual alignment of physical behaviour and unconscious speech patterns (e.g. symmetrical body positions, same choice of words) is a process which is experienced on a daily basis by clients and therapists.

I use the term "suggestive communication" to refer to the refocusing of an interlocutor's attention with a view to changing their thoughts and behaviour, in particular their beliefs. A suggestion is therefore a verbal or non-verbal and conscious or unconscious message aimed at changing an individual's ways of seeing or behaving. Depending on its form, it can involve declarative suggestion, directive suggestion or (indirect) implied suggestion and self-fulfilling prophecies (auto-suggestion), and placebo effects are also widely known phenomena. If we are incapable of not communicating, we are also incapable of not suggesting, and suggestions work outside a hypnotic context too. Therapeutic stories contain suggestive implications which result from the juxtaposition of the content of the story and the client's biographical experience. Unconscious suggestions and autosuggestions are a pervasive feature of therapy, regardless of whether hypnosis is used.

It is therefore apparent that the fundamental building blocks of trance, rapport and suggestion – even in the absence of hypnosis – are everyday phenomena that can be used to achieve clients' goals. It should also be apparent that storytelling automatically deepens trances, strengthens rapport and has an implied suggestive action, and that these effects can if necessary be heightened by means of suitable storytelling methods.

The approach outlined in this handbook uses the everyday forms of trance that occur automatically when listening to stories to achieve therapeutic outcomes. It is therefore useful to identify a number of characteristics of these trance states, which include changes to the following autonomic systems:

- breathing (slower and flatter in a relaxation trance),
- muscular tension (decreased or increased in relaxation),
- heart rate (slower) and blood pressure (lower),
- movements (less frequent, less vigorous, delayed, jerky),
- speech (less frequent, slower, quieter, delayed).

Various phenomena which are familiar from hypnotic work may occur during everyday trance experiences and can be strengthened and made use of for therapeutic purposes by means of suitable storytelling techniques. It is therefore useful to identify the commonplace – and often inconspicuous – forms of these phenomena in order to leverage their benefits for the purpose of therapy. Classical trance phenomena include:

- time distortion (altered perception of time),
- increased suggestibility and ability to learn;
- absence of conceptual barriers;
- interconnected thinking (processing of content on several levels at once),
- positive and negative hallucination (perceiving things that are not present, or not perceiving things which are present);
- amnesia and hypermnesia (inability to remember or increased ability to remember),
- age regression and progression (returning to a previously experienced state or imagining a future state),
- altered physical perceptions in the form of analgesia, anaesthesia, hypersensitivity or hyposensitivity (absence of pain, absence of feelings, reduced or increased sensitivity),
- ideomotor movements (involuntary twitches, arm levitation, automatic writing etc.),
- catalepsy (rigidity of the body) and hypertonia or hypotonia (increased or reduced muscular tension),

- dissociation (uncoupling) and association (recoupling, anchoring) of sensory perceptions, emotions, knowledge and ideas, memories and individual physical and mental functions.

A distinction should be made between partial dissociation, in which the dissociated physical or mental experience is perceived as foreign, and complete dissociation, in which the relevant experience is no longer perceived or remembered (amnesia, forgetting a number, anaesthesia, induction of temporary incapacity to see, hear, move oneself etc.)

Many of the stories utilise everyday trance phenomena for therapeutic purposes.

## The world of dreams

Dreams – which are older than humanity itself – are the prototype of all therapeutic stories, and the most primitive way of bringing order to our mental and social experiences. The cinema in our head helps us to process impressions, reduce stress, clarify goals, examine possible choices and gain motivation to follow the path we ultimately choose.

This handbook is based on the idea that our experiences are fundamentally controlled by our nighttime and daytime dreams, and that therapeutic stories are simply verbalised dreams which both guide us and are guided by us and achieve the same outcomes as nighttime and daytime dreams. The best way to influence attitudes and ideas which originate in the unconscious mind is to copy the mode of operation of the unconscious mind itself.

Therapeutic stories are therefore guided dreams whose purpose is to exert a healing influence on the body, mind, spirituality and social system.

To put it in metaphorical terms, a native Kenyan will probably understand me better if I talk to him in Swahili than if I talk in German or English. He will respond with interest, sympathy and cooperation if he is addressed in his mother tongue; he will be able to concentrate for longer, will enter into a lively dialogue and express many of his own ideas. If I address an individual's unconscious mind in the "dream language" which is its mother tongue, it will respond more enthusiastically than if I use the language of "Psychologese". Dreams are the mother tongue of the unconscious mind, whereas cognitive and analytical discussions are foreign languages to it. Therapeutic stories are so effective because they directly address the unconscious mind (and its enormous capacity for creativeness) in its own language, bypassing conscious thought with its limited capacity for work, scepticism of anything new and attachment to past habits.

People's dreams can be divided into two basic types, which fulfil different functions, namely paradigmatic dreams and metaphorical dreams. Both groups can be subdivided into dreams that stem predominantly from a searching and problem-solving attitude, nightmares that warn against dangers and finally dreams that reinforce past achievements and call for "more of the same". Some dreams prepare the dreamer for an event, some process a past event and some relate to ongoing problems. Many dreams can be clearly assigned to a single category; most people at some point dream of being in a public place wearing no clothes or wearing only underwear, which is a metaphorical warning against giving up protection and an aversive auto-suggestion. Many people revising for exams dream that they are unable to answer any of the questions on the exam paper, which is a paradigmatic warning. Dreaming that you can fly is a metaphorical positive model, dreaming that you are in a war is a metaphorical negative model, and dreaming that you are looking for a street in a strange city is a metaphorical searching model. All realistic dreams, both positive and negative, are paradigmatic dreams, which promote success and either warn against failure or evaluate past failures. I believe that a clear distinction can be made between the fundamental dream types, even though combined forms of these types occur in many different variants.

Dreams and stories are one and the same thing, and so stories can also be divided into metaphorical stories and paradigmatic stories, and then further subdivided into positive models, negative models and searching models. These different fundamental forms serve various therapeutic purposes and represent different goals, namely reinforcing sources of strength, warning against sources of harm and searching for new opportunities.

It often seems as though stories have become a foreign language for us, since the basic language of Western culture is cognitively focused, and therapy work too often relies on conscious, scientific and rational thinking and the promotion of reflection and analysis. In my experience, increased exposure to storytelling encourages the unconscious to seek out more and more stories and incorporate them into the therapeutic relationship; the therapist is barely aware of these processes, just as we are barely aware of the letters we use when we write. The therapeutic conversation becomes a framework for communication between the therapist's unconscious mind and the client's unconscious mind.

Words are more than just letters on a page; provided there is no major internal or external resistance preventing the implementation of what has been said, words provoke what they invoke. Words produce responses in the world of actions which originate in the world of mere possibilities, calling on the hidden depths of the soul, the body's healing potential, a group's unconscious communicative framework and (if truth lies in belief) the individual's spiritual convictions.

Stories too are not merely sequences of words, but a complex fabric of linguistic elements (and also non-verbal elements during the storytelling process). Their network of interrelated meanings generates a network of physical, mental and social responses with unignorable implications for conscious and cognitively focused thinking. Stories impose new priorities in complex ambivalent (polyvalent) systems, which introduce new states of balance (homeostasis). They change the focus of attention of the organic, mental and social system, thereby allowing resources to be balanced and managed differently. Most of the stories we tell address the client's unconscious mind and change its patterns of perception, thinking and behaviour, but to a large extent they also originate from the therapist's unconscious mind. Amid the back and forth of communication and the time constraints imposed by a therapy session, the therapist will be forced to rely on his or her physical sensations and intuition, which are probably a better guide than any cognitive "analysis". As noted above, storytelling therapy for the most part involves the therapist's unconscious mind communicating with his or her patient's unconscious mind, and thus resembles the way in which dreams are communicated, with the sole difference that these are shared dreams that are used deliberately in interpersonal communication to guide an individual's or a group's ways of perceiving, thinking and behaving.

## Structure versus substance

As a general rule, the goal of therapeutic work is to alter recurrent thought, behavioural and relationship structures rather than to influence the ever-changing substance of individual thoughts and behaviours. The stories used in pursuit of this goal must therefore reflect what is going on in the client's everyday life on a *structural* level, revealing the way in which a particular structure (or pattern) influences the client's life and making it possible to identify potentially worthwhile areas of change. One of the fundamental rules that applies to therapeutic work in general also holds true when finding such stories, namely that we should be much more focused on the client's overall patterns of thinking, acting and experiencing than on the individual substance of these thoughts, actions or experiences.

I wish to cite a number of examples to highlight the difference between focusing on structures and focusing on substance. When the Jesus of the New Testament said, "Love your neighbour as yourself," he was referring to a behavioural pattern which brings happiness. If he had instead said, "Give your neighbour Levi ten dinars," he would have been referring to the substance of the problem. When he said, "Your faith has healed you," he was referring to a pattern. If he had said, "You were healed because you thought, 'Jesus will cure me of leprosy,'" he would have been referring to the substance of the problem. He was referring to the substance of the problem when he said, "Go to the village of Bethphage, and at once you will find a donkey tied there. Untie it and bring it to me," but he was referring to a pattern when he said, "If they persecuted me, they will persecute you also."

It is the case for all individuals – and even entire social systems – that the substance of thoughts or behaviours is in constant flux, whereas patterns of thinking and behaving are characterised by extreme stability and regularity of recurrence. We face different sources of conflict every day, for example, but the way we handle these conflicts is always the same. Anyone wishing to influence his or her environment must first turn his or her attention to the interdependencies, relationships and static and dynamic equilibria between humans and objects that have evolved everywhere over time, and observe and shape these enduring patterns rather than their ever-fluctuating substance.

We do not necessarily need to analyse a topic and process it cognitively in order to focus on the underlying structures; we can instead examine patterns intuitively. We need only place ourselves temporarily into the same state we are in during daydreams and try to intuit what might be permanent and recurrent about the stories we tell, and we will be reminded of other people, things, plants or animals in the universe that behave in a strangely similar way, whether or not the outcomes are the same. This forms a good starting point for introducing descriptive images into conversations with clients about otherwise nondescript structures, thereby taking the first steps towards a solution.

## Therapeutic principles

The therapeutic approach behind the stories is characterised by several principles, originating partly from the tradition of systemic counselling and therapeutic strategies developed by Milton Erickson and partly from my own observations.

1.  Counselling is resource-oriented, and as a general rule it prioritises people's opportunities and possibilities and highlights and strengthens their capabilities. Attention is focused away from deficits, and "shortcomings" are regarded as subjective perceptions which may be only temporary in nature and which depend on the interpretations and behavioural patterns of the members of a particular group and the individual's self-image. The ways of seeing and behaving that result in a perception of shortcomings may change at any time, and with them the perceived shortcomings themselves.

2.  Counselling is focused on the future, on goals and on solutions, and aims to identify achievable goals and solutions that increase life satisfaction and to initiate changes in mutual perception and behaviour. "Goal-focused" can also be rephrased as "task-focused"; the therapist firstly determines the desired outcome of the conversation and his or her task in this process, and then performs this task consistently until both parties to the conversation have achieved the goal that was set.

3.  Everything is potentially useful. A client's unique characteristics and abilities, problems, environment and current situation can all be used to achieve his or her goals.

4.  Assume nothing. The therapist does not base his or her therapeutic practice on any particular theories, but instead on the specific situation with

which he or she is confronted. Every client is an individual, and therefore all therapy is individual.

5.  Expect everything. The therapist takes a sceptical view of psychotherapeutic, psychosomatic and psychosocial theories which define what is real and possible in psychotherapy, of theories about clients and their environments, and of the psychotherapeutic literature on the relevant symptom if the constructions of reality embodied in these theories and literature tend to interfere with therapy rather than facilitate it. When confronted with models based on purported certainties about the way in which the human mind works and the way in which psychotherapy works, the therapist asks, "Really?" and "Why not?" When confronted with what are said to be the limits of healing and the alleviation of suffering, the therapist's expectations are positive in the extreme, but this attitude is predominantly conveyed non-verbally and through implications, without giving any verbal promises of success. The therapist is mindful of the possibility of failure to the extent that this is necessary to avoid harm to the client and the therapist.

6.  Everything that is experienced by the mind is based on the imagination and memory of processes which can be perceived by the body; the seeing of imagined pictures, the hearing of internal voices and the imagining of physical feelings. The mental and autonomic processes that occur when imagining these experiences are the same as those that occur during the experience itself, albeit generally in a milder form. Storytelling therapy simulates physical and mental processes at the level of the imagination with a view to deliberately conditioning new response patterns, which then exist in reality.

7.  Physical and psychological experiences are two sides of the same coin, since psychological changes result in specific autonomic changes and vice versa. Anyone who changes his or her breathing, facial expression and body posture or the internal images he or she sees also influences all the associated parameters, for example pulse rate, pain, width of the blood vessels, muscle tone and anxiety. Every physical and mental response can be changed by altering the associated physical and mental responses. Every conceivable physical and mental state of stress or relaxation can be achieved by telling stories that imply a change in individual parameters of this kind.

8.  "All human experience is the result of focusing one's attention." (Gunther Schmidt, seminar discussion 2000). Certain rules apply in this respect, and many apply equally to both physical and mental processes. Similar procedures can be used to cure pain and anxiety, allergies and phobias, tinnitus and compulsive thoughts, cramps and conflicts. The basic features of this focusing of attention are association and dissociation; the client's attention is controlled by highlighting and linking or by ignoring and separating the substance of the story. Stories create new

stimulus–response patterns – new chains of association, new interpretations, new ways of behaving, new physical responses and of course new emotional responses are brought into being through the spoken word. Sensory perceptions and memories that previously produced critical responses are linked to resource-based connotations, interpretations and ways of behaving. Critical stimulus-response patterns and stressful associations are weakened or separated. The conceptual linking and separation of response patterns can then be programmed to appear on a temporary or permanent basis or (as in the case of conditioning) to repeat regularly. As a basic principle, all human experiences at either physical or psychological level can be linked to each other or separated from each other.

9. Therapeutic changes that may potentially have a significant impact are introduced on an experimental basis at first, for example by combining them with a request for the client to test out in practice everything that has been suggested in order to ascertain whether it is useful. If what the client has learned proves to be of value for the unconscious, he or she is asked to continue applying the relevant methods and to reinforce and multiply them insofar as this is useful, and to reject anything that does not prove its worth. This approach to therapy not only avoids resistance on the part of the client and undesirable side effects, but also respects the client's need for security and autonomy.

10. Ways of behaving that benefit not only the person receiving counselling but also any other individuals involved should be prioritised over those that benefit the former and place the latter at a disadvantage. These ways of behaving (competition, non-cooperation, zero-sum games) should only be suggested when solutions of the first kind (friendship, cooperation, non-zero-sum games) are unachievable.

11. The general goal of therapy is to expand the range of possibilities open to the client, and the therapist's task is to offer the client alternative ways of perceiving, thinking and behaving rather than reducing the options available in this respect.

12. A positive attitude on the part of the client is less important than ensuring by all possible means that he or she is placed in a position of power. In this context, the term "power" means anything connected with an experience of bodily and social competence and emotional presence, and the terms "stress" and "weakness" mean anything connected with an experience of paralysis, trepidation, nervousness or diffuse aggression. The therapist can look for evidence of what strengthens or stresses the client by comparing his or her own bodily perceptions against what has just been discussed, at the same time examining the client's facial expressions, position, gestures and voice in order to identify any optical or acoustical signs of power or stress during the relevant part of the discussion, asking the client to give his or her opinion if appropriate.

## Philosophical position

Are we in the world, or is the world in us? Everything we know about the world around us is in us. Our mind holds a record of everything we have perceived, as well as connections between the things we perceive repeatedly (either as cohesive and synonymous or as differentiable and different) and connections between simultaneous perceptions (either as cohesive or random), and all the memories, expectations, interpretations and inferred rules we associate with these perceptions.

If our mind fundamentally shapes all perceptions – current, remembered and fictitious (i.e. experienced as being in the future) – it can also reshape them. Memories, momentary experience and expectations can be modelled both voluntarily and involuntarily, and if the world in which we live is in us rather than us being in the world, then we can change it by shaping what is within us.

In summary, everything we know about the "outside" takes place on the "inside". The way in which the human mind shapes our perceptions varies hugely in terms of the impressions that are retained and their intensity. Memories are particularly liable to be inaccurate and changeable, and our interpretations (beliefs) and expectations of the surrounding world are shaped even more freely by the mind.

The differences between perception and imagination are furthermore slight; anything that takes place split seconds after a perception or later is a memory of this event and therefore imagination, but anything up to a millisecond before a perception is simply expectation. If most of what we experience as perception is imagination, we can only distinguish loosely (if at all) between the inside and the outside and between imagination and reality.

Everything we know about the brain and its perceptions is itself a perception of the brain, or in other words our mind. We can say: our mind claims that there is a brain which creates the mind which claims there is a brain which creates the mind... ending up with a circular chain of reasoning which we can only escape by means of sentences such as the Socratic "I know one thing; that I know nothing" and the Cartesian "I think, therefore I am". What is really real? The boundaries between reality and imagination are fluid and uncertain, and the same applies to our conception of time. When we talk about the past, the present and the future, we are referring to our individual and collectively constructed experience of memory, momentary experience and expectation. In actual fact, however, these three aspects of experience take place simultaneously in our brain and are highly variable in nature, not only in different people but also over the course of an individual's lifetime, and sometimes on much shorter timescales. Memories determine a person's expectations, but are in turn shaped by beliefs and are mouldable and changeable. Memory, momentary experience and expectation are for the most part the product of the stories we tell ourselves about our life. Once again, the boundaries between reality and imagination are fluid.

In my opinion, there are grounds for believing not only that our experience generates stories, but also that the very core of our experience consists of the stories that we tell ourselves and others. Our stories about our world are unquestionably inspired by the reality that underlies them, meaning that we not only construct reality but at the same time analyse it – without being able to distinguish between these two activities.

It is pertinent to ask whether the stories we tell each other are wholly arbitrary in nature, and whether there is therefore no difference between lies and truth or between mistaken and accurate descriptions.

I think that the extent to which a story reflects reality can most readily be measured on the basis of whether it strengthens an individual's self, experienced as his or her body and mind, and whether it promotes relationships within a group (in the opinion of its members). Lies and truth are then merely a question of authenticity, and depend on whether what someone is saying corresponds to his or her beliefs. In the same way that definitions of lies and truth are rooted in a particular context, statements about accuracy or inaccuracy are embedded in stories about patterns of thinking that have or have not proved useful for an individual or a group. Anyone who can open up their mind to new belief systems will discover that the rules of these systems, which dictate whether a statement is accurate or inaccurate, form the basis for consistent models of thinking and acting.

I am of the opinion that we must avoid being too sure of our reality if we want to expand the possibilities of our therapeutic work. Most people in our society take it for granted that the mind is a bodily function. Regarding the body as a function of the mind is an unfamiliar approach, but one which might prove fruitful in the context of therapy. The one-way street of causality from the body to the mind can be replaced on an experimental basis by a model of alternating resonance, and the psychological dimension of the mind can be viewed in the conceptual framework of a (psychoanalytically or spiritually interpreted) collective spirit.

Not only Jesus of Nazareth but also countless rabbis, nuns, shamans, druids and healing women throughout history have regarded it as self-evident that healing has a spiritual dimension. A dialogue between medicine, psychotherapy and religious traditions may open our eyes to new ways of seeing people and expand the different possibilities of physical, mental, social and spiritual healing.

The stories that we tell ourselves and others shape our world. Since healing and problem-solving structures invariably resemble each other, structures that are effective in the context of therapy can be useful when it comes to achieving social and global goals. Further research is needed into theories that postulate that all of the world's living beings can be regarded as the cells of a single organism. To put it in the form of a fable, the toadstools in a fairy ring tell each other that they are individuals, and in a certain sense they are correct. Their mycelium knows that they are a *single* organism, but it keeps quiet about this fact. The toadstools are oblivious to what we know – that they are linked by the network of fine threads which created them and which will outlive them. The collectivistic nature of the tribalism that characterised past ages is no less true than the individualism of modern Western thinking. The idea that every living being is part of a single organism is logically admissible, and – if we can accept it – may also serve as a starting point for healing the global community.

What we suppose to be certainty about what is real and possible imposes limits – perhaps unnecessarily – on what is possible. This handbook invites therapists to take a second look at what they have previously regarded as certain, and its stories encourage them to expand their range of therapeutic possibilities. Many of these stories are based on extensive experience, whereas others are more experimental in nature. Some will provoke welcome criticism, since the handbook is intended as a basis for discussing and in particular trialling new therapeutic methodologies.

I believe that a certain degree of uncertainty over what we suppose to be reality and the blurred boundaries between mere visions of the future and incipient reality must be tolerated in order to endow the stories with the transformative power which my experience has shown rests within them. The *Handbook of Therapeutic Storytelling* is intended to encourage practitioners to start telling stories themselves, and to experiment with the effects of paradigmatic and metaphorical stories both in their work as counsellors and in their own lives.

## Instructions for use

Each story in this book is accompanied by a list of keywords which provide a quick overview of the purposes for which the story can be used, subdivided into the therapeutic topics it covers and the therapeutic interventions it contains. The methodology section discusses various themes by way of example and examines the therapeutic interventions in detail. The index of keywords in the appendix makes it possible to look up stories using the relevant keywords.

A discussion took place among readers of the manuscript as to whether the section on methodology should come before the section containing the individual stories; the counter-argument to this is that reading the stories beforehand makes it easier to understand and conceptualise the methods. The handbook can therefore be regarded as a hermeneutic circle: the methodology section explains the stories just as the stories explain the methodologies. The reader is free to read the methodologies first or to switch back and forth between both sections.

The therapeutic keywords listed alongside the stories and in the index are predominantly symptom-based, that is, problem- and deficit-oriented. This may appear a strange choice in view of the handbook's stated goal of shifting the focus of attention from deficits to resources, and if we had as many words to describe health as we do to describe illness it might have made sense to use an index of resource-based terms. To put a positive spin on the matter, however, a problem-based keyword search reflects the principle of pacing and leading, according to which the therapist (author, trainer, supervisor) should take the other party's current (and often problematic) experiences as a starting point and gradually modify them with a view to optimising resources (i.e. achieving a solution).

The majority of the stories can undoubtedly be used in contexts other than those named, and there is scope in many cases for the addition of extra symptoms and explanations regarding use. The author welcomes readers' suggestions in this respect, as well as feedback on their experiences of using the stories. Contact of this kind (for example via e-mail) will help to make this handbook a more useful work of reference in the future.

# PART ONE

# The stories

# Chapter 2

# Promoting understanding

## Assigning meaning

What meaning does a person assign to his or her life? Goals provide the framework that everyone needs in order to experience their life as meaningful, but a person's fundamental goals in life may change over the course of his or her lifetime, and may be described by that person in dynamic terms as change (or success) or in static terms as happiness (or health, or peace). Although people pursue a wide variety of different goals, everyone – except those who would rather not be here at all – can say what makes their life worthwhile.

### My Aim in Life

The story "My Aim in Life" calls into question the absoluteness of existing life goals, and encourages the listener to formulate his or her own values.

TOPIC: Health, meaning
INTERVENTION: Clarifying goals, externalisation of ambivalence as a dialogue, promoting a searching attitude (example, searching model)

"My aim in life is to leave as much healing and joy in my wake as possible," I said to a friend.
"That's a lofty goal," he said. "I'm happy if I can avoid causing too much harm."

### Renewed Life

The story "Renewed Life" makes it clear that life plans and goals play a vital role in an individual's happiness, health and life expectancy.

TOPIC: Health, life expectancy, meaning
INTERVENTION: Clarifying goals, promoting a searching attitude, promoting positive expectations (metaphor, positive model)

A number of researchers wanted to find out why salmon die after spawning, so they fished a number of specimens out of the river, fitted them with radio transmitters and placed them back into the sea. And what do you think happened? The animals stayed alive.

## Gockle's Good Luck

The story "Gockle's Good Luck" reminds us that we cannot always recognise and accept happiness and that some people have reasons of their own for not improving their situation. It also reminds us that we need goals for which we fight and that unexpected success may overtax our capacities. In conversation with parents, for example, the story can be used to make it clear that children and teenagers should not be allowed to become accustomed to taking an affluent lifestyle for granted, and that they need to experience achieving success and possessions through their own efforts. The story can also be used to alert listeners to the fact that they are taking skills for granted and overlooking opportunities for action, even though – or perhaps because – they are present in abundance.

TOPIC:  Growing up, meaning, success, upbringing

INTERVENTION: Clarifying goals, finding resources, promoting a searching attitude (metaphor, searching model)

> Someone once told me, "When I was growing up my family kept hens and a cockerel named Gockle. The cockerel and the hens ran around in the yard together, scratching and pecking at grains. Once we decided to give Gockle a special treat, and so we picked him up and put him down right in the middle of the box where the grain was stored. That must have been heaven on earth to a chicken! Yet even though Gockle was now standing on thousands upon thousands of tasty grains, he simply looked at us with a surprised expression and did nothing. He did not eat a single grain. Finally we took him outside again, where he scratched and searched for grains like he had before."

## Sacrilege

The story "Sacrilege" illustrates that standing up for your values represents a value in itself. In cases where these values are opposed to the interests of others, it is often necessary to find a balance between defending your ideals in public and taking a less conspicuous approach. The story can also be used to encourage clients not to hide their light under a bushel and to present a self-confident image during interactions with others.

TOPIC:  Belief, identity, self-confidence

INTERVENTION: Finding resources, pattern interrupt by the client (example, positive model)

Someone once told me the following story: "When I visited the Pisa Baptistry close to the city's cathedral, I thought to myself, 'They've turned it into a temple to commerce!' It raised my hackles to pay to enter a church and then find myself surrounded by hundreds of frantic tourists rushing around and taking photographs of everything. Many kept checking their watches, because a singer was paid to perform every hour in order to demonstrate the building's wonderful acoustics. Should a church not be a place of prayer and devotion? After climbing up to the gallery, I thought, 'Surely no one will object if I turn this temple to Mammon back into a house of God.' It took me a while to screw up the courage, but finally I sang the opening line of a psalm loudly and clearly into the open space, 'Laudate omnes gentes, laudate dominum.' The acoustics really were superb. Everything went quiet in the church, and although everyone looked around to find out who was singing, the echoes made it difficult for them to locate me. The security staff searching frantically for the perpetrator also had a hard task on their hands, but by the end of the verse one had spotted me. He waited for me to start singing again in order to catch me red-handed, since it would otherwise have been easy for me to deny my act of sacrilege. I looked around the building in a daze. 'Thank you,' said a woman standing next to me. 'That was wonderful.' I too felt better after having sung the psalm. When the last echo had faded away, I left the house of God, giving a sly grin to the security guard who was still watching me."

## Perception and interpretation

The communications theorist Paul Watzlawick asked, "How real is real?" (also the title of his book, Watzlawick, 1976) and pointed out that reality is constructed differently by all of us. Anyone who talks about reality must therefore also clarify whose reality is meant and (strictly speaking) at what point in time. Reality is always being reconstructed, even within an individual's lifetime. The following paradigmatic stories are intended to challenge our fundamental way of interpreting the world and to lay the groundwork for new interpretations.

### The Creation of the World

"The Creation of the World" makes it clear that all thought systems – and therefore all human ways of interpreting the world – have been devised by humans. We often get the world we think up and believe in; at a personal level, this means that we become what we believe in and what we think, hope and fear.

This rule has far-reaching implications in terms of both our health and our psychological, material, financial and social conditions. We can of course share our individual worlds with others by communicating them verbally and non-verbally, and to a certain extent turn our environment into what we believe it to be. All reality is created on the basis of a communicated and therefore shared world.

TOPIC: Depression, reality
INTERVENTION: Destabilisation through countertheses, finding resources, promoting a searching attitude, trance induction through questions and through stereotype (example, searching model)

> Mohammed created a world. Freud created a world. Tolkien created a world. McKinsey created a world. Bill Gates created a world. Can I too create a world?
>
> The German company Tchibo uses the advertising slogan, "Every week a new world". New worlds are indeed created every week. Most of them are not very original; they swim in the wake of the established worlds and do not gain any traction.
>
> What kind of a world have you created? A philosophical world? A spiritual world? A commercial world? A mathematical world? A social world? An aesthetic world? A material world? A communicative world? A world of fun? An ethical world?
>
> You might be thinking to yourself, "But I haven't created any world at all!" I don't believe that for a second. As soon as you look at something – anything – and inadvertently think something new, you start to create a world.

### The Cave Dwellers

The story "The Cave Dwellers" demonstrates that what we perceive is determined more by our biology and biography than by objective facts, and that the feedback effects from both our sensory perceptions and our interpretations largely drown out what is allegedly real about the world.

TOPIC: Depression, reality
INTERVENTION: Destabilisation through unanswerable questions, promoting a searching attitude (metaphor, searching model)

> She asked her mother, "Mum, mum, mum,
> what is real, real, real?"
> "What do you mean, what is real, real, real?"
> "I mean without this echo, echo, echo."
> "Which echo, echo, echo?
> Right here and now is real, real, real."
> "I see, see, see."
> And then she understood, understood, understood.

### Glasses

"Glasses" is the transcript of a dream. The aim of the story is to make it clear that we often waste time and energy on maintaining counterproductive ways of seeing and experiencing life. Solutions that involve changing the underlying foundations of our way of thinking may be too close for us to see them.

TOPIC: Belief, reality, self-confidence, trauma

INTERVENTION: Finding resources, clarifying goals, destabilisation through unanswerable questions, metaphorical reframing (metaphor, searching model)

Once I dreamt that the left arm of my glasses was crooked, and I wanted to fix it so that the glasses would fit again. I bent it backwards and forwards twice, and then it snapped off. I held it up to the glasses – it had broken off at the hinge, and could no longer be repaired. What should I do?

I put the glasses on in the hope that they might fit somehow, but they hung diagonally across my face. Everything looked distorted through the lenses, and holding them in place the whole time was extremely uncomfortable. Yet opticians are closed on Sundays. What is the best course of action in a situation like this? I thought for a while. Then I remembered – I'd undergone laser surgery over six months ago to correct my shortsightedness. Why on earth was I still wearing the stupid glasses? And I went about my day without them.

### Dot to Dot

The story "Dot to Dot" makes it clear that we construct our own reality, and that different constructions of reality are both possible and admissible. It can be used to encourage clients to be more tolerant, to question their former points of view and to examine new points of view. It also makes it clear that the way in which children see the world and the delusional beliefs of dementia patients (for example) stem from missing information and the use of imagination and emotion to fill the associated gaps.

TOPIC: Belief, compulsion (OCD), delusion, dementia, growing up, reality

INTERVENTION: Destabilisation through unanswerable questions, finding resources, promoting a searching attitude, rhetorical question, trance induction through age regression and through questions (metaphor, searching model)

When I was a small child, I had a colouring book with pictures made up entirely of unconnected little dots. Each dot had a number next to it, and if you joined the dots in the correct order you would discover the picture that was hiding behind them.

I wonder how many pictures might be discovered in these collections of dots if the numbers next to them somehow got lost. If someone had never seen a map of the stars before, which stars would he or she join together to invent signs of the zodiac? How many different night skies could there be? Which world might we be living in if we had been raised by someone else and given different explanations of how the world works?

How many different interrelations or disjunctions might we find between the things that exist in this world? How many terms might we invent for things that are intangible, like peace, justice and identity? In how many ways might we link the frameworks of our values or allow them to co-exist separately? In how many ways might we see a person, and in how many ways might we interpret his or her behaviour? That's why I keep on joining the dots.

## What Does That Make Me?

The story "What Does That Make Me?" encourages listeners to think about the non-absolute nature of the characteristics an individual is assumed to have. It can also be used to illustrate the extent to which purported characteristics depend on how the surrounding context is interpreted. It is impossible to draw any conclusions about a person's real nature from his or her behaviour, even if this behaviour is repeated, firstly because this would preclude the possibility of the person acting differently on a regular basis (otherwise he or she would have different characteristics, that is, be a completely different person, as soon as his or her behaviour changed), and secondly because the characteristics that are ascribed – frugality or stinginess, a scheming mind or an enterprising spirit, heroism or stupidity, stubbornness or strong-mindedness – depend on the observer's own values and criteria.

TOPIC: Identity, prejudice, reality
INTERVENTION: Destabilisation through unanswerable questions, finding resources, real reframing (example, searching model)

Yesterday I went to buy something at a shop in town. The shop assistant was on her own, and she had run out of change. Although we had chatted for a few minutes before I paid, we did not know each other. And yet she placed a 50-Euro note in my hand and said, "Could you please change this for me in the electrical shop next door?" I asked myself whether the woman was irresponsible, careless and naïve for sending a man whom she had never met before out of her shop with 50 euros from her till, or whether she was a good judge of character and trusting, or whether she was warm-hearted and unconventional. I could have left the shop with the money and never returned. Instead, I gave the shop assistant my wallet and said, "Hold onto this until I return." My wallet contained 200 euros, my identity card, my driving licence and my credit card.

What does that make me? One hundred different people reading this study will think that it proves that I am one hundred different people with one hundred or more different characteristics, and yet their judgments have nothing whatsoever to do with me.

## Understanding and misunderstanding

Every individual interprets the world and its various opportunities differently, and our biology and biography have more influence on our beliefs than external parameters. Understanding is a highly subjective and individual matter, which makes it necessary to ask ourselves what "understanding" really means. Perhaps "understanding" means having reached a consensus on a shared view of the world? Yet even this consensus is only apparent, since different people associate different things with the same words and therefore mean different things when they say these words. It is likely that we misunderstand each other constantly at both verbal and non-verbal level, but fortunately most of these misunderstandings merely amount to the mistaken belief that we understand each other. It would appear that successful communication often requires nothing more than for each party in the conversation to have understood something which is compatible in terms of its emotional and practical consequences with what the other party has heard.

### Without Words

The story "Without Words" offers examples of how body language can be interpreted. It can be used as therapeutic homework to provide young people with autism with a new way of interpreting other people's behaviour, and to occupy highly gifted young people with observation tasks as a distraction from provocative or depressive behaviour.

TOPIC: Asperger syndrome / autism, body language, giftedness
INTERVENTION: Homework, increasing complexity, psychoeducation (example / positive model)

While I was driving home I approached a zebra crossing. A pedestrian was walking along the pavement, still a little way before the crossing. I stopped. It is possible to tell whether someone is going to cross the road several metres before they stop or look around, because they make a small turning motion with their body or head, which foreshadows the planned movement.

There are situations in which it can be useful to observe these min-imal movements which anticipate actual movements. When the person leading a committee meeting or seminar asks for a volunteer, for example, a long pause often sets in while everyone waits to see if someone else is enthusiastic enough to volunteer first. And yet the individual who finally volunteers after lots of encouragement is always the one who moved immediately after the request was made – by leaning forwards slightly, by opening his or her mouth briefly, by uncrossing his or her legs, by sighing or by any other movement that might serve as a non-verbal introduction to a spoken contribution. If I want to circumvent this tedious process, I address a direct question to the person who moved first after I asked for a volunteer, enquiring whether he or she would like to take on the task. Experience shows that the answer is always yes.

### Good Morning Everyone!

The story "Good Morning Everyone!" can be used to encourage the lis-tener to adopt a creative approach to gossip. It demonstrates how a victim of gossip can take proactive steps against the "rumour mill" by spreading counterrumours.

TOPIC:  Gossip, rumour, self-confidence
INTERVENTION: Destabilisation through counter-rumours (example, positive model)

> There was once a priest who lived in a small village far out in the country-side in Bavaria. He was a young and good-looking priest who lived alone, which made him a figure of enormous interest for the other villagers. One morning he got up, opened his window, hung out two sets of bedlinen to air – as was the custom in that land – and drank his coffee in peace. Good morning everyone! Now he had plenty of material for his next sermon…

### Theatre Trip

The story "Theatre Trip" demonstrates how other people's words can often be misinterpreted as a result of a guilty conscience or critical inner voices.

TOPIC:  Conscience, reality
INTERVENTION: Inner team, promoting a searching attitude (example, nega-tive model)

> A group of women from the Farmers' Wives Club of Little Middlington were going on a trip to the theatre when the coach in which they were travelling broke down, and the play was in full swing by the time they

arrived. As the group entered the theatre, one of the actors on stage was declaiming, "Who are you? Why do you come so late?" One of the women answered, "We're the Farmers' Wives from Little Middlington. Our coach conked out!"

## The Converter

"The Converter" demonstrates how everyone speaks his or her own language and must learn to speak in the language of his or her counterpart, using the examples of men and women and different professions.

TOPIC: Misunderstanding, reality, relationship
INTERVENTION: Circular reasoning (example / metaphor, searching model), mirroring, psychoeducation, suggestive question

An unemotional technician and a romantically inclined office worker came for relationship counselling with the hope that I could help them understand each other better. I explained that people – and in particular men and women – are never able to understand each other.

"I understand," said the technician. "We need a converter which transforms my language into my wife's language."

"That's a very clear way of putting it," I replied, and then asked, "What's a converter?"

# Chapter 3

# Promoting health

## Heart, circulation, bleeding and blood flow

Metaphors are often used in hypnotherapy to bring about changed bodily reactions, for example in relation to the distribution of energy and other resources and the discovery of new healing opportunities. These effects are often achieved by stories which facilitate a new way of seeing the world. This is because storytelling produces a natural trance, during which the story's implications are interpreted and examined by the unconscious mind as instructions for how the body should act, and in many cases also implemented.

Heart rate, blood pressure and blood flow can be influenced within this framework, that is, by expanding and constricting blood vessels in the body as a whole or in individual body parts, which has a major effect on many organic and psychosomatic disorders; for example, it is often possible to stop a nosebleed or bleeding from a wound or surgical incision. Circulatory disorders, for example problems caused by various body parts "going to sleep" or sensations of cold, can also be treated using suggestive stories, as can blushing and (indirectly) erythrophobia, which itself causes the suffer to blush in many cases and results in a vicious circle. There are even indications that the blood's ability to clot is open to influence.

### Nosebleed

The story "Nosebleed" is a basic intervention which can be varied in many different ways, and which serves as an example of the effectiveness of hypnotic suggestions in everyday life outside an explicitly therapeutic context. I have used the technique described below on five people, four of whom were children. In four cases the bleeding stopped within one to three minutes, and in one case there was no significant improvement. The valve should be turned to the right or left depending on the symptoms (to the left in order to increase blood flow). The suggestions are unambiguous, despite being phrased in an indirect and non-directive manner.

Karen Olness and Daniel Kohen write about a ten-year-old boy brought to a doctor with a severe nosebleed: "Lower nasal plugs on both sides failed to improve the situation. The doctor decided to try hypnotherapy in addition to rear nasal plugs. He suggested to the patient that he could stop the bleeding himself and that he should tip his head right back and relax. Within a few minutes, the bleeding stopped and the young boy could breathe easily again. [...] The next morning the parents reported that there had been no further bleeding." The authors believe it is a good idea to use similar suggestions with any person suffering from life-threatening bleeding from any part of the body (Kohen & Olness, 2011: 277).

The story can be used not only for somatic complaints, but also for patients suffering from erythrophobia (fear of blushing or compulsive blushing), as well as for patients with "bad" habits and other (chronic) psychosocial symptoms in order to highlight the power of the mind to eliminate a certain symptom without further ado. In such situations it is recommended that further episodes of the story be told, explaining how individuals simply "turned off" a problem or symptom (e.g. a red-hot oven ring, a garden hose or an annoying radio). Since most symptoms are involuntary and are defended by clients as occurring "not on purpose", I would advise against discussing the content of the story on a cognitive level. Nevertheless, when eliminating symptoms it is always necessary first to ask oneself and the client, "What purpose does this symptom serve?"

TOPIC: Angina pectoris, bleeding, blood flow, coronary heart disease (CHD), phobia (erythrophobia), haematoma, hypertonia, peripheral artery disease (PAD), prolonged reversible ischemic neurological deficit (PRIND), transient ischaemic attacks (TIA)

INTERVENTION: Trance induction through eye fixation and through questions, using connotation (example / metaphor, positive model)

They met by chance on a grassy field. The old man was exercising his dog, and the young man was simply going for a walk. They recognised each other because they belonged to the same chess club, and so they started chatting. Suddenly the old man hesitated. He took out a packet of tissues, pulled out a few and held them in front of his face. His nose wouldn't stop bleeding.

"Can I show you how to stop the bleeding?" said the younger man. "Look around you. Can you see anything red?"

"That tree over there has red berries," said the older man.

"That's right. Berries as red as blood. Can you imagine a valve on a water pipe in the same red colour?"

"I can."

"Does it look more like the red handle on a tap, or a large red stopcock of the sort you sometimes use to turn off the water supply to a house?"

"A stopcock."

As they stood next to each other and talked, the younger man stretched out his arm in front of him and kept turning his hand to the right as though he was closing a big valve.

"You can put your tissues away again now," he said.

### Manta Ray

The story "Manta Ray" outlines an intervention for impending heart attacks and asthma attacks, and was inspired by a patient who had suffered a heart attack but who amused the ambulance crew, paramedic and himself with jokes and anecdotes to relax both them and himself and to keep his blood vessels open, based on the principle that anxiety narrows the blood vessels, whereas relaxing images and thoughts widen them and thus increase the chances of survival in a threatened or acute heart attack. Similarly, anxiety during an asthma attack makes it harder to breathe and results in exactly what the patient fears. The metaphor incorporates suggestions for relaxation of the emotions and muscles, regulation of the frequency and intensity of the heart rate and breath and widening of the vessels (warm water), since the simulation of these autonomic states by the imagination stimulates a matching state in the body. Prior mental training is necessary to ensure that these images are called to mind automatically during a heart attack or asthma attack. If necessary, the manta ray should start flapping his fins with "fast and irregular beats", which then gradually become slower. When the story was told to a patient suffering from palpitations (sinus tachycardia), a reduction in pulse rate and a significant improvement in the accompanying symptoms were observed afterwards. The story can be modified to feature an electric ray that generates electrical pulses while he moves, in the same rhythm as his heart beat. As ever, it is important to use these methods to complement traditional medical treatments rather than as an alternative to them. Further stories that can be used on heart diseases are found in Hammel, 2011: 67, 162. Stories and narrative interventions for asthma patients are found in Hammel, 2011: 70, 171 and in Hammel, 2017:120.

TOPIC: Acute coronary syndrome, angina pectoris, anxiety, asthma, bleeding, blood flow, breathing, coronary heart disease (CHD), exam nerves, heart attack, hyperventilation, migraine, stage fright, pain, premature labour, tachycardia, trauma

INTERVENTION: Imagined rapport, stimulation through simulation (metaphor, positive model)

While the paramedic hurried over and the ambulance crew shouted instructions to each other, I imagined a large manta ray gliding through the warm water, with strong calm flaps of his majestic fins, noiseless and beautiful, the embodiment of calm, the embodiment of calm, the embodiment of calm … a truly wonderful creature!

## Placebo I

The case study "Placebo I" illustrates how blood pressure can be regulated by imagining blood pressure tablets. The story could also end: "Your body knows it so well that it will do what it needs to do even if you simply draw a white circle on every page of your presentation to remind you of the blood pressure tablets." Further interventions on stage fright and exam nerves can be found in Hammel, 2017: 103.

TOPIC: Hypertonia
INTERVENTION: Unreal placebo (example, positive model)

"I used to get terrible stage fright every time I had to speak in public," said the man. "My blood pressure shot up, I got palpitations and my breathing became rapid and shallow. But then my wife gave me these tablets to lower my blood pressure, and I've not had any problems since then."

"Can I tell you a secret?" replied the other man. "Every time you take a tablet, your body knows that it needs to reduce its blood pressure – it knows what it has to do in response to the tablet. It knows it so well that it will do what it needs to do by itself, even if you just carry the blood pressure tablet with you."

## Placebo II

The case study "Placebo II" demonstrates a similar procedure for sluggish circulation, in which the patient imagines a Kneipp hydrotherapy treatment.

TOPIC: Blood flow, hypotonia
INTERVENTION: Unreal placebo (example, positive model)

"My feet often feel as cold as ice," said the man. "That's why I catch so many colds. I used to have Kneipp treatments and that really helped, but I can't do that everywhere."

"Let me tell you a secret," said the other man. "An imaginary Kneipp treatment will work just as well if you imagine it hard enough."

## Steam Engines

The story "Steam Engines" can be used to regulate blood pressure and breathing and to reduce stress, as well as to equip patients to handle stressful emotions more easily.

TOPIC: Aggression, asthma, borderline personality disorder, chronic obstructive pulmonary disease (COPD), heart attack, hypertonia, impulse control, mania, stress

INTERVENTION: Ambiguity, metaphorical reframing (metaphor, positive model)

> Steam engines hold a particular fascination for many people and exert a special attraction over both young and old. Anyone who owns such a precious machine must handle it very carefully. The most important thing that a steam engine does is to regulate pressure. It is vitally important for the steam pressure valve to open in good time and reliably discharge any excess pressure. It is also important to ensure that steam engines are only heated to a moderate temperature, particularly if they are already well advanced in years. They need regular breaks, proper oiling and expert maintenance. It is a huge mistake to overheat a steam engine, and a mistake that will only be made by an amateur. A good technician knows what his treasured engine needs, and always drives it at a moderate pressure.

### The Eagle's Journey

The following story was designed and tested for the purpose of reducing and stabilising the pulse and blood pressure, and can also be used to stabilise a patient's breathing rate at a low level and reduce the frequency, duration and intensity of muscle contractions, for example during premature labour. It is also suitable for reducing panic attacks; when used in this connection, the start of the story must be told in a flustered or panicky manner (principle of pacing and leading). In slightly modified form, the story can also be used for dental treatment, for example in connection with a dental phobia, in which case the eagle should see a chain of snow-capped mountains a long way off which might bear a vague resemblance to a row of teeth for some people, but the eagle has a sharp beak and is not worried about such things...

TOPIC: Acute coronary syndrome, angina pectoris, anxiety, asthma, coronary heart disease (CHD), dental treatment, exam nerves, heart attack, hypertonia, hyperventilation, panic disorder, premature labour, sleep, stage fright, stress, treatment phobia

INTERVENTION: Ambiguity, imagined rapport, metaphorical reframing (metaphor, positive model)

> Imagine you're an eagle flying over the Alps. You're flying in the direction of the midday sun, towards the place where the land known to humans as Italy lies far behind vast mountain ranges. You can see towering mountain peaks and cavernous valleys. You pass through a storm, with flashes of lightning electrifying the air and squalls of wind making you flap your wings more vigorously. There is no question of coasting on air currents here – you need to use your wings, and you also need to use them to make it safely over the summit of the Bernina Pass. Once you are over

the summit, the mountain peaks gradually get lower, and the weather gets calmer and more pleasant. As you fly onwards, the landscape turns into a patchwork of hills and then into a series of gentle undulations, before finally levelling out almost entirely. You reach the sea. Its waves are smooth and flat, and it stretches out before you like a giant mirror. You fly out over the open sea. For a long time you fly towards the rising sun, then again towards the midday sun, until you reach land again – the Sinai Peninsula, which is a desert. Once again you fly towards the rising sun, before finally catching sight of a broad and smooth expanse to your left – the Dead Sea, the calm surface of which is completely unbroken by waves. You fly there, towards an oasis you have spotted behind it. The Jordan River is small and surrounded by green trees and bushes. You alight on its bank and take a drink from its water, finding a shady branch to sit on if you like. Take a minute to look around. You are at the lowest point in the world. The calm, smooth mirror of the Dead Sea lies four hundred metres below sea level. Enjoy the peace and quiet as you sit on your branch, and take anything which has proved useful with you when you fly back home.

## Infections, allergies, autoimmune diseases

The stories in this chapter are aimed at strengthening the immune system and preventing it from responding inappropriately or excessively. Declarations and implications that highlight, describe and praise the strength of the immune system can be used to strengthen it, and it can also be useful to imagine medicines and forms of treatment that boost the immune system.

A basic intervention for allergies and non-infectious inflammation is to explain them as a misunderstanding, thereby acknowledging the body's protective response as essentially useful. This acknowledgement that the responding part of the body has "good intentions" makes it possible to use the "goodwill" behind the bodily function for healing purposes. Negotiations can be held with the unconscious with a view to abandoning or reversing the problematic bodily response on an experimental basis, with the agreement that the new response will be intensified and continued if it proves useful and that the previous response can otherwise be restored. These negotiations with the unconscious can take place either directly and openly or metaphorically; in both cases, however, it must be remembered that the unconscious – which represents both a psychological and a physical function – is also listening and responding.

Allergies are "phobias of the body." They can be systematically and gradually desensitised using an approach that is widespread in behavioural therapy and which is also popular (in an imaginative form) among hypnotherapists; the client is put into a state of relaxation and, while remaining in this worry-free state, asked to imagine situations that trigger his or her allergy first to a minor extent and then ever more severely, attempting at all times to stay relaxed. If this is not possible, the patient should stop imagining the relevant situation and return to a state of relaxation, only imagining the critical situation in such a way and to such an extent that he or she remains free of anxiety and symptoms. The ultimate aim is to imagine a situation triggering a severe allergy while remaining in a state of deep relaxation and free of all symptoms. As homework, the client is set the task of returning to exactly the same state whenever he or she is exposed to the "allergen", noticing any difference between his or her current and former experiences, and of practising ever deeper relaxation whenever he or she encounters it (in-vivo desensitisation). In more precise words, there is no such thing as an "allergen" in the sense of a substance which attacks the body; instead, the body incorrectly identifies a substance as a threat, just like Don Quixote tilting at windmills or a soldier suffering from combat PTSD who is afraid of loud noises (when it is not the noises which are potentially harmful but his or her reactions to them). The very concept of "allergens" may therefore unintentionally encourage the body in its misconceptions.

As a general rule, a mild allergic reaction is triggered if a sufferer merely imagines the relevant allergen, for example when looking at a photograph of trees in bloom, listening to the pollen count report on the radio or talking about the allergy. It is helpful to alert clients to the fact that they showed the symptoms of the allergy while they were talking about it during the anamnesis discussion prior to treatment, for example by scratching their skin, blowing their nose, rubbing their eyes, clearing their throat etc., and that at the end, after performing a series of imaginative exercises, they were free of all these symptoms even while focusing their attention much more intensely on the allergens that previously triggered a response. I give clients the post-hypnotic order that this change (which is easy for them to verify) is just as applicable to real meadows with real trees, and they should therefore look forward to the next meadow they visit.

### Morbus Feivel

In my experience, anyone who regularly makes the apparently nonsensical claim that he or she is suffering from infectious health, as described in the story "Morbus Feivel", is more likely to remain healthy during an outbreak of infectious disease. At the same time, some people appear to respond to the warning, "Watch out! I'm suffering from infectious health!" by recovering more rapidly from an illness. The story is based on a Polish-Jewish narrative tradition popularised by Isaak Bashevis Singer (Singer, 1968). The idea of infectious health also appears in Hammel, 2012b: 51.)

TOPIC: Cold, flu, gastroenteritis, immune system, infection, compulsion (OCD / washing), reality

INTERVENTION:  Unreal reframing (example, positive model / searching model)

The city of Chelm once became the breeding ground for a strange epidemic, and this is how it happened. So many people in the city were falling ill that Doctor Feivel thought to himself how much quicker and easier it would be to stop examining the city's residents to find out what illness they were suffering from, and instead to find out who had been infected by health and what kind of health it was. He diagnosed healthy bones in a patient who had no broken legs, a healthy heart in another patient, a severe case of healthy skin in a third and so on. When Schlemihl came to see him, he diagnosed uninflamed health of the gums. When Schlemihl asked him what he meant, the doctor – who had already started examining his next patient – muttered, "Morbus Feivel, advanced stage of severity." Schlemihl did not really understand what he meant, but did not wish to admit his ignorance and so did not query the diagnosis. When he arrived home and his wife asked him what the doctor had said, he answered curtly, "Infectious health." Schlemihl's wife wondered how it could be possible that she and the children still had a cold when they lived in such close quarters with Schlemihl. When she asked Doctor Feivel, he explained, "It's because of the incubation time. The proper symptoms only appear a few days after transmission of an infection of this kind."

And by the next day Schlemihl's wife and children were indeed feeling much better. "We're suffering from infectious health," they explained to their neighbours. "We caught it from Schlemihl."

The neighbours were also infected with health over the next few days, and soon Morbus Feivel had spread like wildfire throughout the entire city. Before long the residents of surrounding villages came to infect themselves with Schlemihl's epidemic, and eventually the entire country was infected with it – at any rate according to Schlemihl's version of the story.

### Risk of Contagion

A variation on the intervention in "Morbus Feivel" can be seen in the story "Risk of Contagion". The story externalises the problematic bodily experience into the glass and gives implied instructions to the immune system to switch from a defensive to an offensive position.

TOPIC:  Cold, cold sores, gastroenteritis, flu, immune system, infection
INTERVENTION: Preventive suggestion, unreal reframing (example, positive model)

I recently visited my sister and her family. Right at the start of my visit I took a drink of water out of a glass which was standing in front of me.

"You didn't drink out of that, did you?" asked my sister. "That glass belongs to Luise, and she's highly contagious."

I bent over the glass and spat the following words into it: "Make sure you don't catch the Stefan disease!"

Then I drank all the water in the glass. And nothing else happened – at any rate not to me.

### Illness on Order

The story "Illness on Order" illustrates how believing that "anyone who calls in sick must really be sick" can result in real illness, and how pretend or inconsequential illnesses can develop into real ones. The story can also be used as a metaphor for mental and social blocks.

TOPIC: Anxiety, bullying, compulsion (OCD), conscience, immune system
INTERVENTION: Aversive suggestion (example / metaphor, negative model)

> A doctor once told me, "Once I decided to spend part of my working day at home so that I could make headway on a mountain of paperwork. I hung a 'Closed due to illness' sign on the door of my practice – and fell ill straight away. Yesterday I told my daughter-in-law about it. 'I know just what you mean,' she said. 'I fall ill every time you give me a sick note as a favour.'"

### A Jarful of Allergies

"A Jarful of Allergies" outlines a method of metaphorically instructing the body to cure an allergy.

The story is inspired by the story of an eleven-year-old girl who had learned self-hypnosis reported by Karen Olness and Dan Kohen. The girl once asked, "Can hypnosis also help with hay fever?" The immune response which causes hay fever was then explained to her in medical terms. "She gave the very logical response, 'So I need to hypnotise myself to keep the histamines in the mast cells and not allow them into the bloodstream?' Somewhat surprised by this matterof-fact analysis, I [the doctor treating her] agreed. She thanked me and left. Several months later, Sarah's mother told me that her daughter's symptoms of hay fever were mild despite the high pollen count, and that the swelling of her eyes and mucous membranes was so minor that she no longer needed any medication." (Kohen & Olness, 2011: 266)

The end of the story uses a quote by the hypnotherapist Maria Freund. Freund writes, "A few years ago I suffered from a severe allergy to early blossoming trees. The solution I found was to start taking a naturopathic remedy before the trees came into blossom, and at the same time to repeat the following sentence to myself like a mantra whenever I was outside, and in particular when I passed trees in blossom: 'I used to need hay fever, but I don't any more.' It really worked, and after a while I only needed the sentence and could stop taking the naturopathic remedy. I didn't experience any further symptoms in following years, and if I ever do feel a trace of anxiety again when I look at trees in blossom, I repeat the sentence to myself a few times in my head." (e-mail message, 2008).

Further stories and narrative interventions on allergies can be found in Hammel, 2011: 70; Hammel, 2014: 80, 169; Hammel, 2016: 39, 43, 47; Hammel, 2017: 120.

TOPIC: Allergy

INTERVENTION: Anchoring, externalisation of a problem as an object, post-hypnotic suggestion, unreal reframing, visualisation (metaphor, positive model)

> Imagine that the histamines triggered by your allergy are all stored in a glass jar. How big is the jar? What shape is it? What do the histamines look like? Are they in powder or liquid form? Do they look like small creatures, or maybe like a fog? How full is the jar? And how empty would you like it to be? Remember that your body can produce more of these substances whenever you need them. If you'd like the jar to be completely empty, take it to a place where you can tip out the histamines. Notice the movements of your hands while you are emptying the jar. Whenever you make a similar movement, you'll remember – either consciously or unconsciously – how you tipped out the histamines. And every time you remember, you'll feel safer and safer, and you'll know for sure; I used to need my allergy, but I don't any more.

### The Way to the Meadow

"The Way to the Meadow" provides a brief demonstration of how allergies can be systematically desensitised in the imagination, and how the result can be anchored using post-hypnotic suggestions in the form of declarations and implications. The final sentence implies completeness by alluding to the end of the creation story, "And behold, it was very good." (Genesis 1:31).

A method of systematically desensitising hay fever through hypnotic suggestion can also be found in Hans A. Abraham, based however on the medicinal desensitisation of allergies, that is, an unreal placebo, rather than the desensitisation of phobias. Gibbons suggests that the very small quantities of pollen present in the air or on objects during the colder months of the year act as a desensitising vaccination for the client (Abraham, 1990).

TOPIC: Allergy

INTERVENTION: Post-hypnotic suggestion, systematic desensitisation (example, positive model)

Imagine that you're in a cold, clear place on a winter's day. You take deep, calm breaths and enjoy the crisp, fresh air. Time passes, and now it's spring. Keep breathing steadily and carry the pleasant sense of calm with you. Imagine that you're breathing deeply, calmly and with pleasure, since you know that you're safe now and will remain safe. It does you good to breathe so calmly and peacefully. Imagine that it's spring, and you're walking in a meadow past blossoming birch trees with the same sense of calm and the same deep breaths, and perhaps you're even surprised that you feel so good. You breathe deeply and steadily. You feel no fear, and you enjoy this feeling. Imagine walking up to a birch tree, and having the wonderful idea of hugging it – and behold, it is very good.

### The Recovery Game

"The Recovery Game" demonstrates how the immune system can be strengthened through suggestion during a time of illness; it can also be used (in slightly modified form) to prevent illness. The story is one of a whole genre of therapeutic stories which involve inventing computer games or similar games of skill, and which can be designed to boost performance at school, to increase self-confidence or for many other purposes. They are ideal for use with children and young people in the context of joint storytelling.

TOPIC: Cold, flu, immune system
INTERVENTION: Mental game, preventive suggestion, unreal reframing (metaphor, positive model),

Paul was lying in bed and feeling bored. He longed to feel well again. "Can't someone do something to speed things up?" he asked.

"It just takes time," came the answer. "Although there is a computer game... unfortunately we don't have it, but I'm sure you can imagine it... it works like this; your body's police force is on patrol, searching for criminals in the blood vessels and throughout the entire body. The police officers look like large spheres, with eyes and sharp teeth. The criminals are little spheres which try to hide. When a police officer has eaten five of the little spheres, he has enough health points to split into two police officers. Then they hunt as a team of two, and soon as a team of four, eight and so on. The game can be played at different speeds, and of course the aim is to make the police officers as fast as possible while still catching all the criminals without whizzing past any by mistake. If you're successful, you can set it to go even faster. The game has ten different skill levels, and you should make sure that you start on a level where you have a good chance of winning. The final thing it is important to know is that the game has a sophisticated graphical design, which means that you can choose how it looks. The police officers can whizz through the body's blood vessels – both the small ones and the large ones – or through a kind of sewerage system which looks like a large and complicated system of water slides. They can roll like marbles along a marble run with lifts and moving staircases, or they can travel at supersonic speed in spaceships zooming through the air in a huge inter-galactic system of tunnels. Choose the version you'd like to play first, and press the start button – now!"

## Placebo III

The story "Placebo III" demonstrates how the placebo effect can be actively used to heal a cold, even if the relevant medicine is not currently available and has never been taken by the patient before.

TOPIC: Cold, immune system
INTERVENTION: Stabilisation through praise, unreal placebo (example, positive model)

> Someone once told me the following story; "I was visiting my sister. My niece was getting confirmed, and my brother-in-law had a terrible cold. He was sneezing, sniffing and coughing, and clearly felt terrible. 'The homeopathic remedy Schuessler Salt No. 3 would help,' said my sister. 'But we don't have any in the house.'
> "'That doesn't matter,' I replied, and turned to my brother-in-law. 'Say to your body, "Dear body, please check whether Schuessler Salt No 3 would help, and if it would then respond as if you had taken it."'
> "'But he's never tried it before,' objected my sister.
> "'That doesn't matter either,' I replied, citing as evidence the case of a patient treated by some doctor or other. In the meantime, my brother-in-law had stopped sneezing and sniffing and looked a little better in general.
> "I cried out, 'Great job! You must have an incredibly powerful sub-conscious – that's truly impressive! Brilliant! What a feat of the subconscious – and you managed it so quickly! I think Schuessler Salt No. 3 has done you a lot of good! You're doing a brilliant job...'
> "My brother-in-law gave a lopsided grin and looked a little embarrassed, but his symptoms had reduced significantly, and stayed like that all day."

## Placebo IV

The story "Placebo IV" uses the technique of focusing the body's self-healing capacities on a region of the body in cases of inflammation. The body is addressed very directly and reminded of what was useful in an earlier situation. Imagining a medicine prompts the body to behave in the way that it would normally behave in response to that medicine. The body is told to do "more of the same" if this behaviour is helpful.

TOPIC: Inflammation, phlebitis
INTERVENTION: Test suggestion, unreal placebo (example, positive model)

> My foot had been hurting for weeks. What on earth could be wrong with it? I remembered feeling something similar when suffering from phlebitis many years ago. A homeopathic remedy called Lachesis had cured the problem back then.
>
> "Dear body," I said, "please check whether Lachesis would help. If you think it would, please behave as if you had taken it." Was that the right thing to say? A momentary shiver ran over my skin, which I decided must be my subconscious responding to the idea. The symptoms vanished overnight and did not return.

## Call-Out

The story "Call-Out" is another intervention which can be used to heal inflammation, and which can be used (like the following story) to strengthen the immune system, cure or reduce the severity of allergies and autoimmune diseases and cure inflammation. I have used the story for patients suffering from conditions including inflammation and Crohn's disease. For patients suffering from bowel conditions, I refer to the fact that the hoses are stable and made from strong, fireproof materials.

One client responded to this story with a similar tale; "Once I was called out with the volunteer fire brigade, and we set out with sirens blaring. We arrived at the scene of the fire and extinguished it. While we were driving back, the sirens were still sounding."

TOPIC: Allergy, appendix, colitis, Crohn's disease, phobia (erythrophobia), exam nerves, Graves' disease, Hashimoto's disease, immune disease, immune system, inflammation, lupus erythematosus, sarcoidosis, stage fright
INTERVENTION: Metaphorical reframing, prioritisation, using connotations (metaphor, searching model)

> The alarm bell rings. The pounding of rapid footsteps can be heard, mingled with the sound of people calling to each other and then the creaking of protective clothing being pulled on quickly. Rapid footsteps can be heard once again. Within less than a minute, the firefighters are in the fire engine and driving away, accompanied by the deafening sound of the siren. They arrive at the scene of the fire. Smoke is billowing out of a third-floor window. The officer-in-charge gives the commands.

The fire engine driver raises the ladder, two firefighters get the hoses ready and another two run to the front door of the apartment block. A window opens.

"Hello, what's going on?"

"Fire! Stay where you are! We'll rescue you!"

"But I don't need rescuing! The room next door is my kitchen – the cake I was baking started to burn while I was out at the shops, so I opened the window to get rid of the smoke. Why don't you come in and have a cup of coffee? I'm sure you won't mind the smell of smoke."

The firefighters are taken aback at first, but then they laugh. "Mission abort!" calls out the officer-in-charge. "False alarm!"

The hoses are rolled up again and the ladder lowered. The men at the entrance to the apartment block stroll casually back to the fire engine, grinning. They take off their helmets and protective clothing and place them in the fire engine. Then they go upstairs, where mugs of hot coffee are already waiting for them.

"I think you should *overhaul your alarm system*," says the owner of the apartment. The officer-in-charge nods. The alarm system needs an overhaul.

"We review every call-out, particularly call-outs of this kind," he says with a wink. "We'll tell the control room so that the same thing doesn't happen again in the future. Great coffee though!"


### The Villa

The case history "The Villa" illustrates the technique of influencing an immune disease or other somatic disorder through metaphorical instructions which imply progress alone and exclude any possibility of relapses. It is also useful for promoting the healing of wounds or bone fractures.

The story relates to a case from 2004 (thirteen-year catamnesis). The metaphor largely excludes the possibility of relapses. Once the brain has accepted the image as being fundamentally relevant to the way in which the body is viewed, it excludes any bodily behaviour which is incompatible with the metaphor. The architect's profession is used as the source of the metaphor; as illustrated by the story "Sorting Screws", images and tasks which pick up on aspects of the patient's identity are more powerful than those that are externally dictated.

On the topic of wound healing and the accelerated healing of bone fractures through auto-suggestion, Milton Erickson describes the case of the US psychiatrist Robert Pearson, who healed his own broken skull completely within a single week. (Rosen, 1982) Erickson refers to studies carried out by a surgeon and psychiatrist who used hypnosis to promote wound healing in every second patient on whom he operated. These patients' wounds healed more rapidly. (Zeig, 1985: 222).

TOPIC:   Allergy, bone fractures, colitis, convalescence, Crohn's disease, immune disease, immune system, inflammation, sarcoidosis, wound healing

INTERVENTION: Metaphorical reframing, utilisation of the client's professional experience (metaphor, positive model)

I once had a patient who was an architect and who suffered from Crohn's disease, an inflammatory bowel disease.

The cortisone preparations and surgical interventions used to treat it had placed an enormous strain on her body. After attending a number of therapy sessions, the disease seemed to have remitted somewhat. I said to her, "Imagine your body is a magnificent old house awaiting renovation – what does it look like?"

She described a Wilhelminian-style villa surrounded by lush greenery, with exquisite stucco work, superb wallpaper and elegant furniture. The house appeared to have been neglected for many years. Wherever the eye turned, there were traces of water damage, cracks in the walls and crumbling plaster. Many of the formerly beautiful features now looked neglected and derelict.

"What does the restoration team need to do?" I asked.

She listed a number of jobs, and we discussed the order in which they should be done.

I asked for an update on the renovations at each of the following therapy sessions, and was always told that the workmen had made progress. What choice did they have? After all, renovations go forwards, not backwards.

Once the woman told me, "The original features in this room have been damaged to the extent that the workmen are unable to restore them faithfully. They replace what is missing to the best of their ability, and try to make it look like it might once have done." After another few weeks she told me that the renovators had finished their work, and that the villa had been fully renovated.

That was around thirteen years ago, and her state of health has been significantly better ever since.

## Skin and hair

Many skin conditions such as acne, eczema, warts and neurodermatitis can be influenced by suggestion. Acne and certain rashes and facial eczema can be treated by asking the patient to spend several weeks in an environment without mirrors. The procedure is effective because it diverts attention away from the symptom (defocusing) and because the patient will touch his or her face with his or her fingers less frequently, avoiding the associated inflammation, cracked dry skin or greasy skin. (A related case study by Erickson can be found in Rosen, 1982. Further explanations of Erickson's approach are given in Short & Weinspach, 2007: 106.)

### Wart Remedy

There are various suggestive procedures for removing warts. The dialogue "Wart Remedy" combines several intervention types.

The described method has proved its value on numerous occasions, and works even if the patient does not imagine any medicine, since it shifts the focus of attention to the removal of the wart. The action carries the implication that the wart is equivalent to a fingernail, or in other words that it turns into keratin. Positive connotations are also ascribed to the wart by incorporating it into a cosmetic routine.

A four-year-old boy discovered an effective way of removing a wart by telling it angrily to, "go jump in a lake!" In methodological terms, he was addressing his body with a directive suggestion, and externalising and visualising the wart.

Crasilneck and Hall treat a wart by suggesting that it is becoming colder and colder, or in other words by constricting the blood vessels and reducing the circulation. (Crasilneck & Hall, 1985). Gibbons uses a suggestion of heat concentrating in the wart and triggering the incipient healing (Gibbons, 1979; several similar techniques can be found in Kohen & Olness, 2011: 272, 397).

TOPIC: Cosmetic concerns, warts
INTERVENTION: Ritual for healing, painting, connotation, unreal placebo (example, positive model

> "What are you doing?"
> "I'm painting my wart with nail polish."
> "Do you think that will work?"
> "It worked last time. I imagine to myself that it's the same medicine from the pharmacy that my friend uses."

### The Lipoma

Women in Germany continued the traditions of medieval folk medicine by "charming" or "talking away" warts until just a few decades ago (and in rare cases even today). The procedure, which is described in the story "Lipoma", originates from this practice.

TOPIC: Lipoma, warts
INTERVENTION: Cosmetic concerns, real placebo, reversing the focus of attention, ritual for healing, magic spell (metaphor, negative model / positive model).

> Many years ago I had a small round bulge on my thigh, which I ignored for around eighteen months. Then I happened to be visiting my GP, and asked him what it was.
> "It's a lipoma," he answered, "a fatty lump. Keep an eye on it. If it doesn't change it can stay, but if it grows it will have to come out." I kept

a close eye on the lipoma, and it started to grow, for the first time in eighteen months. I went back to the GP, who removed it surgically.

Years later I told someone this story in order to highlight the fact that noticing something makes it grow; a small problem can turn into a large one if you pay it a lot of attention. I don't know whether it was because of this conversation, but two weeks later the lipoma reappeared, at the same spot where a scar indicated that its predecessor had been removed.

"If the lipoma can grow by suggestion, it can also shrink by suggestion," I thought. I remembered the wart charmer's old folk remedy; "Rub the wart with spit three times every morning and every evening, using a different finger each time, and repeat three times: 'Wart, wart, rub away.'"

I wondered to myself whether the same would work for a lipoma, and decided to try. The lipoma had disappeared after three days.

### Keep All Cells Alive

An experiment is supposed to have been carried out in the 1960s (apparently successfully) to find out whether blisters could be imagined into existence. I have not been able to find a source for this experiment, but it served as inspiration for the reverse experiment which is described in the story "Keep All Cells Alive". The modified suggestion "keep all healthy cells alive" can be used during radiation therapy.

TOPIC:  Burning, freezing, irradiation
INTERVENTION:  Preventive suggestion (example, positive model)

> By the time he realised that the melted cheese was far too hot it was too late to spit it out. An intensifying sensation of pain radiated around his mouth. "Keep all cells alive! Keep all cells alive!" he thought suddenly, in the midst of the pain, as though he was calling loudly to his mouth. He repeated the entreaty again and again in his thoughts; "Keep all cells alive!" The pain finally abated, and he probed his mouth with his tongue. Everything felt exactly as it had before – soft and supple. His body had followed his instructions.

### The Silent Hand

As a story or a practical exercise, the story "The Silent Hand" represents an intervention for reducing skin moisture, or in other words for regulating the formation and absorption of oil and perspiration, and reducing the production of dandruff. During therapeutic work with bulimia and emetophobia (fear of vomiting and vomit) the story can be used to teach clients that they have involuntary control over their excretions, even their sweat. For patients suffering from colds (including blocked-up ears), the story can be used meto-nymically (as an example of an adjacent phenomenon), since it is associatively linked with the idea of reducing the swelling of the mucous membranes and the production of secretions. Finally, the story can be used to teach clients how to influence the production of endogenous substances through suggestion, for example a change in the quantity of tears secreted in the case of patients suffering from dry eyes. The story also illustrates how events experienced by the therapist can be turned into a third-person narrative – which is automatic-ally more detached than a first-person narrative – using the phrase "my friend Peter" (the "My Friend John" technique).

TOPIC:  Acne, bulimia, cold, cosmetic concerns, dandruff, phobia (emetophobia),
    eye liquid, hyperhidrosis, oily skin, rhagades, sweating, tears
INTERVENTION:  Metonymy (example, positive model)

My friend Peter belongs to an African drumming group led by a Congolese drummer. The leader was teaching a piece to the group which ends by getting quieter and quieter until the music stops entirely and the drummer's hand is lying motionless on the drum. The leader lifted his hand away from the drum without making a sound. The other drummers copied him, but each of them made an audible squelch because of the sweat and oil on the skin of their hands. They tried repeatedly to lift their hands soundlessly, but time and time again the leader lifted his hands in complete silence while audible squelches could be heard from the others. In his thoughts, Peter said to his hand, "Dear hand, please absorb all the oil and sweat which is currently on your surface." Seconds later, he lifted his hand in absolute silence. "How on earth did you manage that?" the others asked hm. Within a matter of seconds, they too could regulate the sweat and grease on their own hands.

## Muscular tension and relaxation

Although trances often involve an experience of general muscular relaxation, sometimes they can also involve extreme muscular rigidity (catalepsy). The level of muscular tension is influenced not only by the trance itself, but also by suggestive content, for example by imagining images which imply a high or low degree of muscular rigidity.

### The Worry Catapult

"The Worry Catapult" is an intervention which can be used at a somatic level to avoid or reduce stress-related facial wrinkles, at an emotional level for relaxation and at a social level to practise new behavioural patterns for dealing with interpersonal stress. The procedure is similar to the "clenched fist" technique, a "method which can be used by a child to 'throw away' tension and problems by clenching [and then relaxing] his or her fist" (Kohen & Olness, 2011).

TOPIC: Aggression, anxiety, Bell's palsy, body language, burnout syndrome, cosmetic concerns, facial wrinkles, muscular tension, self-confidence, teeth grinding, work/life balance

INTERVENTION: Unreal reframing (example / metaphor, positive model)

> One of the games we used to play at school was to stretch a rubber band between two fingers of one hand and then shoot folded bits of paper at the other pupils, or even at the teacher when his back was turned at the blackboard. It was against the school rules, of course, but it was still great fun and a good way of keeping boredom at bay. A sawn-off forked branch and a rubber ring from a preserving jar could be used in a similar way to make a stone catapult, and even now I still often think of these different kinds of catapaults.
>
> Sometimes wrinkles appear on my face because I am afraid, annoyed, sympathetic or troubled. I know that if they become a fixed part of my repertoire of facial expressions, in a few years' time these expressions will turn into basic facial characteristics that determine my neutral appearance regardless of my mood – wrinkles and all. This is not what I want, and it is also not what I need.
>
> My face muscles are like a worry catapult which is stretched between my ears. Whenever my skin tenses up in one spot and forms wrinkles in another, and whenever a particular level of tension has been exceeded, the catapult goes "pop" and the muscles relax. All the worries, all the annoyance, all the anger – catapulted away into time and space. Sometimes they are fired into nothingness, and sometimes they are sent to someone who – unlike me – will give them a good home. The only thing left on my face is a smile, as I know that the worry wrinkles have not made a home for themselves this time.

### Arm Wrestling

"Arm Wrestling" describes a method of muscular stiffening with simultaneous analgesia. The general trance phenomenon of catalepsy is heightened and strengthened by an additional visual/imaginative suggestion, and a similar procedure is followed for the numbing of any pain; as well as the fundamental anaesthetic effect of trance-induced relaxation, it is implied that a steel girder cannot feel pain. There are certain risks and side effects involved with this story; it took three weeks for the damaged muscle fibres in my arm to heal and the pain to disappear.

TOPIC: Competitive sport, pain, success, tension

INTERVENTION: Catalepsy (example, positive model / negative model), hypnotic anaesthesia

"Fetch Timo!" shouted all the children. Up until then challenging my Year Six pupils to arm wrestling matches had been good fun, but Timo – a member of the other Year Six class who had now appeared in my classroom – was built on an entirely different scale to your average Year Six pupil. He looked at me through his thick glasses with a friendly gaze, sat down opposite me and held out a giant paw. I could think of little worse than being beaten at arm wrestling by a Year Six pupil, but could not help wondering whether there was any way for me to win. I did not want to lose, but there was no avoiding the situation when his arm was already stretched out in front of me. What should I do? I imagined that my arm was a large steel bracket, welded and bolted like the massive steel roof girders which tower over vast railway station concourses. I no longer saw an arm; I only saw a girder staying rigidly in position up in the roof. Timo pressed his hand against the steel girder for a long, long time. When his arm finally trembled, I very slowly tipped the girder over and let it topple under its enormous weight, burying Timo's arm below the roof of the station concourse. I had won.

### If You Can Manage...

"If You Can Manage..." demonstrates how symptoms which occur spontaneously can be eliminated by an attempt to induce them intentionally (symptom prescription).

TOPIC: Hiccups
INTERVENTION: Paradoxical intervention, reward and punishment, symptom prescription (example, positive model)

"If you can manage to hiccup another ten times, you can have an ice cream," said Nikolas to Vita and started counting, "1 – 2 – 3 – 4 – 5 – 6 – 7 – 8 – 9..." He never reached 10, but she got the ice cream anyway.

### The Frozen Hiccup

"The Frozen Hiccup" illustrates another effective method of curing hiccups. The voluntary suppression of the blinking reflex acts as a kinaesthetic/figurative instruction to the subconscious to suppress the hiccupping reflex in the same way, with simultaneous distraction effects and the induction of a trance as an essentially symptom-free state. The trance is induced through eye fixation and cataleptic rigidity, and through overburdening with a challenging task. The intervention can also be used auto-suggestively as an exercise in front of the mirror. The intervention is based on one by Gerald Mozdzierz (Mozdzierz, 1990).

TOPIC:  Hiccups, nervous muscle twitching

INTERVENTION:  Mental gymnastics, metonymy, trance induction through eye
fixation, utilisation of a bodily function (example, positive model)

> A short while ago I went to stay with some friends. When I was leaving,
> the hostess got a bad case of hiccups. "Look into my eyes for one minute
> and don't blink," I told her. "Thank you," I said once the minute had
> passed. The hiccups had vanished.

## Bodily sensations and the perception of pain

There are many different ways of influencing the experienced quality and
intensity of bodily perceptions, and the many different methods of hypnotic
anaesthesia are particularly relevant for therapeutic purposes. Many of these
techniques are used intuitively by people in everyday life; if you ask people
how they behave while undergoing treatment in a dentist's chair, you will often
find that they focus their attention on internal and external triggers which
help them to ignore what is currently happening and concentrate on areas of
experience which involve no pain. A small number of patients concentrate
directly on what is happening, allowing them to experience volition and control and avoid the fear of helplessness which can intensify pain. Other people
clutch someone's hand, a tissue or a solid object to divert their attention at
a somatic (kinaesthetic) level. Similarly, runners and gym goers who listen to
music are doing so to produce an anaesthetic trance.

### Of Pain and Lice

The story "Of Pain and Lice" illustrates how hypnotic anaesthesia can
be prevented. We activate and reinforce anything we address and request,
whether pleasant or unpleasant, and the only logical purpose of asking
for something we do not want is therefore to pick up on an experience we
have already had and turn it into something different and positive. What
patients refer to as "distracting themselves" and "thinking about something
else" can be a very effective form of anaesthesia, and their efforts can be
promoted by the medical and care staff who engage in small talk with them.
Erickson and Rossi refer to "iatrogenic [medically caused] disorders and
diseases arising as a result of a physician's poorly disguised concern and
distress over his patient. Iatrogenic illness has a most tremendous significance because in emphasizing that there can be psychosomatic disease of
iatrogenic origin, its converse cannot be overlooked: that iatrogenic health is
fully as possible and of far greater importance to the patient. And since iatrogenic pain can be produced by fear, tensions and anxiety, so can freedom
from it be produced by the iatrogenic health that can be suggested hypnot-
ically" (Erickson & Rossi, 1979: 96).

TOPIC: Attention, pain

INTERVENTION: Pacing and leading, psychoeducation, reversing the focus of attention (example, negative model)

> I waited in the doctor's office and wondered how I could distract myself from the treatment I was about to undergo by focusing my attention on something else. The doctor came in, greeted me and started the procedure. "Does that hurt?" he asked. He could have achieved a similar but more pleasant result if he had said, "The patient before you had lice. I hope you're not feeling itchy?"

### Go Away

The following stories demonstrate various techniques for hypnotic anaesthesia. The case study "Go Away" involves taking the pain as a starting point and then rapidly minimising it through a plausible chain of associations. It illustrates a typical feature of verbal pacing and leading, namely that the pain (the problem) is referred to directly at the beginning, but only mentioned indirectly as an "inconvenience" by the end. If the patient is in a great deal of pain, it is often important to recognise and acknowledge the pain before reducing it by telling it to "go away" ("pacing and leading" principle). The principle is based on one of Milton Erickson's methods (cf. Short & Weinspach, 2007:108).

TOPIC: Pain

INTERVENTION: Hypnotic anaesthesia, pacing and leading, reversing the focus of attention (example, positive model)

> A woman attending a psychotherapy session suddenly developed a bad headache. She explained that it was linked to a problem with her cervical vertebrae for which she was undergoing medical treatment. Her face was screwed up in pain, and it was clear that she was struggling to focus on anything else. I told her, "That must really hurt. It must hurt a great deal, and you must be wishing that it would go away soon, that it would perhaps go away in three minutes or in two minutes, or that it would go away in one minute or in half a minute, or perhaps even sooner. When do you think this inconvenience will go away?"
>
> "It has almost gone already," she answered very calmly.

### Mr Peabrain

"Mr Peabrain" demonstrates a way of externalising pain by handing it over to a fictitious character, following a similar procedure to that described in the introduction for sending away hay fever.

TOPIC: Aggression, pain

INTERVENTION: Externalisation of a problem as an object, hypnotic anaesthesia, invisible friends, trance induction through confusion, unreal reframing, visualisation (example, positive model)

"Does it still hurt?" I asked my niece.

"Does what hurt?" she replied.

"If you don't know what I mean, then I guess it can't still hurt."

"Are you talking about my headache? I gave it to Mr Peabrain. He can do what he likes with it."

"Who's Mr Peabrain?" I asked.

"I don't know. I only just met him."

"And now he's gone?"

"Yes."

"You could have asked Mr Peabrain to give you something you need in return," I suggested.

"Oh no," she replied. "Mr Peabrain doesn't give things – he only takes them."

## Selling Pain

The case study "Selling Pain" shows how pain can be numbed by the continual interspersal of anaesthetic implications into a conversation. In order to optimise the effect, the anaesthetic metaphors are adapted to the patient's metaphorical language and career history. Stubbornly talking at cross-purposes with the client's interests serves as an irritating factor which defocuses his or her attention from the pain. The interspersal technique shown here was developed by Milton Erickson, who anaesthetised one patient and helped another with urinary urge frequency and incontinence with a psychosomatic origin to hold urine for longer periods by means of a conversation on tomato plants (O'Hanlon & Hexum, 1991: 71).

TOPIC: Pain

INTERVENTION: Externalisation of a problem as an object, hypnotic anaesthesia, interspersal technique, invisible friends, visualisation (example / metaphor, positive model)

I met the old lady in the corridor of the X-ray department, lying on a bed among other patients and surrounded by the normal bustle of a hospital; nurses rushing back and forth, porters pushing beds and so on. She was waiting, so we had plenty of time to talk.

"I've broken my hip, and it hurts so much. I bet no one would want to buy this pain off me!"

"Who do you think should buy it?"

"Not you. You're a good person."

"Who else then?"

"Not a good person. Maybe a bad dog. But even a good dog wouldn't want it. It hurts so much, and as if that were not bad enough I'm hungry too. The food is horrible in the old people's home where I live. I could cook nicer food myself."

"I'm sure you must have been a fine housewife."

"Not quite – I worked in a shop."

"Really? What did you sell?"

"It was a gift shop selling different works of art and antiques."

"You could wrap up your problems in gift paper and sell them there."

"I don't work there any longer."

"But if the worries were a gift being sold in the shop, what would they be? An antique, made of ceramic or earthenware maybe?"

"Oh, I love earthenware – one sees such wonderful pieces!"

"I'm sure you used to enjoy selling gifts."

"I certainly did! I got to know so many of my customers – lots of them were American. Thank you for talking to me. My hip has already stopped hurting as much."

"Perhaps you would like to sell your pain to me now?"

"I'm not sure – if you really want…"

"I'll stick it in my hair, then I won't feel it. And you can stick the rest of your problems in your hair, too. Or just give them to me. I'm going now."

"Don't forget to throw them away!"

"I will do – into the next bin I find. Goodbye!"

### Crossed Out

"Crossed Out" demonstrates a negative kinaesthetic hallucination technique. Instead of focusing attention away from the part of the body that hurts, attention is focused onto the pain, together with a targeted suggestion that the pain will disappear.

TOPIC: Itching, pain

INTERVENTION: Action as a metaphor, hypnotic anaesthesia, painting (example, positive model)

The fourteen-year-old Luise told me, "Recently I was bitten by a mosquito. I kept on scratching the bite, and it itched like mad. I looked at the bite, and then I used a biro to draw a circle around it and to cross it out. The itching stopped and did not come back."

### The Disconnectable Body

"The Disconnectable Body" can be used in connection with medical interventions or as mental preparation for sport. Sportspeople must however be particularly aware of the risks of anaesthetising oneself while training. Care must be taken to avoid any possibility of injury or the worsening of physical conditions as a result of eliminating pain signals through suggestion.

One of Milton Erickson's patients said, "Just before you arrived, I developed another horrible attack of pain. So I went into a trance, got into my wheelchair, came out into the living room to watch a television programme, and I left my suffering body in the bedroom." And she pleasantly and happily told about the fantasised television programme she was watching. Another such patient remarked to her surgeon, "You know very well, Doctor, that I always faint when you start changing my dressings because I can't endure the pain, so if you don't mind I will go into a hypnotic trance and take my head and feet and go into the solarium and leave my body here for you to work on." (Erickson & Rossi, 1979: 100; in the same vein, cf. O'Hanlon & Hexum, 1991: 65).

TOPIC: Competitive sport, pain
INTERVENTION: Dissociation of body parts, hypnotic anaesthesia, inner team, unreal reframing (example, positive model / searching model)

> I once knew a man who had a very strange talent; he could simply unscrew the lower part of his body from the upper part whenever he went for a walk – like unscrewing the lid from a jam jar or vice versa. Then the lower body would walk alongside the man while his upper body supervised from above. Sometimes the legs, stomach and backside would move a couple of hundred metres away from the upper body, but they never ran away and always came back. At the end of the walk, the upper body and lower body would screw themselves tightly back together again. Then the head would say, "What a good job I didn't have to listen to the legs moaning all the time on our long walk." And the legs would say, "What a good job that we didn't have to listen to the head's unkind warnings and pep talks." Everyone would be happy and content, and they would sit down together for a cup of tea and a chat about the different things they had seen during their walk.

### Pirate Anaesthesia

The story "Pirate Anaesthesia" demonstrates a series of methods that all involve simulating states which are wholly or predominantly incompatible with pain, and can also be used to produce a temporary paralysis of the leg. I first told it during a conversation with a group of children. One of the group, a twelve-year-old named Sarah, asked me afterwards, "How did it go again?" I repeated the story, and three weeks later she told me, "I told the story to my gran, and she couldn't move her leg at all afterwards. It gave her quite a shock!"

TOPIC: Pain, sleep, treatment phobia

INTERVENTION: Ambiguity, avoiding resistance, catalepsy, dissociation of body parts, hypnotic amnesia, hypnotic anaesthesia, seeding, trance induction through description of a trance situation, trance induction through suggestion of trance characteristics and trance phenomena (metaphor, positive model)

Imagine that you're a pirate, with a wooden leg made from strong and solid old oak and a black eye patch – or perhaps without the eye patch? Either way, a pirate has a lot to do on a big old pirate brig – with all its lines, sails and masts, the goods it is carrying and all the other pirates. The pirate is always worn out by the time evening comes and he settles down for the night in his cabin on the swaying, rocking ship. Of course the pirate has to unstrap his wooden leg before he goes to sleep so that it doesn't bother him during the night. The wooden leg is attached by four long leather straps. He undoes the first, then the second, then the third and then the fourth strap, and then he removes his wooden leg and put it down close to his bed before going to sleep. He dreams of the hard, rigid oak leg floating across the sea with a hoisted pirate sail. It sails ever onwards until finally it becomes a dot on the horizon and disappears out of sight, floating on into a distant, unknown world, with its whereabouts completely unknown to the pirate.

### Peace Settlement with a Tooth

The story "Peace Settlement with a Tooth" demonstrates how certain symptoms can disappear if the patient recognises the body's underlying good intentions, tells the body that the symptoms are no longer required and (if necessary) sends them back to the time when they had a useful purpose. It also incorporates the story of the sleeping dog, which contains metaphorical instructions and is suitable for curing phantom pain, post-operative pain and hypersensitivity. The integrated story of the sleeping dog can also be useful for patients suffering from pain, aggression and anxiety disorders in response to traumatic events.

TOPIC: Aggression, amputation, anxiety, dental treatment, hypersensitivity, narcosis, operation, pain, phantom pain, series of stories, trauma

INTERVENTION: Age regression, hypnotic anaesthesia, positive connotation, sending symptoms back into the past, stabilisation through praise (example, positive model)

One of my molar teeth had become sensitive after a trip to the dentist, and for weeks it twinged painfully at every blow of air or the slightest touch. And yet the treatment had gone so well! The anaesthetic had worked perfectly, and I'd experienced almost no pain at all while I was in the dentist's chair.

"Perhaps the nerve needs to come out. That's what happened to me," explained a friend.

"I hope not!" I answered, then considered what to do instead.

"Dear molar tooth," I said to my tooth. "I'd like to tell you a story.

" 'A burglar wanted to break into a villa which was guarded by a large and ferocious watchdog. He decided to solve this problem by throwing a piece of meat laced with anaesthetic into the garden. After the dog had eaten it and fallen into a deep sleep, he broke into the villa and stole everything which caught his eye. When the burglar had gone, the dog woke up. He caught the scent of the fugitive and barked and barked … but the burglar was long gone. The owner of the house heard the dog barking and came to see what the matter was. He praised the dog for his loyalty and reliability and talked in friendly and appeasing tones to him until the dog also started to calm down, until the dog's barks reduced in frequency, until the dog's barks became quieter and quieter, until the dog finally stopped barking, until the dog finally quietened down altogether, and until the dog finally went to sleep. He knew he was a good watchdog. Now he could rest easy.' "

When I'd finished the story, I continued talking to my tooth, "Dear molar tooth, you're right to tell me if something is troubling you, but your job is to hurt when you are injured. The sensations you're producing at the moment are inappropriate because they belong to an earlier time. Picture that dental treatment very clearly in your mind for one last time, and take the pain which you are now producing back there. Experience it once more intensely in your memory, and then leave it in that situation, which you experienced once but which is now in the past." The tooth did what I asked and gave me no trouble from then on.

### The Good Gel

The case study "The Good Gel" can be used in supervision to increase awareness of placebo effects and their possible uses. It can also be used to encourage clients and patients to boost the effect of medical remedies through auto-suggestion. The story illustrates the fact that belief in (therapeutic, professional, private) success plays a key role in achieving goals; furthermore, people can to a large extent decide to believe in their goals.

TOPIC: Medicine, pain

INTERVENTION: Hypnotic anaesthesia, real placebo (example, positive model)

I didn't use to believe in placebos. Then one day I needed some painkillers for a patient I was treating in my doctor's practice, and left the room briefly to fetch them. When I came back, the woman had vanished without any pain relief.

A few weeks later, she returned and asked, "Could I have some more of that wonderful gel, please?"

"What did she take with her the last time she was here?" I asked my assistant.

"The conductive gel we use for ECGs."

"Then give her some more of that."

### A Walk Along the Beach

The story "A Walk Along the Beach" illustrates another simple method of hypnotic anaesthesia. The problem is not that it is difficult to induce an anaesthetising trance, but that we often do not believe that everyday trances can fulfil the same role. What is more, we do not generally notice that our pain has disappeared when we are either in a pain-free trance state between painful waking states or at a later stage (because we are absorbed by something else, and because the change from a trance state into a waking state is associated with amnesia).

TOPIC: Amputation, anxiety, operation, pain
INTERVENTION: Age regression, hypnotic anaesthesia, unreal reframing
(example / metaphor, positive model)

A doctor had to carry out an operation to remove a patient's large toe-nail, but the patient could not tolerate painkillers.

"What should I do?" he asked her. "I'd feel like I was torturing you if I operated on you while you were still fully conscious!" The patient shrugged her shoulders.

"Where do you most like going on holiday?" he asked.

"The Baltic Sea," she answered. "My husband and I have had some wonderful walks along the beaches there."

"Tell me about them, and immerse yourself in the tale," said the doctor. "Dive deep down into your memories and describe everything you see, hear, feel, taste and smell on your walks there."

The woman started her story and kept on going. "Now a storm is brewing," she said as the doctor began the operation. She saw the storm approaching but remained quite calm.

### Expanding Time, Contracting Time

The following example demonstrates a method for mentally anaesthetising pains which only occur intermittently, for example pulsating pains. The story is based on an autobiographical experience. The pains stayed away from then on (nine-year catamnesis). The reference to a friend changes the story into a third-person narrative. Milton Erickson treated pulsating or intermittent pain by teaching patients to distort time. The procedure involves setting the speed at which time is experienced to "very fast" during periods of pain, and "slow" during periods which are comparatively pain-free (O'Hanlon & Hexum, 1991).

TOPIC:  Grief, labour pains, pain

INTERVENTION: Hypnotic anaesthesia, time distortion (example, positive model)

> My friend Peter had suffered from pulsating pains in only his right foot for many years, even though as far as he could tell he used his right foot in exactly the same way as his left. The only explanation he could find was that he had suffered two torn ligaments in his right knee when he was much younger, one of which had not been treated operatively. Now he said to his body, "I'm sure you remember how some lessons in school used to pass very slowly and some very quickly, and how very rapid events can sometimes seem to occur in slow motion while much longer periods of time pass in the blink of an eye. Please try greatly contracting the time during which you experience pain and greatly expanding the pain-free intervals. Only contract and expand time for bodily experience, and let time pass as normal for the other senses." After a few minutes, the periods during which he experienced pain had become noticeably briefer, and a short while after that they had gone for good. On the few occasions when he felt a slight twinge of pain, he said, "Dear body, don't forget to expand and contract time."

## Sense of sight

Vision disorders are similar to disorders that affect an individual's hearing and sense of balance in that they are sometimes psychogenic rather than somatic, and storytelling interventions can be used to achieve a significant improvement of perception in such cases. Even if there appears to be little doubt that responses are "psychosomatic", however, consideration should always first be given to whether medical treatment is necessary.

### Blinded by Love

The story "Blinded by Love" is an example of a minimal conversion disorder, and can be told, for example, to people experiencing a psychological crisis and suffering from symptoms relating to perception or mobility.

Williams and Singh report on "the hypnotherapeutic treatment of an eight-year-old girl with conversion amblyopia [psychogenic reduction in visual acuity, editor's note]. Two hypnotherapeutic sessions over a period of three days resulted in the complete recovery of her vision, with no regression over the next 14 months" (Williams & Singh, 1976).

TOPIC:  Conversion disorder, eyes, psychosomatic disorder, visual impairment
INTERVENTION:  Anamnesis questions, shifting the focus of attention from the body to the mind (example, positive model)

> As I walked through the pedestrian zone, I wondered why I was finding it so hard to see things. What could be wrong with me? A delayed effect of the laser eye surgery I had undergone last autumn? My vision was normally 20/20, and I couldn't understand it. When I was driving on the motorway that evening, I strained my eyes to peer through the windscreen and find the best angle of vision. Where had all the cars gone? What on earth was going on? The answer was supplied by my friendly unconscious. I had just spent three days at a conference on trauma which had involved a lot of biographical work, and I had also fallen for a woman who was not interested in me. As soon as I asked myself, "What am I finding so difficult to look at?" the visual impairment disappeared. Things like this happen, and more often than you might think.

## Christmas Bell

The story "Christmas Bell" can be used to illustrate the phenomenon of "institutional blindness" or to highlight the fact that the unconscious mind tends to provide the conscious mind only with new information or information associated with a message of some kind (a warning or the answer to a question).

TOPIC: Attention deficit disorder (ADD / ADHD), habit, reality, self-perception
INTERVENTION:  Paradox ("Perceive what you are not perceiving!"), promoting a searching attitude (example, searching model), reversing the focus of attention

> On one of the last days of April I took down a Christmas bell which was hanging from a hook on the ceiling. I had got so used to seeing the bell as part of my surroundings that I had not noticed it at all during all the months which had passed since Christmas. I had simply no longer perceived it. It was the last of the Christmas decorations – or was it?

## Crooked and Straight

"Crooked and Straight" highlights the fact that the unconscious mind – unless it is too busy looking for mistakes and aiming for perfection –ignores any errors which exist in reality and sees what was intended to be there in their place.

TOPIC: Compulsion (OCD), forgiveness, perfectionism, reality
INTERVENTION: Promoting a searching attitude (example, searching model)

> I was recently hanging up a poster when I noticed that it was crooked and straightened it.
> "Why are you adjusting the poster?" asked a cleaner who was watching me.
> "It's crooked," I answered.
> "That doesn't matter," she said. "Your eyes will straighten it out."

## Sense of hearing

Storytelling methods can be used in connection with the sense of hearing to help patients suffering from tinnitus, psychogenic forms of hearing impairment, attention focus problems (concentration) and the social effects of organic hearing impairment.

For example, many tinnitus sufferers can identify fluctuations in the volume and experienced intensity of the hallucinatory noises they perceive, and are aware that they notice the noises more at certain times than at others. Hypnosis-based tinnitus therapy takes advantage of this fact and incorporates lessons learned from pain therapy.

Experience in the field of anaesthesia has shown that a reduction in the intensity of sensory stimuli can most easily be achieved if a patient focuses his or her attention on pleasant experiences, whether real or imagined (cf. "Of Pain and Lice"). Questions such as "Does it hurt?" are much less effective than questions such as "Are you ok?" or "Does it feel better now, or not quite yet?" that is, questions targeted at a low-symptom or asymptomatic state. Tinnitus patients should therefore only be asked about the volume of the noises at the start of the session (if at all), with reference being made thereafter only to the level of silence and ways in which this can be increased. As soon as the listener learns to search consistently for silence rather than noise, the silence will multiply until it drowns out the previous noise.

### The Hindenburg Path

"The Hindenburg Path" describes a dialogue which appears to make no sense because one of the interlocutors is hard of hearing. People suffering from a hearing impairment may seem odd (unapproachable, indifferent, arrogant etc.) and be treated accordingly, which may mean that they increasingly grow to resemble the mistaken image which others have of them. The same applies to people who find it difficult to communicate because they grew up speaking a different language. In the situation described in the story, the problem is probably a result of the man's efforts to avoid loneliness by attempting to communicate in spite of his hearing impairment. The story reflects the general principle that "odd" behaviour often turns into "ordinary" behaviour once we are aware of its context.

TOPIC: Hearing impairment, misunderstanding
INTERVENTION: Psychoeducation, promoting a searching attitude (example, negative model / searching model)

> Mr Neumann greeted Mr Krauss, an elderly man who lived nearby.
> "Hello, Mr Krauss."
> "Hello ... and where have you come from?"
> Mr Neumann pointed in the appropriate direction and replied, "From down there."
> "Oh, the Hindenburg path."
> "The Hindenburg path? Why's it called that?"
> "It's so steep you can't go up it."
> "I see. But what does that have to do with Hindenburg?"
> "Haven't you ever heard of the enormous Hindenburg airship...!"

## Hearing Difficulty

The story "Hearing Difficulty" picks up on the fact that tinnitus sufferers often focus their attention on the wrong thing. It can be used not only in connection with tinnitus, but also as a metaphor for many other internal and external conflicts.

TOPIC: Attention, compulsion, forgiveness, perfectionism, tinnitus
INTERVENTION: Paradox ("Don't perceive what you are perceiving!") (example, negative model), reversing the focus of attention

> I remember a particular teacher who taught me when I was at school and whose lessons seemed to me both easy to follow and informative. Then one day another pupil pointed out how often she ummed and ahhed while she was talking, and that ruined everything. Up until then I had been able to listen to her words and had not even noticed the hesitations, but from then on I could only hear, "um... ah ... um." The words that she said were nothing but pauses between the sounds.

## Taekwondo

In the intervention "Taekwondo", a properly functioning auditory cortex teaches and sets a good example to its nonfunctioning counterpart. The story is an abbreviated description of the procedure and outcomes of a trial involving the use of mental training to treat tinnitus, which took place in cooperation with Peter Schneider on 24 January 2007 at the MEG laboratory of the Heidelberg Head Clinic. Measurements were carried out using software that played sounds of different tones and volumes to the test subject so that he could compare them to the frequency and volume of the tinnitus sounds he heard (Schneider, 2009; cf. Hammel, 2009; the experiment was based on the findings of Schneider et al., 2009). Before the 90-minute training session, the test subject rated the tinnitus sounds at a level of 11 dB above the audible threshold. After the trial, the rating had sunk to 0 dB. During the conversation, the test subject was repeatedly asked to rate the "level of silence" on a ten-point scale. As a further intervention, he was placed in a "silence lift" in which he could travel to different floors of a ten-storey tower block of silence, with the tenth floor representing complete silence. Before the final measurement, he decided that the roof terrace should be the eleventh floor (Hammel, 2009).

The story "Learning to Walk" brings the two sides of the body into a similar dialogue of teaching and learning.

TOPIC: Attention, tinnitus

INTERVENTION: Dissociation of body halves, imagined rapport, promoting a learning attitude, reversing the focus of attention (example, positive model)

"Do you do any sport?"
   "Taekwondo."
   "Which belt?"
   "Second dan."
   "That's quite an achievement! Now imagine that your left ear, the ear which is good at listening to silence, is the master. Your right ear, which suffers from tinnitus, is the student. What can the master teach his student, and what would the student like to learn from his master?"
   "Concentration."
   "That's right. Listen to the master for a while, and watch how he instructs his pupil. Watch the pupil listening to his teacher and following his instructions. What do you notice?"
   "Everything has gone quiet."

## Sense of balance

The symptoms of travel sickness and sea sickness, and potentially also other balance disorders, can be relieved through suggestive metaphors or through breath pacing and the refocusing of attention to the sense of hearing. Ongoing or recurrent feelings of dizziness may indicate the presence of a disease that requires treatment and should therefore always be investigated by a neurological expert.

### The Sailor on Shore

The story "The Sailor on Shore" provides patients with instructions on how to deal with dizziness by optimising their sense of balance, for example if they are suffering from seasickness or travel sickness. A spirit level can be used as a metaphor in place of the nautical instrument referred to in the story.

TOPIC:  Sense of balance, travel sickness

INTERVENTION:  Reversing the focus of attention (example / metaphor, positive model)

> "I've just come off a ship after spending five days out at sea," explained the woman. "My head is trying to make me believe that I'm still out on the waves. Everything is swaying and rocking from side to side."
>
> "I once visited a naval museum," answered the man. "I saw a candle-holder there which was specially designed to hold candles upright all the time, even out on the open sea. It consisted of three interlocking rings which were connected to each other but which could each rotate independently of the others. The outer ring hung on a chain and was positioned vertically, and the next ring was also positioned vertically, but at right angles to the first. The last and innermost ring was positioned horizontally, and supported the actual candle holder, whose centre of gravity was below the ring. No matter how much the ship swayed and rocked, the rings moved in such a way that the candle stayed upright."
>
> "I'm not dizzy any more," said the woman.

### Hypnotising Dogs

The story "Hypnotising Dogs" is also designed to cure the symptoms of travel sickness, since what's good for dogs is also good for humans. The method involves refocusing attention from bodily experiences to the hearing, relieving anxiety and stress through a relaxation trance, and producing heart and breathing rates that are similar to those experienced during sleep and are wholly dissimilar to those experienced during attacks of nausea. The procedure is also suitable for infants, dementia patients, coma patients, people with severe mental disabilities and other people with whom verbal communication is not possible.

TOPIC:  Disability, chemotherapy, dementia, vomiting, sense of balance, coma, travel sickness, infant, nausea

INTERVENTION:  Breath pacing, shifting the focus of attention from feeling to hearing (example, positive model)

I recently took a coach trip with a group of family members, including Luna the labrador.

"She feels sick," said my sister-in-law. "She's already retched several times. She doesn't like travelling by car because it sometimes makes her vomit. Can't you hypnotise her so that it doesn't happen while she's in the coach with us?"

I talked to Luna for a while and then asked my nephew Nikolas: "Would you lend Luna your MP3 player? Find some peaceful music – a lullaby or something similar. Set the volume very low, and place the headphones on Luna's ears."

Nikolas found a band whose music was suitable and put the headphones over Luna's head. After half a minute or so, Luna relaxed and lay down, and was soon asleep. Her symptoms of nausea did not reappear.

## Speech

Speech is a complex phenomenon; the problem to be overcome in the first story is organic and has far-reaching psychological and social consequences, whereas stammering is primarily of psychomotor origin.

### The Pruned Tree

The case study "The Pruned Tree" investigates how people can come to terms with losing their voice. The story can, however, also be used in other situations such as amputations and surgical interventions of all kinds, in particular mastectomies, the operative removal of sexual organs and sterilisation. In these cases the metaphor expresses the idea that the removal of the body parts that symbolise fertility (or the loss of their functionality) furthers goals aligned with fertility. Fertility is reframed as innovative energy and creativity, and the parts of the personality associated with the body part are asked to consent to the operation and to reconcile themselves with the consenting personality parts.

TOPIC: Amputation, aphasia, cancer, convalescence, fertility, hysterectomy, larynx, mastectomy, oophorectomy, operation, orchiectomy, prostate, sexuality, sterilisation

INTERVENTION: Metaphorical reframing, painting, positive connotation, dissociation of connotated notions, utilisation of side effects and consequences of treatment (example, positive model)

I recently met a Russian man in hospital who had undergone a laryngectomy. His son had painted him a picture of a tree bearing red apples, with the following caption in big letter; "The tree was pruned, and now it bears more fruit than ever. Dear father, we loved your voice. But we love you much more!"

The following stories can be used to establish helpful inner figures within the framework of stammering therapy with children. When treating patients who suffer from stammering, it is useful to identify settings in which the problem disappears or reduces in severity, for example when singing or in certain low-stress situations. As a general rule, I would only mention this at the very start of the course of therapy, and then talk about stammering less and less, because simply talking about stammering increases its frequency. One possibility is to hold a light-hearted discussion with the child about how he or she learned to stammer, and to praise – with a wink of the eye – his or her skill in learning a "foreign language" before his or her "mother tongue". This implies that stammering is useful in some way and that it is actively produced, which means that it can be actively influenced. It furthermore implies that the child's mother tongue can also be actively learned, which in turn implies that a distinction must be made between the two languages, and that it is not necessary to forget how to stammer, but merely to learn another language as well, leaving stammering as a fallback option for any time when it appears necessary. I avoid the words "stammerer" or "stutterer" because they describe the symptom not as an action (which can be replaced by another action) but as an identity (with the implication that this identity will be difficult or impossible to change). It is conceivable that a child with siblings who are more advanced in terms of cognition and communication may use stammering as a way of gaining time to "catch up" mentally or demand attention. Stammering may also act as a symbol of the child tripping up while trying to catch up and draw level with grown-up family members and elder siblings who have set off quickly and are hurrying on ahead. Another option is to establish two figures who represent two parts of the self, for example using stuffed animals, glove puppets, painted or imagined figures or two protagonists in a story.

### Mrs Flow

The story "Mrs Flow" personifies therapeutic goals and resources in a fictional character, and at the same time distracts the patient from any stressful real-life experiences that might block the work.

TOPIC: Stammering

INTERVENTION: Imagined rapport, mental gymnastics, pacing and leading, paradox ("Imagine a flat staircase!"), promoting a learning attitude (example / metaphor, positive model)

> Mrs Flow builds staircases. She builds wooden staircases, marble staircases, and even glass and rubber staircases and spiral staircases. She builds staircases that go up and staircases that go down, and she has invented a new type of staircase that goes up and down and up and down and up and down. She has invented a staircase that can be folded up, a

staircase that can be pushed together and a staircase that is completely flat. I don't quite understand how it works, but experts have assured me that it really does exist – a completely flat staircase. Mrs Flow also works together with a colleague to build escalators. The interesting thing about these escalators is that they start off as a not-staircase, gradually turn into a staircase, become less and less of a staircase and then end up as a not-staircase.

When I was a child, I always wondered where escalators come from and go to. Once I saw an escalator at an airport without any steps at all. You could build a hill into a step-free escalator of this kind so that it changed from a flat treadmill into an escalator going up, then an escalator going down, and then a flat treadmill again, maybe with a higher level in between – up the staircase, flat for a while and then down the staircase, or the same thing but going down instead of up. The luggage carousels at the airport are just like flat staircases that go around lots of corners. Some of them bring the luggage up a steep slope, a luggage staircase or a luggage lift first before it starts going around the carousel. There's a great deal of flexibility when it comes to designing these staircases and luggage carousels, and Mrs Flow is an expert on the matter.

### Mrs Sing

The story "Mrs Sing" can be used in the same context as the previous story, and is also likely to be useful for singing-based speech training after a stroke-related loss of speech and motor functions.

TOPIC: Aphasia, stammering, stroke
INTERVENTION: Imagined rapport, pacing and leading, promoting a learning attitude, shifting the focus of attention from a deficit to a resource, systematic desensitisation, utilisation of the symptom, utilisation of connotations (example / metaphor, positive model)

Mrs Sing is an exceptionally talented singer, and she is also talented at reciting poetry and giving speeches. Mrs Sing is Mrs Flow's singing teacher, because one of Mrs Flow's ambitions is to learn how to sing. There are many different styles of singing, including opera and gospel, pop songs and folk songs, whisper singing and spoken singing. Mrs Sing is teaching Mrs Flow to sing in many different styles.

She is also teaching her something she has discovered during her many years as a singing teacher, namely that the boundary between singing and speaking is fluid rather than fixed, or in other words a transition rather than a boundary. Some singing is sing-sing-sing-sing, some singing is sing-sing-sing-speak, some singing is sing-sing-speak-speak, some singing is sing-speak-speak-speak and some singing is speak-speak-speak-speak.

Some people think the last of these is not singing at all, but everything is singing in one way or another after you have learned to sing in this way – even speaking becomes a kind of singing with less clearly defined notes.

Mrs Flow starts by learning sing-sing-sing-sing, then sing-sing-sing-speak, and so on. After that she works her way backwards, all the way through to singing.

It's also important to remember that every room has slightly different spatial qualities, with a different echo and different acoustics. Mrs Sing teaches Mrs Flow to sing and sing-speak in different rooms so that she can adjust her singing, sing-speaking and speaking to whichever room she is in.

Singing, sing-speaking and speaking is different in a church and in a kitchen, in a toilet and out on the street, on a staircase and on a market square, in complete silence and in a ship's engine room and so on and so on.

Any kind of singing, sing-sing-sing-speaking and sing-sing-speaking must take into account the surroundings and the audience. And when you have learned to sing, speaking is just singing with fewer notes. You simply imagine you are singing, and leave out the notes – almost imperceptibly to begin with, but more and more as time goes on. The sound is still special, because the voice of anyone who has learned to speak while imagining that they are singing – a skill that will become automatic and effortless after a while – will be a treat for the ear and mesmerise those who hear it. Mrs Flow is no longer really interested in singing for its own sake; she wants a voice that soothes the ear, regardless of whether she is singing or sing-speaking, and whether she is in a church or on a staircase.

## Memory and access to skills

Memory training can be important for various reasons. When revising for exams, the primary task is to build on existing resources; in this context, memory training involves firstly the (re)construction of mental structures in the form of comprehensible and easily retrievable associative chains, and secondly exercises to increase self-confidence and reduce exam nerves, with the overall aim of giving students confidence that they can retrieve what they have learned.

Memory training for dementia patients may be aimed at mitigating the organisational and social problems associated with slowly progressing memory loss, potentially lengthening the period during which a good quality of life is possible.

There is much controversy over whether lost memories relating to traumatic events should be retrieved. If attempts of this kind are undertaken, they must be incorporated into a solid therapeutic structure with precautions against retraumatisation and the potentially hazardous consequences of these memories. Work to recover lost memories may be useful in the event of amnesia after a stroke or coma.

It often makes little difference to the therapeutic approach whether the patient is recovering memories or skills, such as the ability to move a particular body part. In both cases the patient has lost access to mental resources which were once gained and are presumably still present in the brain, even though they cannot be accessed at present.

In order to motivate clients, I tell them that every time they imagine a movement they used to be able to perform and want to be able to perform again, they are activating and strengthening the part of the brain responsible for this movement. I tell them how Milton Erickson, when he was paralysed as a child, first started by imagining movements, then made movements that were so small as to be invisible and then gradually increased the range of these movements (Short & Weinspach, 2007:17) and that the constant repetition of the imagined movement brings them closer to the real movement. The same applies to the recovery of memories. Since the memories themselves have not been lost, merely the routes that lead to them, it is useful to approach these memory gaps from many different directions and to search for the routes that still remain, both in conversation with others and in your own mind, in order to open up pathways to new areas of memory – a task which is similar to finding the correct path through a maze with many dead ends.

If the part of the brain responsible for processing speech is affected by a stroke to the extent that the patient no longer understands the words people say to him, it is almost impossible to instruct and motivate the patient to carry out training using a conventional style of communication. The problem is compounded by the fact that the inability to communicate or understand can isolate the patient, who will normally respond by falling into a depression, further reducing the motivation to engage with training.

In situations such as these, metaphorical substitute communication must be established using all possible methods, for example by depicting the patient's resources and aims in pantomime language, using picture stories, comics, videos, music and sensory experiences. The aim is to activate the patient's ambition, patience and perseverance, to promote healing and to demonstrate to him or her that he or she can still communicate, regardless of whether or not he or she can speak.

### *Pantomime*

The case study "Pantomime" shows what communication of this kind might look like and the effects it can have. Interventions of this kind can also be used to utilise the behaviour of a person suffering from mutism for the purpose of establishing rapport.

TOPIC: Aphasia, body language, language and speech, learning, memory, mutism, stroke

INTERVENTION: Mental    gymnastics,    pantomime,    promoting    positive
expectations, utilisation of rapport (example / metaphor, positive model)

"Hello. My name is…" he began.
"She can't talk," the nurse told him. "She's had a stroke…"
The young patient's helpless gestures told him that she could not
even understand what he was saying, with the exception of a few words
to which she replied with a nod or a shake of the head. How can one
communicate in such a situation? He used gestures to outline a steep
staircase with high steps in the air in front of him. He sighed; too steep,
too high! He shook his head in disappointment. Then he gestured with
his hands to indicate a staircase with shallow steps, and he walked up
the entire staircase with his fingers. The woman watched attentively
and nodded. He used hand gestures to outline a high mountain in the
air. A climber (represented by two fingers) wanted to reach the top, but
kept falling back down. Then he found a less steep route which zig-
zagged upwards with many twists and turns, and he followed this path
to the top. The woman's eyes began to light up, and the pantomime
continued.

"Never losing sight of your goal" and "strength" were the next ideas to
be expressed. The movements of a long-distance runner and a raised fist
encouraged her to persevere and develop a fighting spirit. A clock with
a ticking hand told her that it would take time. He continued the game
of charades by placing his hands to the side of his head and pretending
to fall asleep and wake up, fall asleep and wake up, over and over again
until she had reached her goal, which he demonstrated by shading his
eyes with his hand, peering out and pointing into the distance. He used
his hands, his feet and his whole body to demonstrate how her children
would support her on the left and her parents on the right, and how they
would all complete the long journey together. He stretched his fist up to
the sky once again; she would have to put all her strength into the fight.
Three days later he came back to visit the patient again, and the patient
in the neighbouring bed spoke in her place.

"She's been here for four weeks now, and before you came she wasn't
improving at all. But over the past three days she's made enormous
progress."

He spoke to the patient, and this time she understood every word.
Then he said goodbye.

"Goodbye," she said. That was the first word she learned to say again.

## After the Storm

The story "After the Storm", like the following three stories, is an intervention
which can help a patient to recover missing words and skills if he or she has
the necessary level of understanding. The stories refer implicitly to the fact

that the relevant information is not lost in the brain but merely inaccessible, and can therefore be found again.

TOPIC: Convalescence, grief, learning, memory, stroke, trauma
INTERVENTION: Ambiguity, metaphorical reframing (metaphor, positive model)

> The storm has wrought havoc. Fallen trees are strewn throughout the forest. Their trunks are blocking the paths and roads. No traveller can pass. Yet the time after the storm is the time when the lumberjacks start work. They use their saws to open up the paths, move the blockages and clear the roads, starting at the outer edge of the forest and moving right to its very interior.

## The Keys

The story "The Keys" can be used in the same context and can also be used to improve levels of retention and retrieval when revising for exams.

TOPIC: Convalescence, learning, memory, stroke
INTERVENTION: Metaphorical reframing, promoting a searching attitude (metaphor, positive model)

> Was I dreaming? Or was it real? I walked through the building, with countless doors on my right and left. I tried their handles, but almost none of them opened. The rooms were closed off to me. I sat down and cried.
>   "Why are you crying?" someone asked.
>   I pointed to the locked doors.
>   "Have you forgotten?" he asked, and pointed to my coat pockets. "You've got the keys!"
>   I reached into my pockets and pulled out hundreds and hundreds of keys in different shapes and sizes, all attached to two large rings. But how could I tell which of the keys matched which of the many rooms?
>   "You just have to try them all," my new friend encouraged me. "Take all the time you need. You have all the time in the world. Try all the doors, and try all the keys. Gradually you'll open more and more doors. Keep on going. Don't give up. You'll become freer with every room you open, and one day you'll know which door belongs to every key and which key belongs to every door."

## Africa

The story "Africa" uses implication to take advantage of the fact that the shape of Africa on a map resembles the shape of a skull. The gradually explored interior of the continent corresponds to the brain in metaphorical terms.

TOPIC: Convalescence, exam revision, learning, memory, stroke
INTERVENTION: Metaphorical reframing, promoting a learning attitude, promoting a searching attitude (metaphor, searching model)

People have been making maps for millennia, but there are major differences between the maps of earlier centuries and today's maps. For example, a map of Africa published three hundred years ago featured large blank areas labelled "terra incognita". Few such areas could be found on the coast, but the interior of the continent was almost entirely blank. Over the years that followed, however, many explorers travelled into the heart of Africa and recounted everything they saw there to cartographers, who eagerly drew it all down. Routes by land were discovered, as were routes by water. The twists and bends of every river were explored and drawn in. The names of the settlements were noted down, as well as the names of the tribes. The blank areas on the maps became smaller and smaller. The parts of the continent that could be described grew larger and larger. Finally the blank areas disappeared altogether. All of Africa had been mapped.

### Memory

The case study "Memory" illustrates a procedure for learning to remember things again. Single associative connections are useless if they are disrupted; instead, a larger network of links is communicated so that individual functioning associative connections within this network can help to reactivate others or reconstruct the context.

TOPIC: Convalescence, learning, memory, stroke
INTERVENTION: Psychoeducation, promoting a learning attitude, promoting a searching attitude (example, positive model)

"After my stroke," he said, "people knew *me* but I no longer knew them.
    'I'm Peter!' one of them said.
    'Which Peter?' I replied.
    'Don't you remember me? We went to school together, we did our apprenticeships together, we worked side by side...'
    'I'm sorry, I don't remember you,' I said.
    'But we went on holiday together,' he continued, 'and you gave my daughter Julia this funny teapot.'
    'Are you Julia's father?' I asked with surprise. 'He was called Peter and went to school with me. Is that you?'"

### The Archivist

"The Archivist" serves as a metaphor for cooperation between conscious and unconscious thinking, and for the way in which memory works.

TOPIC: Convalescence, exam revision, memory, stroke
INTERVENTION: Hypermnesia, metaphorical reframing, promoting a searching attitude, promoting positive expectations, psychoeducation, trance induction through alternation of the familiar

Do you sometimes find yourself trying to remember a name that is on the tip of your tongue? And then later on, when you're doing something else entirely and have stopped thinking about it, the name will suddenly pop into your head, even though you weren't thinking about it... Isn't it strange that you didn't find the solution when you were looking for it, and only *afterwards*? Why is that? There is only one possible explanation...

A friendly archivist is working in your brain and managing the archives of everything you know. He sits at the information desk, which is located on the ground floor near the lobby. He has arranged all the books and files that are required most frequently around him in an orderly fashion. Those required less frequently are stored on long shelves in the basement. It sometimes takes him a while to find things if a book has been moved or if your query does not quite match the information in his records. Since you're not used to waiting, you might think that he's forgotten you. But an archivist would never do that; they are experts at customer service and painstakingly careful in their work. Holding your request in his hand, the archivist moves through all the rooms in the basement.

He searches and searches, and finally he cries out, "Got it!" He comes back up the stairs with the book in his hand. He brings you what you have been looking for.

### Learning to Talk

The intervention "Learning to Talk" can be used to help stroke patients recover lost words, and also to relearn movements and other lost skills. It can be told in two different forms, both of which are combined here. The first describes all of the things a person has already learned over his or her lifetime which seemed difficult at first but then became easy, before pointing out that the same will be true of the challenge he or she now faces.

Erickson describes how a child learns to stand and to walk, and emphasises that these tasks represent a much greater challenge than many of those we later fear (Rosen, 1982: 55). He says: "When you first went to [...] grade school, this matter of learning letters and numerals seemed to be a big insurmountable task. To recognise the letter A [,] to tell a Q from an O [,] was very, very difficult. But you learned to form a mental image of some kind. [...] You developed more and more mental images [...] Now you can go anywhere you wish, and transport yourself to any situation." "You imply that just as you overcame difficulties in the past, so you will now" (Erickson et al., 1976).

In the second variant, the therapist reminds a mother that she has taught her children how to talk (walk, etc.) and can therefore also teach herself. In a modified form of the second variant, reference can be made to the work done by teachers, child care workers, trainers etc. This follows the same principle as the story "Sorting Screws", namely that patients are motivated by references to jobs and areas of interest in which they were successful before their stroke.

TOPIC: Aphasia, convalescence, language and speech, learning, memory, stroke
INTERVENTION: Age regression, imagined rapport, promoting a learning attitude, promoting positive expectations, psychoeducation (example, positive model)

> When your daughter was very young, you helped her learn how to talk. You probably had to repeat some words to her two or three times before she could understand them and pronounce them correctly, but finally she managed it. Later she even learned English and French... as second languages, of course. German was and still is her mother tongue. And your parents also helped you learn how to talk. Like all children, you couldn't understand anything to begin with – that must have been a difficult task! And yet you finally managed it. Gradually you learned more and more words, a whole world of them. Now you are grown up. You are no less clever than you were then, and you must perform the same task. With one difference; this time you understand a lot of what you are learning, and you can draw on many valuable experiences from your past. Most importantly, you know that if you've learned it once, you can learn it again.

### Learning to Walk

In "Learning to Walk", the side of the body which still functions correctly is referred to as the teacher while the nonfunctioning half of the body is referred to as the pupil. A discussion is then held on what the teacher teaches the pupil and what the pupil can and wants to learn from the teacher (cf. the story "Taekwondo").

TOPIC: Convalescence, learning, paralysis, stroke
INTERVENTION: Age regression, dissociation of the two sides of the body, imagined rapport, mental gymnastics, promoting a learning attitude (example, positive model)

> Imagine that your left-hand side, the one which can move, is a mother, and your right-hand side, the one which can't move quite so well, is her young daughter. The mother wants to teach her daughter how to walk. Both of them need a great deal of patience to achieve this task, but luckily they have this in abundance. The woman repeatedly takes her

child by the hand. They practise and practise, over and over again. She explains something to her daughter, and the daughter replies. What are they talking about?

## Sorting Screws

The case study "Sorting Screws" makes it clear that the training provided to stroke patients should be based on activities which played a significant role in their former life.

TOPIC: Convalescence, learning, paralysis, stroke
INTERVENTION: Promoting a learning attitude, promoting a searching attitude, utilising rapport (example, positive model)

> He had survived two major strokes. He had undertaken the tough and painstaking work involved in regaining all his former skills, not just once but twice. Some time later, he founded a self-help group for stroke patients and their relatives. He wanted to show them how they could recover their lost knowledge and skills.
>
> "How do you go about doing that?" I asked him.
>
> He replied, "I might ask someone, 'What did your husband used to do?' If she says, 'He was a carpenter,' then I answer, 'Let him practice moving his hand and arm by giving him a box containing a mixture of screws and nuts for him to sort out.'"
>
> He looked at me and said, "If you want patients to be more ambitious, you have to give them something to do which fits their lives."

## Shifting Interests

The story "Shifting Interests" makes it clear that people often have hidden skills which remain unknown to their nearest and dearest, sometimes for decades. It is impossible for us to tell what another person cannot do or does not know, and we are only aware of a small fragment of what he can do and does know. This is particularly true when working with children with behavioural problems or persons with mental health problems or disabilities.

TOPIC: Attention, dementia, disability, memory
INTERVENTION: Promoting a searching attitude (example, positive model)

> After spending a long time in a coma, Dennis returned to the land of the living with reduced mental functions. He had forgotten many things, and was apathetic about most of the rest. Yet he often pointed to the sky and said, "Look, an F-14 Tomcat plane!" or "Wow, an Apache

helicopter!" and described the engine types, performance, carrying capacity, cockpit equipment, crew and weapons of the aircraft he saw flying past.

"He fought in the Korean War," said his wife. "But I had no idea he still remembered all of this. We've been married for thirty years, and he's never shown any interest in aircraft."

## The Nail

"The Nail" encourages listeners to influence the quality of a chronic disorder before influencing its quantity, that is, to focus more on the "how" of the symptoms before attempting to influence their intensity with a shift to "whether" and "how much". The story suggests that even small changes in this respect serve as a useful starting point and have implications for the "whether" and "how much" of the problem. With patience, even microscopically small changes can act as a foundation for larger alterations in terms of both quantity and quality.

The story can be used in the context of child and family therapy as well as parent coaching in order to encourage family members to pursue their goals (parenting, gaining independence) with tenacity and unwavering patience. The story can be used as an aversive suggestion for therapeutically treatable forms of hair loss, particularly if the symptom has become symbolic of an internal experience (conversion symptom). In this context, the story describes the active pulling out of hair in metaphorical terms and thus provokes resistance against the loss of hair, just as the loss of hair previously expressed resistance against whatever was associated with the hair (e.g. the time during which the hair was growing). When treating psychogenic hair loss, the trauma or other triggering event should be treated therapeutically in order to prevent the regrown hair falling out again at a later date.

The story is contraindicated for patients who have previously had a fingernail or toenail removed.

TOPIC: Chronic disease, depression, growing up, hair loss, multiple sclerosis, pain, parenting, stroke
INTERVENTION: Aversive suggestion, mental gymnastics, promoting positive expectations (metaphors, searching model)

After packing up the last of my belongings in preparation for moving house, I walk through the empty rooms one last time to say goodbye. When I reach the bedroom, I stop in my tracks and stare. A nail is poking out of the wall right in front of me – just where the head of my bed had been. I can't leave the apartment looking like that. I need to remove the nail. But the apartment is empty, and I have no pliers. I walk over and pull at the nail. Nothing happens. I wobble it. Nothing happens. But is that really the case? Nothing seems to be happening to the nail. Yet something is happening in my head; I start to think about how long I will have to wobble this nail just to get it to move sideways, let alone forwards. Days, months, years? Surely not! I pretend to myself that I can move the nail sideways and wobble it back and forth, back and forth. It only takes around a minute. Then I notice an almost imperceptible movement to the side. After another two minutes of lateral movements, the nail moves noticeably to the side. After another few minutes, it makes the first small jerk forwards. After ten minutes, I have it in my hand. It's out. I close up the hole with some filler.

## The Left-Handed Person

The story "The Left-Handed Person" demonstrates an intervention for reorganising neurological functions, particularly in the case of left-handed people who have been taught to use their right hands.

TOPIC: Left-handedness
INTERVENTION: Test suggestion (example, positive model)

For many years I wondered why I had always used scissors with my left hand, even scissors for cutting paper which have a special ergonomic design for right-handed people and are extremely uncomfortable to use with the left hand. I used my right hand to do everything else. Was it possible that I could be left-handed without knowing it?

"You fell over more than any child I've ever known while you were learning to walk," my father told me. I have a motor control disorder that affects my coordination. Could this have concealed the fact that I'm left-handed?

"Dear brain," I said, "please check and see whether I'm left-handed or not. If I am, please sort out everything which is in the wrong place. Shift everything which should be done with my left hand to the left, and everything which should be done with my right hand to the right. If it works please keep it that way, and if not change it to how it was before."

I had the sensation that something was buzzing and working away in my head. Over the weeks that followed, my thoughts and working processes seemed to be better organised. My overall mood was lighter and more cheerful, I seemed to have fewer mood swings, and my previous episodes of depression seemed to have disappeared. There was one very obvious change; ever since I have lifted heavy objects with my left hand, waved with my left hand and automatically used my left hand for tasks that I had previously performed with my right hand. At the age of 38 I had discovered that I was left-handed.

## Excretion

Enuresis and encopresis in children can take various forms and have various causes, and organic causes should be excluded before any psychotherapeutic treatment. A distinction should be made between a child who has never been dry or clean and a child who regresses at a later stage; similarly, a distinction should be made between cases in which the problem occurs only at night, cases in which it occurs only during the day and cases in which it occurs at any time. If the child has a dry night, is it because he or she has avoided having anything to drink in the evening and managed to hold on until morning? Or has he or she woken up and used the toilet in the middle of the night? If the child has previously been dry, it is important to establish when the regression first occurred and which stresses were present in the preceding months, since the symptom may be a reaction to a loss or a traumatic experience. The therapist can explain to the child that this situation is now in the past, and that his or her parents or other carers will look after him. If the child talks about what happened and cries about what he or she has lost, the bedwetting may become unnecessary. A farewell ritual can also be carried out by painting a picture of what has been lost, folding it up into a paper boat and floating it down a river towards the sea. If the child is being raised within a religious tradition, he or she can also light a candle in church and place a slip of paper underneath with the following words: "Dear God, please take good care of..." It is important for the child himself or herself to decide on the best course of action.

Consideration should be given to the protective role which the symptom may perform for the child. Some children suffering from daytime enuresis or encopresis are expressing their resistance to subjectively or objectively intolerable power relationships or living conditions. Consideration should also be given to the possibility that these children are offering resistance to previous or ongoing sexual abuse.

Incontinence in adults may have several different causes, and the extent to which it is or can be psychologically influenced may also vary greatly. It should not be assumed that incontinence with a purely psychological cause will be easy to treat therapeutically in every case; equally, however, incontinence with clearly organic causes is not always impossible to treat by means of talking interventions.

### Continent Eyes

The case study "Continent Eyes" highlights the widespread phenomenon of conversion disorders. Simply alerting clients to the possible existence of a conversion disorder may cure it; alternatively, speculation that the incontinence might be a conversion symptom can also cure disorders which can be influenced through suggestion, presumably through a type of placebo effect.

TOPIC: Cancer, conversion disorder, eyes, incontinence, prostate, psycho-somatic disorder, sexuality, tears

INTERVENTION: Shifting the focus of attention from the body to the mind,· paradoxical intervention, psychoeducation (example, positive model)

A man once came to see me because he was still suffering from continence problems after undergoing prostate surgery, even though his doctors had told him that there was no longer any organic cause for his incontinence. During his third therapy session, he told me that he had recently cried for the first time in years when a doctor told him that all of his symptoms were perfectly normal, and that he would in all likelihood become continent again.

"Have you ever heard of a conversion symptom?" I asked him. "Maybe your excretion organs are incontinent because your eyes are continent. Your bladder has taken on the role of your eyes or vice versa, depending on your point of view. I wouldn't be at all surprised if you became incontinent in an unexpected way in the near future."

When I next saw the man, he said: "I don't know whether it's because of what we discussed, but now I only need to use one third as many incontinence pads to stay dry."

### Soiled Underwear Again

The case study "Soiled Underwear Again" demonstrates a symptom prescription in the form of homework to carry out a ritual. This paradoxical intervention follows the Milan tradition of systemic family therapy. The young boy soiled himself exactly once in the following week. Later the frequency increased again, and his mother stopped bringing him to therapy.

TOPIC: Encopresis

INTERVENTION: Homework, paradoxical intervention, symptom prescription utilisation of the symptom (example, positive model)

Paul was six years old. Almost every day he waited until he was alone, found a quiet spot in the house where he could hide in peace and take his time, and then soiled his underwear. His excuses were many and varied, and often he had none at all. He only used the toilet reluctantly and under protest. None of the doctors who had examined him had found any problems. His mother had tried both being patient and being strict.

When I met Paul and his mother, I asked him whether he thought he could deliberately soil himself on a particular day. He responded in the affirmative, both to this question and to the question of whether he could deliberately not soil himself on a particular day.

So I came to an agreement with Paul and his mother that he should deliberately soil himself, today if possible, and that his mother should allow him to do so. Tomorrow could then be the day when he deliberately did the opposite. Or he could soil himself today and tomorrow, with his mother's express permission; what mattered was that he had soiled himself at least once before our next meeting. He could tell his mother beforehand or afterwards, or simply let her work it out for herself. And I discussed the details with Paul; on how many days of the following week he would soil himself, and on how many he would not. His mother offered to note down every time when he soiled himself on the calendar so that I could see whether he had done his job properly. The young boy protested that he would never soil himself again. I made a point of telling him that it was much too early to be thinking about that. I implored him to try and soil himself at least one more time.

### The Bladder Alarm Clock

Children sometimes wet the bed because they have not yet learned to wake up when their bladder is full, and have not realised that it is a straightforward task to instruct their brain to wake them. The approach followed in the case study "The Bladder Alarm Clock" resembles that in the interventions "Alarm Clock with a Snooze Button" and "Breathless" in the chapter on sleep disorders. After the therapy described in "The Bladder Alarm Clock" no further treatment was necessary. Olness and Kohen summarise case descriptions and studies concerning the use of hypnotherapy to treat children suffering from enuresis (Kohen & Olness, 2011: 170; cf. Kohen, 1990: 489; Mrochen, 2002: 117; Trenkle, 2002: 124). The behavioural therapy approach involves the use of a bedwetting alarm which is triggered by moisture. The intervention described here avoids potentially humiliating the child and increases his or her sense of autonomy.

TOPIC: Bedwetting, sleep
INTERVENTION: Anamnesis questions, conditioning of sleeping behaviours, metonymy, psychoeducation (example / metaphor, positive model)

Daniel's mother brought him to therapy because the nine-year-old was still wetting the bed three or four times a week. I talked to Daniel about how his excretory organs worked, and how the brain worked together with them. When I asked him whether he sometimes woke up in the night to go to the toilet and empty his bladder, he answered in the negative. He explained that he was not allowed to drink anything after six in the evening. If his bed stayed dry, it was because he had been able to hold on until the following morning.

I asked how he woke up in the morning. He responded that his mother usually woke him up. When I asked whether he sometimes woke up earlier and went back to sleep, he replied that this happened quite often.

"Then that makes our job a lot easier," I said with relief. "Like many people, you have an internal alarm clock in your brain. And this is no ordinary alarm clock, but a bladder alarm clock. You can say to it, 'Dear alarm clock, please wake me up as soon as my bladder is nearly full, and make sure that I can get out of bed and reach the toilet in time. Only let me carry on sleeping if you know that my bladder can wait until the morning.'"

When Daniel came to a therapy session eighteen days later, he had only wet the bed once.

"Great job!" I said. "And what do you think went wrong on the night when you did wet the bed?"

"I forgot to set my alarm clock the evening before," he replied.

I said to Daniel, "It's true that some alarm clocks need to be set every evening, but I have an alarm clock which I only have to set once. After I've set it, it keeps on waking me up every night or every morning in the same way until I change it. Your alarm clock also works like that. Say to it, 'Wake me up every night when my bladder is nearly full, just like we agreed, unless I say otherwise.'"

The course of therapy lasted 90 minutes, split over two sessions. I said to Daniel's mother, "I'll charge you for two hours. Let me know if you need the extra half hour at any point in the future."

## Sleep

Many sleep problems can be influenced by conditioning. As was the case in the story "The Bladder Alarm Clock", when an agreed circumstance occurs the client is prompted to wake up or do something specific while remaining asleep. The client can practise this behaviour by reaching an agreement with himself or herself before going to bed every evening, and checking every morning that it has worked; after he or she has repeated this procedure a few times, it will become an automatic habit.

### Alarm Clock with a Snooze Button

The story "Alarm Clock with a Snooze Button" represents a basic intervention for handing over control of sleep from the conscious to the unconscious, and for suggesting that it is safe to do so because the unconscious knows that it can easily handle the task. The alarm clock story can be used for patients who find it difficult to fall asleep or stay asleep, for patients who repeatedly oversleep and for patients who are worried about waking up too early from an anaesthetic or not waking up at all. It can also be used for all sleep disorders that can be prevented by waking up in time, such as bedwetting, sleep apnoea and snoring, as well as for nightmares. The story embodies the basic suggestion that control is retained even during sleep, and can therefore be used to make it clear to patients with a compulsive and controlling personality that they can stay relaxed while remaining fully in control.

TOPIC: Compulsion, control, enuresis, narcosis, sleep, waking up
INTERVENTION: Conditioning of sleeping behaviours, psychoeducation (example / metaphor, positive model)

"My body has an internal alarm clock," one friend said to another. "Before going to sleep, I tell myself: 'Tomorrow morning I'll wake up at ten past six.' And then the next morning I'll wake up at exactly ten past six. Yet recently I woke up at ten past six and did not get straight out of bed. I went back to sleep again and overslept."

"That could never happen to me," answered his friend. "My internal alarm clock has a snooze button. Before going to sleep, I tell myself: 'Tomorrow morning I'll wake up at ten past six, and then I'll wake up every five minutes after that.'"

## My Right Eye

"My Right Eye" demonstrates how an intervention of this kind can be used to interrupt nightmares. In the following intervention, the conditioning of sleeping behaviours is linked to the technique of producing psycho-autonomic states by highlighting one of their features until the remaining aspects of the mind–body experience align themselves accordingly. Eyes which are open rather than closed are one of the typical features of the waking state, and they therefore prompt the body to align the remaining aspects of its autonomic state by waking up. This method is similar to "leading" in hypnosis, which involves aspects of the desired state being demonstrated by the therapist and copied by the client, with the organism adjusting to a new psycho-autonomic balance that corresponds in psychological, social and autonomic terms to the modified aspects. Other psycho-autonomic aspects which can be easily influenced and which influence wakefulness (alertness, trance, sleep) include breathing rate, the focus of attention (internal or external), movements and body position. The method can be described as stimulation through simulation or as self-pacing and self-leading (pacing and leading in self-communication). On the simulation of altered psycho-autonomic states through the demonstration of individual elements of these states, consider the intervention "Manta Ray". Note also the procedure for producing sleep through breath pacing and breath leading in the story "Instead of a Lullaby". Similar conditioning is possible in connection with sleepwalking; Olness and Kohen asked a young boy who suffered from sleepwalking to, "programme himself to stay in bed

during this transition phase [between REM phases and non-REM phases].
He practiced the exercises every night before going to sleep. The sleepwalking
decreased in frequency immediately [...] and had disappeared entirely within
two months." (Kohen & Olness, 2011).

TOPIC: Dream, night terrors, nightmare, sleep, sleep apnoea, sleepwalking
INTERVENTION: Conditioning of sleeping behaviours, stimulation through
    simulation (example, positive model)

> I used to have bad dreams occasionally which bothered me greatly. So
> I told myself, "From now on, whenever you start to have a bad dream,
> open one eye. Keep it open until you wake up. Then close it, carry on
> sleeping and dream something else instead."
>
> Even I was a little surprised when I kept on finding myself awake
> because my right eye (it was always the right) had opened while the left
> remained closed. Upon waking, I would ask myself, "What's wrong?"
> Then I would answer myself, "Another bad dream – lucky for me that my
> method works so well." I would close my right eye again and continue
> sleeping peacefully.

### Breathless

The story "Breathless" is intended to change sleeping habits in patients
suffering from sleep apnoea. Further narrative interventions on sleep apnoea
can be found in Hammel 2011: 95 and Hammel, 2015: 54.

TOPIC: Breathing, enuresis, falling out of bed, sleep, sleep apnoea, sleepwalking
INTERVENTION: Conditioning of sleeping behaviours (example, positive model)

> Yet again I had forgotten to breathe! And every time it happened, I would
> wake up feeling scared. There didn't seem to be anything I could do about
> it; when I was asleep I didn't notice that I was holding my breath, and so
> I couldn't start breathing again until I had woken up.
>
> When I spoke to my friend about it, he expressed his surprise, "Haven't
> you realised? Even when you're asleep, your brain is still awake. How
> else could you wake up to go to the toilet when your bladder was full?
> And why don't you fall out of bed? Your brain says, 'Turn over, you've
> reached the left side of the bed.' Your brain must also notice when you
> stop breathing."
>
> "So why don't I just keep on breathing?"
>
> My friend shrugged his shoulders. "At least your brain tells you to
> wake up."
>
> "Good point," I replied. "Dear brain," I said that evening. "There's
> something I'd like to ask you. Whenever you notice my breathing getting

shallower, please take a really deep breath before I stop breathing altogether, and then keep on breathing normally."

I woke up a few more times that night – but it was the long deep breath I had just taken which woke me up rather than the fact that I had been holding my breath.

## Stop

The dialogue "Stop" uses the brain's ability to respond while the body is asleep to help spouses or partners stop each other from snoring. It is however necessary for the intervention to be perceived by both spouses or partners as originating from a desire to work together to solve the problem (rather than a desire to lecture and insult the other party). The intervention can be used in a similar fashion to reduce teeth grinding and nightmares.

TOPIC: Nightmare, relationship, sleep, snoring, teeth grinding
INTERVENTION: Conditioning of sleeping behaviours in a partner (example, positive model)

"I don't snore," says the man.

"I can prove that you do snore," said his wife. "Tonight I'll hold your hand, and every time you start snoring I'll press it until you stop."

She pressed her husband's hand multiple times that night. The following night she had to press his hand less frequently, and for shorter periods of time. And on the third night the snoring stopped entirely, but she kept on holding his hand – to show how much she loved him.

## Snoring

The story "Snoring" is another intervention which relates to the same topic.

TOPIC: Sleep, snoring
INTERVENTION: Conditioning of sleeping behaviours (example, positive model)

Recently I stayed at a friend's house. "You snored all night long. It woke me up and I couldn't get back to sleep for over an hour," she told me the following morning.

"Wake me up if it happens again tonight," I said.

"Did I snore last night?" I asked the morning after, although I had slept all night without being woken.

"No, not at all. I don't understand why," she answered.

"I told myself not to lie on my back at any point during the night, and instead only to move from my left side to my right side."

### Boat Ride by Night

"Boat Ride by Night" is a metaphorical intervention for snoring and teeth grinding. It incorporates instructions for curing sleep apnoea and for transforming some of the energy stored as muscular tension in the jaw into useful tension in the soft palate in order to prevent snoring. The metaphorical procedure can be supplemented by addressing the body directly and ordering it to move muscular tension from the jaw into the soft palate, and the story can also be used to reduce jaw clicking. It may be a good idea for the client to tell or read the story to himself or herself on a regular basis over a period of time before going to sleep. The metaphor can also be used in other contexts where flexible changes in muscular tension result in the disappearance of symptoms.

TOPIC:  Clicking jaw, encopresis, incontinence, mitral valve prolapse, muscular tension, sleep apnoea, snoring, teeth grinding
INTERVENTION: Conditioning of sleeping behaviours, utilising ambiguity (metaphor, positive model), using connotations

> Perhaps it's not something you've ever noticed; when you fall asleep, the cavity of your mouth turns into an ocean, with a boat gliding across it with well-trimmed sails. Is it a fishing boat? I know from the song "Fishermen of Capri" that fishermen stay up all night and work when the rest of the world is asleep. They put just the right amount of tension in their sails so that the wind pushes the boat smoothly into the waves, carrying the fishermen onwards. These fishermen are experienced sailors. They know how to steer their boat. Nothing ever rattles or flaps. The ropes and sheets are tightly stretched and firmly lashed in place, but they're still flexible enough for the fishermen to make slight changes to the tension as soon as the wind turns. The fishermen know their boat. They know how to handle it so that the energy of the breaking waves – which might otherwise damage the hull – is transferred partly to the sails and partly to where the boat needs it most. And from what I've heard, there is always a fresh breeze at sea. The wind never stops. It blows ever further and ever onwards, coming and going in waves, changing all the time and yet always remaining present.

### Cow Bells

The story "Cow Bells" can be used to teach clients or supervised students how to prevent insomnia caused by a snoring spouse or partner, loud traffic or other sources of noise. The story also illustrates how noises which make it difficult to concentrate can be incorporated into an imaginative soundscape which is henceforth experienced as pleasant rather than irritating. This can be particularly useful for those suffering from attention deficit disorders. Emotionally stressful noises (for example, the drill of a dentist) can also be rendered less stressful if they are incorporated into a pleasant fictional soundscape.

Daniel Zelling told the following bedtime story to patients attending therapy sessions whose sleep was disturbed by snoring; "Have you ever been on a beautiful, ocean-going sailing vessel with the sting of a salty spray on your face? I want you to imagine [...] that you're on a beautiful, large sailboat [...]. You hear the gulls and the creaking of the wooden mast under a full load of canvas: The clatter of the rigging; the squeak of the boom – all the sounds of the ocean and the sailboat. [...] It is so relaxing... so peaceful... the wind in your face; the salt spray from the ocean; and you are lulled to sleep... You can use this image at night. At night when you go to sleep, the noises that surround you can fit into this image." (Zelling, 1986)

TOPIC:  Attention deficit disorder (ADD / ADHD), falling asleep, noise, sleep, snoring

INTERVENTION: Conditioning of waking behaviours, unreal reframing (example / metaphor, positive model)

"I do like living on an Alpine meadow," the woman said. "And it's nice that the cows have bells. It's just that it's very hard to sleep when they lie next to my house all night long and ring their bells in time as they chew the cud. Being a musician doesn't make it any easier. In many ways it just makes it more difficult."

"Once you told me about a conservatoire in Utrecht where people learn to play the carillons in church towers and town halls," I replied. "Imagine that you are there now, and that three students are practising different Baroque pieces at the same time. Try to work out which pieces they are playing, and fill in the missing notes."

"That reminds me," she said. "I once helped my mother with a similar problem. She couldn't sleep because her neighbour had left a hay blower running in his barn. I told her, 'Imagine it's a brook rushing down the mountainside.' From then she had no problem sleeping. I look forward to trying out your idea with the carillons tonight."

"How were the carillons?" I asked her the following morning.

"I slept through it all," she said. "And I was so looking forward to the bells."

### Releasing the Spring

"Releasing the Spring" is a story which instructs patients who suffer from nocturnal teeth grinding to relax their tense jaws on a regular basis in response to a signal they have previously agreed with themselves, and to overcome mental and emotional problems without tensing the body. (On forms of suggestive therapy for asthma, cf. Kohen & Olness, 2011.)

TOPIC: Asthma, body language, cosmetic concerns, falling asleep, muscular tension, sleep, teeth grinding

INTERVENTION: Ambiguity, promoting a searching attitude, rhetorical question, trance induction through questions and through confusion (metaphor, searching attitude)

> A watchmaker was repairing an exquisite and very valuable watch. The inner workings of the watch included a cylindrical spring box which she needed to open. The coiled spring in this housing was under great pressure. The watchmaker wanted to release this pressure in order to fix a problem with the watch. Using a special tool, the watchmaker expertly loosened a tiny screw and relieved the tension in the spring, not too quickly and not too slowly, but just enough that the spring could properly relax. Then the watchmaker mended the watch and closed it back up again, and from then on the watch worked perfectly. Or had it always done so, and this whole story merely draws attention to a tiny detail which might be very useful?

### Instead of a Lullaby

The story "Instead of a Lullaby" demonstrates one way of encouraging an infant to fall asleep. A sleeping state is stimulated by simulating the relevant breathing pattern and other aspects of the associated bodily behaviours. The procedure can also be used on adults and animals.

TOPIC: Falling asleep, infant, sleep

INTERVENTION: Breath pacing, pacing and leading, using rapport (example, positive model)

> Someone placed the six-month-old Manuel in my arms and asked me to hypnotise him so that he would finally go to sleep. I started talking to the baby, using a deep voice to ensure that I had his full attention. I copied his fidgeting movements, and when we had fidgeted together for a while I started to reduce the frequency and amplitude of the fidgeting; I gradually moved more slowly and calmly, making sure that I didn't rush and that he was copying my pace of movement. My voice also gradually became quieter and calmer. Then I began to breathe loudly at the same rate that he was breathing, before letting my breath slow down; he copied me, and was asleep within three minutes.

## Sexuality

Many sexual disorders have a compulsive element and can be treated using the methods described in the chapter on "Compulsion". For certain sexual problems such as erectile dysfunction, the client can be asked what he could do to maintain the symptom, make it persist for longer or even worsen it. It is likely that the client will express a number of fears, warnings and compulsive thoughts. All of the client's statements in this respect can be interpreted by the therapist as the efforts of a member of his "inner team" to protect him, and the therapist can highlight and praise the good intentions of this team member. He can ask the team member certain questions which the client should answer on his behalf. He can then ask the parts of the client's personality who are trying to protect him (and thereby causing the problem) whether they would be prepared to try doing less of what they have previously been doing or even doing the opposite. And he can ask whether they would agree to do "more of the same" as long as this new behaviour (inaction, thinking, silence) is of benefit to the client whom they wish to protect, making it clear that they will be able to return to the old pattern at any time if the new behaviour is not useful.

Another approach involves activating and linking erotic resources by connecting a highly connotative story with the client's reality through multiple suggestions, ensuring that the matching real-life experiences are imbued with ever more erotic connotations.

### Snail Race

The story "Snail Race" can be used with patients suffering from various sexual dysfunctions, although it is recommended that the text be adapted to the relevant situation. The accumulation of suggestions through semantic field associations and ambiguity is unmistakable.

TOPIC: Erectile dysfunction, premature ejaculation, sexuality, vaginismus
INTERVENTION: Ambiguity, interspersal technique, using connotations (example, positive model)

> The snails are having a race. A group of birds who are watching are open-mouthed – or rather open-beaked – at the length of time taken by these moist creatures to make progress, and how slowly they expel slime as they moisten the ground over which they glide. They make steady progress, but it takes them a very long time to reach their goal. Yet a snail race is enormous fun for those who know how to take their time. There's a lot to see; how the snails strain forward to make progress! How they straighten their smooth, solid feelers, and stretch them out towards their goal! How the sides of their body move with a wave-like motion in order to push them onwards! Someone once said that if only we could learn to experience slowness, we would see how snails really lean into the corners. And it's true; anyone who wants the snails to go faster can simply experience everything more slowly. Then a snail race will be just the right place for him, and he will see how fast they are. When the snails race each other, they are full of movement. From their feelers to their slime glands and from their mouth to their tail, everything moves forward. They are experts at rationing their strength. And when the time comes, they accelerate for

one final spurt on the home stretch until they finally cross the finishing line, panting with exertion.

### How to Handle Sexual Assault...

The case study "How to Handle Sexual Assault..." discusses the possibility of protecting oneself against sexual harassment.

TOPIC: Aggression, exhibitionism, sexual harassment
INTERVENTION: Catalepsy, destabilisation through irritation, disruption of rapport, pattern interrupt by the client, trance induction through confusion (example, positive model)

A colleague recently called me for some advice. A female friend of hers was being sexually harassed on a regular basis by a neighbour who engaged in exhibitionistic behaviours towards her while he was in his garden, and sometimes also made lewd comments on her figure and her clothes.

We discussed possible solutions together, and decided that the police would probably not be much help in a case like this. In my colleague's opinion, the next time it happened her friend should look over and comment wearily,

"Not exactly well endowed, are you?" I for my part thought that the woman should keep a pile of water bombs made from balloons filled with tomato juice ready in her garden. Alternatively, a blowpipe filled with cherry pits should also do the trick – simply aim at his manhood, and one hard puff! A friend who was listening in on the conversation suggested that the woman should carry a digital camera around with her and take a photo the next time it happened. Even if the photo didn't show much, the neighbour would be in a very awkward position as soon as the flash had gone off – not only because it might be shown to the police, but also because he would have to live in permanent fear from that moment onwards that the offending image might be posted on the Internet, "liked" by friends and neighbours and go viral. "You'd be better off with a video," suggested someone else. "Then you'd have sound too!"

My only fear is that these brilliant ideas were never used; once the woman had these tricks up her sleeve, her behaviour would have altered and the neighbour would probably have intuitively stopped the harassment.

## Eating behaviours and addiction

The issue of addiction has close connotations with trance. When working in this area, it is particularly important to, "avoid being hypnotised by the client"

(Gunther Schmidt, seminar discussion, 2000), or in other words to avoid situations in which an empathy-induced consonance of experience paralyses the therapist, or in which a compassionate therapist takes action while the client's level of passivity remains the same or even increases. The therapist must occasionally take the lead, albeit while ensuring that the client follows him or her along the chosen path. This may sometimes mean imposing conditions, and therapists must therefore have a good sense of the conditions which clients are likely to accept. The following paradigmatic stories focus on a number of aspects of addiction therapy.

### The Fat Woman and the Thin Woman

The story "The Fat Woman and the Thin Woman" was developed while working with anorexic patients, and takes as its starting point the idea that even patients suffering from anorexia have a part of their personality which knows that they are underweight and which can engage in a conversation with the other part of their personality. The story is also based on the idea that the therapist should avoid representing the viewpoint "you are too thin", and should instead represent the ambivalence between the outer world, which assumes that the patient is "too thin", and the client's inner world, which assumes that she is "too fat". The task pursued in therapy is to initiate an inner dialogue between both viewpoints and parts of the personality, with the ultimate aim of negotiating a middle road and a "third way".

TOPIC: Anorexia, body dysmorphic defect, self-perception
INTERVENTION: Ambiguity ("exchange" as "communicate" or "swap roles and places"), destabilisation through multi-partiality, externalisation of ambivalence as two persons, inner team, interspersal technique, reversing the focus of attention, trance induction through stereotype and through confusion, visualisation (metaphor, searching model)

> There is not just one world, but two different worlds. This must be the case, because we are not talking about the same world. We are talking about different worlds.
>
> The fat woman lives in the inner world. The fat woman is not very popular. Everyone in the inner world despises her, and everyone in the outer world refuses to believe that she exists. The thin woman lives in the outer world. The thin woman is also not very popular, because everyone in the outer world worries about her, and no one in the inner world believes in her. The fat woman from the inner world does not believe in the thin woman from the outer world. She can't work out why the people she meets claim to meet the thin woman every day. The thin woman from the outer world does not believe in the fat woman from the inner world either, and she can't work out why the person most affected by all of this

claims to see the fat woman every day. Who is right? Those who believe in the fat woman, or those who believe in the thin woman?

Both the thin woman and the fat woman live in people's heads – but in different worlds. They live on different planets. Now that we have entered the age of technology, visiting other planets is simply a question of deciding on a means of transport. I can imagine boarding a special capsule which would take me out of the inner world and over to the outer world for a limited period of time. That might be quite pleasant, since I'd get rid of the fat woman on the way there, and I've needed a break from her for a long time. The price I'd have to pay when visiting the outer world is that I might meet the thin woman, even though I don't believe in her and perhaps don't want to believe in her. And apparently she doesn't look too great, but who knows. I can also imagine that at the same time as me, in exchange so to speak, a second spaceship would launch off from the outer world and fly to the inner world for a holiday in the fat women's world. Then they'd know what it was like living with her day after day, and would no longer deny her existence.

I wouldn't go on this journey very often – why bother? Later I will send the fat woman herself on a journey to the thin woman, so that they can exchange experiences and learn from each other. I want the fat woman to learn from the thin woman, and the others want the thin woman to learn from the fat woman. I'll stay at home and take a break from the fat woman.

### The People of Lensland

Like the previous story, the metaphorical story "The People of Lensland" can be used for patients suffering from body dysmorphia, in particular anorexia. It can however also be used in relation to hypochondria and the exaggeration (or downplaying) of illness in order to help the unconscious set a more realistic benchmark for the assessment of symptoms.

TOPIC: Anorexia, Asperger syndrome / autism, body dysmorphic defect (BDD), hypochondria, self-confidence, self-perception, shyness
INTERVENTION: Promoting a searching attitude, reversing the focus of attention (metaphor, searching model)

The people of Lensland are born with binoculars in front of their eyes. Most of them are born with binoculars which are the wrong way round, and everything they see looks very small. Whenever they meet someone, they might think, "Aren't they a long way away!" "Aren't they small!" or "Aren't they thin!" However a few people are born with binoculars which are the right way round. Whenever they look down at themselves, they might think, "Aren't I long and wide!" The people of Lensland find it very hard to agree amongst themselves. Yet once upon a time a woman living there made an incredible discovery...

## A Good Reason to Stop Therapy

The case study "A Good Reason to Stop Therapy" illustrates how aversive suggestions can sometimes be used to prevent self-harming behaviours. For example, intelligent, ambitious and self-aware anorexic patients can be shown autopsy images of the brains of women who have died from the disease, and told that these brains were eaten up and consumed by the patients' bodies as a source of fat until they resembled "holey cheese", like the brains of patients who have died of Alzheimer's disease.

TOPIC: Borderline personality disorder, bulimia, double bind, self-harming behaviours, vomiting
INTERVENTION: Aversive suggestion, destabilisation of behaviour through the prefigurement of negative consequences, pattern interrupt by the therapist

Once I received a phone call from a former patient.
"I stopped attending therapy six months ago because I was annoyed with you," she said. "But I think something you said helped me after all. Now it's stopped working, and I'd like to come and see you so that you can help me again."
"Of course," I replied. "What would be the purpose of the therapy?"
"During one of the sessions you scared me by telling me that some people get oesophageal cancer as a result of vomiting too much."
I remembered that I had told the client about these tracheotomised patients and about the course of their treatment, how they responded to this treatment and how difficult it was for them to communicate. I had also told her about the difference between a cannula for respiration immediately after the operation and a cannula for speaking, the gurgling noises when the patient coughs or tries to speak, the phlegm and blood which come out of the tube and the way in which the liquid is suctioned out.
The woman continued speaking, "After my last therapy session I was unable to make myself vomit, and that meant that I could no longer binge on food. After a while I noticed that my self-confidence was improving, and I started to like myself more. Then my father became ill with cancer and died. After six months without bulimia I've started to relapse. I'm not afraid of cancer any more, but I'd like to be afraid of something so that I can be free again."

### Outbreaks

"Outbreaks" can be used not only for patients suffering from bulimia, but also for any other reactive disorders. The story can be associated with a symptom prescription by therapeutically prescribing vomiting as a modified ritual (cf. the story "Grunting"). Every excretion, including breathing out, sweating and the loss of dead skin, can be viewed as a release of psychological stress, even during times when the patient is healthy.

TOPIC: Anxiety, breathing, bulimia, colitis, compulsion (OCD), dandruff, depression, excretion, fever, gastroenteritis, hyperhidrosis, sweating, throat clearing, tics, trauma, vomiting

INTERVENTION: Utilisation of the symptom or a bodily function (example, positive model)

> Whenever something happens to me which I find unpleasant, I have the habit of asking, "What purpose can it serve?" I once fell ill with a stomach bug. I woke up one morning and knew with absolute certainty that I would be sick sooner or later. I would probably be sick several times, and maybe even lots of times. What purpose could this vomiting serve? I devoted each trip to the bathroom to an experience, a time or a person that had injured me. I can still clearly remember the powerful, liberating sensation of these outbreaks of vomiting.

### Compass and Magnet

The story "Compass and Magnet" can be used for cases of alcoholism and alcohol abuse. At the start of the story, symbols of alcohol consumption alternate with symbols of orientation and control. The rule of alternation ensures that the magnet is associated with symbols of alcohol by the unconscious. The watch with a stopwatch function is a reference to the task of ending alcohol-induced disorder. The prompt to clear out the drawer is only insinuated, and can be made more explicit if necessary.

TOPIC: Addiction, alcohol, attention deficit disorder (ADD/ADHD), depression, grief, neglect, order (tidiness), prioritisation, trauma

INTERVENTION: Externalisation of ambivalence as two categories of objects, promoting a searching attitude, visualization (metaphor, positive model / searching model)

> A drawer in one of my cupboards was full of all sorts of odds and ends: a compass, a water bottle, maps, a corkscrew, a GPS device, a bottle opener, a watch with a stopwatch function and a magnet.
>
> "Are you sure you want to keep a magnet in there?" asked a close friend after looking into the drawer when it was open one day. "It will wreck your compass!"

He was right – the compass needle was pointing continually at the magnet instead of due north. I took the magnet out of the drawer and looked at it. It was a strong magnet, which I had originally used to retrieve screws and other bits and pieces which had rolled into a crack in the workshop floor. I'd been living somewhere else at the time.

"Here, have it as a present," I said to my friend. "I don't need it any more."

My friend took it. When he left, I returned to the cupboard. I hadn't noticed before how much of a mess it was in, but now I noticed. I took the compass in my hand. The needle settled down and pointed due north again.

### Language Rules

The story "Language Rules" is an effective way of supporting the withdrawal process. The language used by an addict reveals a great deal about whether he or she is truly committed to the goal of surviving withdrawal and the likelihood that this goal will be achieved. The negotiation of new and helpful "language rules" can increase this likelihood; for example, a relapse can be interpreted (or reframed) as a temporary interruption to an addiction-free life instead of a continuation of the previous addicted life, and linked to the question of how long the interruption should last.

TOPIC: Addiction, self-communication, smoking, withdrawal
INTERVENTION: Clarifying goals, externalisation of ambivalence as a dialogue,
   framework suggestion, psychoeducation, reversing the focus of attention
   (example, positive model)

"I could stop smoking whenever I wanted," she said.
   "What you *could* do is irrelevant to what really happens," he pointed out.
   She hesitated, and then said, "I'll stop smoking tomorrow."
   "If you can tell me what you'll start to do when you stop smoking, I'll believe you," he replied.
   "I'll start not to smoke."
   "I think that's how everyone originally starts off – everyone is born a non-smoker, and everyone dies a non-smoker. Some people take a break in between until they find their way back to their real identity. And so if you were to relapse and stop being a nonsmoker for a while, you wouldn't have started smoking again, you would simply be a non-smoker who was taking a short break. Do you agree?"
   "I like that idea."
   "You've only told me what you'll start not to do. I'm much more interested in what you'll start to do."
   "I'll start to love myself for my soft skin, for my willpower, for my new-found freedom, for my sense of smell and taste and for my prospects of a long and healthy life. Is that good enough for you?"

"I think it will be good enough for you," he answered.

## Dry

The story "Dry" is an example of an intervention which produces internal images acting as metaphorical instructions for a life without alcohol. The metaphor of the rose of Jericho can also be used to reassure cancer patients that they can survive radiation therapy and beat their cancer.

The man in the case example abstained from alcohol for three years after the therapy session. The procedure is based on an intervention by Milton Erickson. A client once visited him and said that he wished to stop drinking. He and his entire family were alcoholics. Yet he had only a very short amount of time available for therapy, because he was in the process of moving to a different state. Erickson sent him to the Desert Botanical Garden in Phoenix and told him to look at specific plants which could survive for several decades without water. Years later, a young woman visited Erickson and explained that she wanted to meet the man who had cured her father and mother of alcoholism by sending her father to the Botanical Garden – and she added that her father had not relapsed (O'Hanlon & Hexum, 1991: 10).

TOPIC: Addiction, alcohol, cancer, irradiation
INTERVENTION: Action as a metaphor, homework, object as a metaphor, pilgrimage (example, positive model), ritual

> "Take this desert plant with you," I said to the man. "It's a rose of Jericho. It can survive unharmed for 50 years or more without a single drop of water. When you're ready, bring it back and tell me what this plant has in common with your life. I'm also going to give you some homework – I'd like you to go on a pilgrimage to atone for the wrongdoings you've committed while drunk. When you're ready, tell me where you intend to go on your pilgrimage."
>
> The man nodded. When I met him again a few months later, he had stopped drinking. "I've already booked my flight," he said. "I'm going on a solo meditation retreat for two weeks. In the Sahara."

## The Cart, the Mud and I

"The Cart, the Mud and I" illustrates how an attitude of resignation can turn a relatively minor accident into a disaster.

TOPIC: Addiction, depression, habit, motivation, neglect, relationship
INTERVENTION: Aversive suggestion, destabilisation through the prefigurement of negative consequences, paradoxical intervention (metaphor, negative model)

When I forgot to steer the cart around the mud, I said to myself, "It's too late to do anything now", and I waited to see what would happen.

When I pushed the cart right into the mud, I said to myself, "It's too late to do anything now," and I waited to see what would happen.

When the cart sank in the mud and I sank along with it, I said to myself, "It's too late to do anything now," and I waited to see what would happen.

When the cart disappeared in the mud, and I disappeared along with it, I knew what I had always known.

# Chapter 4

# Promoting wellbeing

## Resource orientation and positive thinking

What is a resource? What is positive thinking? The science of physics tells us that our basic resources are time, space, energy and matter. We experience time and space as movement and change, which means that all of a person's skills and opportunities that relate to movement and change can be regarded as resources. All the objects, powers and thoughts that expand our opportunities are resources, and all those that limit them are restrictions. Our basic emotional resources are love, joy, pride and thankfulness, but much less widely appreciated feelings such as fear and anger are also resources insofar as they help expand the individual's capacity to experience and act. Behavioural biology suggests that humans are pack animals; from a systemic perspective, therefore, all the current or potential interactions within a social system which expand the ability of its members to act are resources.

### Noah's Brothers

The world can always be viewed either from a positive perspective, or in other words one which focuses on opportunities, or from a negative perspective, or in other words one that ignores opportunities. Yet although this fact is widely known, people are not necessarily mindful of it on a day-to-day basis. "Noah's Brothers" reminds them to focus more often on the positive aspects of their lives.

TOPIC: Crisis, depression, faith, finding resources, self-communication, survival
INTERVENTION: Metaphorical reframing, positive connotation (metaphor, negative model / positive model)

> The flood has receded. The ark has run aground on Mount Ararat. A new morning has dawned. The door of the ark is opened, and the animals are allowed to leave. Noah's brothers also disembark from the ship. They look around – nothing but mud and stones, as far as the eye can see.

"Stupid flood! What are we supposed to eat now?" the younger brother asks Noah, stirring up a muddy puddle with his foot.

"Safe at last, thank the Lord!" the elder brother says to Noah, blinking into the morning sun. A rainbow arches through the sky over both of them.

### A Glance into the Garden

The story "A Glance into the Garden" can be used in similar contexts as the previous story.

TOPIC: Depression, relationship

INTERVENTION: Externalisation of ambivalence as a dialogue, finding resources, metaphorical reframing (example / metaphor, negative model)

"How wonderful the flowers are looking," said Mrs Hinze.

"How terrible it all looks! Everything is overrun with weeds!" said her husband.

They were talking about the same garden.

### Of Cars and Men

The story "Of Cars and Men" illustrates how we can look at people and objects in terms of their resources and make use of their best qualities as a basis for any improvements required. Anything that is intact and successful can be used as a model for the desired final state, and as a benchmark for an appropriate amount of effort. This principle can be used as a basis for all constructive criticism, all training, all medical treatment and all therapy.

The story implies that suffering or absence of suffering by clients should not be judged solely on the basis of what the counsellor or other people would find difficult to bear. It is more important to learn what the client has been accustomed to since his or her childhood, and therefore regards as normal. "According to Erickson, a doctor examining a patient who has sprained their left ankle should first look at the right ankle [...]. When he then goes on to examine the sprained ankle, he will be able to identify not only everything that is wrong with the sprained ankle, but also everything that is right with it." (Short & Weinspach, 2007:111)

TOPIC: Criticism, depression, health

INTERVENTION: Changing punctuation (example, positive model)

I recently took my car to the garage. "There's a scratch on the right-hand door," I said. "How much will it cost to fix?"

The car mechanic looked at the car from behind, then from the left and then from the front.

"The scratch is on the right-hand side," I said.

"I always look at a car from its good side first," he answered. "Then I get a feel for its value, and I can decide how best to deal with the damage."

"If he takes that approach to everything in life, he's a wise man" I thought.

## Life as a Sinus Curve

A life is described as happy or otherwise not primarily because of the actual events which occur during it, but because of the way they are arranged in the individual's memory. Many life stories stop at an unhappy ending rather than continuing to the subsequent happy ending. In order to achieve a "happy" biography, the stories told by a person about his or her life must end with events that were experienced as positive, and also start with such events if possible. Like the following stories, "Life as a Sinus Curve" encourages the listener to structure biographical stories in such a way that they end with positive experiences of this kind.

TOPIC: Biography, crisis, identity, motivation, success
INTERVENTION: Changing punctuation (metaphor, positive model)

> If we imagine that life's ups and downs resemble a sinus curve, we can draw this curve in two different ways. We can start the curve at its highest point, trace it down through its lowest point and then return to its highest point – or we can do the opposite, and draw the curve from its lowest point, through its highest point and back to its lowest point. In mathematical terms, it is exactly the same curve.

## From Oasis to Oasis

Like the previous story, "From Oasis to Oasis" illustrates how a positive or negative interpretation of life is a question of punctuation. The story contains a metaphor to help patients during radiation therapy. It can also be useful in therapy with clients who suffer burnout or bullying at work but have to continue going to work till a better solution is found.

TOPIC: Bullying, burnout syndrome, cancer, crisis, cyclic illness, depression, grief, hope, irradiation, motivation, vision
INTERVENTION: Changing punctuation (metaphor, positive model / negative model)

> When the Bedouins travel by camel from oasis to oasis, they look forward to reaching the lush green foliage of the next watering hole while they are

packing up and leaving the one before. A European traveller once met up with a group of Bedouins at a meeting point between two oases and travelled with them for a few days. The European rode from desert to desert, occasionally passing an oasis on the way. He longed for shadow and water, and admired the Bedouins for the sense of calm they exuded. They rode from oasis to oasis, constantly reassured by thoughts of the next oasis as they journeyed through the desert.

### Dinner for One

"Dinner for One" illustrates how memories, momentary experiences and future expectations influence each other, and how concentrating on negative memories can have a particularly negative effect on future expectations and the very nature of the future. It encourages the listener to distinguish between memories that should continue to be used as a basis for expectations, and those that should be ignored when developing a personal vision of the future.

TOPIC: Depression, hope, vision
INTERVENTION: Dissociation of mental functions, inner team, promoting positive expectations, dissociation of connoted notions, (example, positive model)

Last Sunday, while sitting in my consultation room, I thought to myself, "I need to see a therapist."

"But you are a therapist," said my inner voice, "and this is your consultation room."

"Well, if you say so…"

Three glasses were standing next to a half-full bottle of apple juice. I filled up the glasses, and invited everyone to attend a family therapy session; the I of memory, the I of momentary experience and the I of expectation. All three took their seats, and I asked for their permission to drink from each of the glasses in turn on their behalf. I led the conversation.

To begin with the three almost got into an argument, because Expectation I believed that no one was taking any notice of him and that Memory I – who had nothing positive to say – was getting all the attention. I asked Expectation I how the situation could be improved, and I asked Momentary Experience I to give his opinion on the relationship between Expectation I and Memory I. I also asked Memory I for his opinion on what had been said, remaining neutral and acting like a good family therapist should.

Each of the three had some good ideas. They suggested that a distinction should be made between pleasant and unpleasant memories, and that only the pleasant memories should be used as a basis for developing new and more heartfelt expectations.

When everyone was happy and the bottle of apple juice was empty, I thanked them, dismissed them and ended the session. This therapy session had a long-lasting effect on me, and put me in a very optimistic mood...

### November Blues

The intervention "November Blues" is particularly effective for patients suffering from mild depression.

TOPIC: Depression, hope
INTERVENTION: Stimulation through simulation, mental game, unreal reframing (example, positive model)

> Does bad weather sometimes get you down? Try imagining, just for fun, how it would feel if you were someone with exactly the opposite problem – if you were slightly manic and overactive, and if you found it hard to hide your gradually intensifying lust for adventure, which fascinates some of the people around you but which irritates others. Just for a while, pretend that you were like that too. Imagine that the sun is shining very brightly, and the only reason you can't see that right now is because you're wearing sunglasses or special tinted lenses to protect against the glare of the sun-light. Perhaps it's spring, which would explain why you're starting to feel the familiar rush of spring energy and an onslaught of high spirits – at such an inconvenient time! But there's really not much you can do about it, and you and the people around you have no choice but to learn to deal with this thirst for action. Simply think yourself into this state of mind wherever you are, and notice the difference that it makes.

## Attack and defence

This section covers methods for handling one's own aggression and possible responses to bullying, teasing, physical threats and double bind messages.

It also contains strategies that vulnerable people can use for emotional self-protection or defence, as well as examples and metaphors for conversations with an individual believed by other group members to be guilty of teasing others, plotting intrigues or sabotaging procedures. The aim of the stories is to encourage the individual in question to show solidarity with weaker members of the group, or (where applicable) to warn him or her of the possible consequences of his or her actions. It is often useful to assume that all the parties involved are pursuing goals they believe to be beneficial in some way (or which are beneficial without them being aware of this fact), and in most cases these positive intentions can be easily reconstructed by everyone. Realising and recognising that the opposite side is neither crazy, stupid nor evil, but merely pursuing different yet comprehensible goals (albeit with an unsatisfactory outcome) often results in a noticeable reduction of conflict within a group.

In the event that the therapist is working with only one member of a group in a conflict situation, that individual's resources must be strengthened so that they can defend themselves and attack if necessary. Priority should always be given to deescalating strategies over escalating strategies, but it should not be forgotten that defensive behaviour can in some situations have an escalating effect, while offensive behaviour may have a deescalating effect. Asymmetric conflict escalation involves one party becoming more aggressive as the other becomes more defensive and vice versa.

### Finding Treasure

The story "Finding Treasure" prompts the listener to use aggressive and auto-aggressive impulses as a springboard for progress towards a genuinely rewarding goal. Unpleasant feelings such as anxiety, aggression or loneliness can only be put to good use if they are dealt with from a resourced-focused perspective.

TOPIC: Aggression, anxiety, success

INTERVENTION: Externalisation of a problem as a person, pattern interrupt by the client, promoting a searching attitude, visualisation (metaphor, searching model)

> This is something I was taught by Fedor the Magician. Many have tried to find the treasure by attempting to kill the dragon who guards it. They were fools who sacrificed their lives to a plan which was doomed to failure. If you tame a dragon by meeting him without fear, he will use all his powers to help you – and it's a lot easier to find gold with a dragon by your side than to steal it from him!

### The Bulls Are Coming

"The Bulls Are Coming" is a story that was told to me by a mother of two children, and which demonstrates a strategy for overcoming an all-powerful opponent (whether internal or external). In bullying situations, the story can serve as a prompt to explore ways of putting up resistance. In the case of traumatised or depressed patients or patients suffering from other forms of auto-aggression, it can be illuminating to divide the personality into attacking, vulnerable and protecting personality parts. This metaphorical externalisation can promote anamnesis and the clarification of goals, using the following systemic questions based on the metaphor; what approach is followed by the internal attackers? Which patterns of behaviour and which internal voices correspond to these attackers? What approach is followed by the protecting parts? Where can they find help, or maybe they don't need any? How can the vulnerable part make a useful contribution?

TOPIC: Aggression, anxiety, bullying, compulsion (OCD), cutting, depression, family, immune disease, neurodermatitis, parents, self-harming behaviour, siblings, trauma, violence

INTERVENTION: Externalisation of ambivalence as two (or more) persons, inner team, visualisation (metaphor, positive model / negative model)

> My children and I were enjoying a picnic. Sarah was eleven at the time, and Thomas had just turned four. Our little dog Woyzeck was also there, and we sat and ate in perfect harmony. Yet we hadn't noticed that there was no fence between us and the herd of bulls grazing in the meadow behind the woods where we were picnicking – and suddenly the bulls started to thunder towards us. I grabbed the dog and ran until I was safely behind the fence. The children didn't make it as far as me. "Get behind me!" yelled Sarah, positioning herself in front of Thomas.
>
> Stretching her arms out wide, she confronted the galloping bulls, who screeched to a halt. For a while the bulls and the girl stared at each other. Then the herd turned around.

### The Power of Thoughts

"The Power of Thoughts" illustrates that other people's aggression can often be prevented simply by assuming a position of internal defence against them. This story too can be used in relation to both internal and external opponents (Hammel, 2008).

TOPIC: Aggression, bullying, school, self-communication, violence

INTERVENTION: Externalisation of ambivalence as two (or more) persons, inner team, visualisation (example, positive model)

> I was once waiting at a bus stop together with some young boys, who were really getting on my nerves by repeatedly tugging on my bobble hat. "If you don't stop that, the bobble will fall off!" I snapped at them. I asked them to stop over and over again, but they ignored me. I then thought to myself, "The next person who tugs on my bobble hat will get a hard kick in the shin!" But no one did.

### Nails Make the Man

This approach is reinforced through external symbols in the story "Nails Make the Man".

TOPIC: Aggression, bullying, school, self-confidence
INTERVENTION: Pattern interrupt by the client, psychoeducation (example, positive model)

> A young girl once told me, "There are lots of people at my school who go out of their way to annoy me every day, in particular a group of young kids from Year Five and a number of people in my own year. One after-noon last week a friend and I tried out some different nail polishes. When she left, she took the nail polish remover with her. Two of my nails were still painted black, and I had to go to school like that the following day. That day I wasn't bothered by any of the Year Five pupils who had always pestered me in the past. And so the next day I painted all my nails black, dressed myself in black and put on a studded belt. Once again, I wasn't bothered by any of the Year Five pupils or anyone in my own year. It was absolutely incredible. Nico, a boy who had always given me a hard time before, opened his mouth as if to say something scornful, but then looked up at me, closed his mouth, turned around and walked away. Today I only wore the studded belt and a black jacket, but the effect was the same."

### Life as a Game

"Life as a Game" outlines a basic model for infinitely variable stories which can be developed spontaneously. The method of integrating the desired suggestions into a fictitious computer game is used here in the context of shyness and teasing at school. I developed the story for a young boy who was being teased by his classmates and his sister, and would burst into tears straight away rather than defending himself. The problem disappeared within some weeks.

TOPIC: Aggression, bullying, school, self-confidence
INTERVENTION: Externalisation of a problem as a game, mental game, unreal reframing, visualisation (metaphor, positive model)

> Imagine that your life is a computer game. While you're practising karate or playing football, or doing any other activities which you're good at and which you enjoy, you collect health and skill points –brightly coloured little spheres that help you to level up in the game.
> While you're walking around at school, there's an invisible glass shield in front of you, which protects you against attacks by other pupils who are trying to shoot at you with brightly coloured little spheres just like yours. Sometimes you open your glass shield very briefly at exactly the right moment in order to defend yourself and attack the other players, by shooting at them with the brightly coloured little spheres which you collected while playing football and practising karate. As you get better at

the game, the attacks reduce in frequency. When they disappear altogether and you're completely calm, you've won the game.

### Peer and Rasputin

"Peer and Rasputin" shows how children (and adults too, of course) can use invisible friends to learn new skills. The story demonstrates the hypnotherapeutic technique of inventing and anchoring animal helpers so that their effects can be experienced in everyday life. After the story has been told, the child can be helped to identify his or her personal protective animal, and to make a pretend Rasputin or other protector to take to school. This approach can also be used for children who are afraid of monsters (ghosts, burglars), by developing a personal protective monster who is stronger than the scary creatures. I developed this story when I was contacted by a parent whose child was incapable of self-defence (Hammel, 2008). On the use of the story with children who are scared of monsters, cf. the comments on the story "The Gang of Pigs".

TOPIC: Aggression, anxiety, bullying, monsters, school, self-confidence
INTERVENTION: Invisible friends, unreal reframing (metaphor, positive model)

Peer is six years old. He lives in Lillebløm in Elkland and is in Year One at school. When he first started school, Peer was afraid of the older pupils because they had beaten him up twice on the way to school. Then he got to know Rasputin, and Peer and Rasputin became friends. Rasputin is a forest troll. Rasputin went to school with Peer for a few months, and no one dared to beat Peer up while Rasputin was there. But then came winter – hibernation time for trolls. Rasputin said goodbye to Peer and promised to be back after the winter. What should Peer do? "I know just what to do," he thinks. Now when he goes to school, he pretends that Rasputin is still with him, and he holds his head high and acts as though he feels safe and strong. This was hard for him at first, but then he simply imagined to himself that Rasputin was still there. If anyone tries to annoy him, he looks over at where Rasputin is standing in his imagination, and then he feels safe. The funny thing is that no one ever bothers him any more. I wonder why that is?

### Thank You

The brief dialogue "Thank You" shows how a surprise can stop aggression in its tracks. A similar use of non sequiturs in conversation with people who habitually ignore the contributions of other participants (which is true for many patients suffering from schizophrenia or personality disorders) can make it possible to hold a coherent conversation. The therapist takes the side of the symptom in order to allow the client to perform a behaviour that matches that of the therapist. In therapeutic terms, this equates to use of the symptom or to the delegation of patterns of behaviour and the assumption of one side of an ambivalence by the therapist.

Erickson quotes a letter from a former student: "I had a rather paranoid patient in the room. All he wanted to talk about was **his** ideas. I tried to get his attention but couldn't. Then I thought about the unexpected, so I said, 'No, I don't like eating liver either.' The patient paused, shook his head, and said, 'Usually, I like chicken.' And then the patient began talking about his real problems." (Rosen, 1982: 222)

TOPIC: Aggression, bullying
INTERVENTION: Catalepsy, destabilisation through irritation, pattern interrupt by the client, rapport disruption, trance induction through confusion (example, positive model)

"A woman just bawled me out because I turned my car around in her driveway."
"What did you say to her?" I said.
"Thank you – you've made me sad, and I'm very happy about that. Then I drove away."

## The Spanish Conquistadors

The story "The Spanish Conquistadors" demonstrates how well-established patterns of attack and defence can continue even after the situation that gave rise to them has disappeared. Depending on the context and the approach taken, this can open up new opportunities but also be highly destructive.

TOPIC: Aggression, bullying, burnout syndrome, goals, relationship, responsibility, success, trauma, violence, work/life balance
INTERVENTION: Expanding resources (metaphor, searching model)

It had taken them a hundred years, but they had finally arrived in Gibraltar. The Reconquista was over, and the Spanish had reconquered the entire Iberian Peninsula from the Moors. Then someone asked, "And what happens now?" The truth of the matter was that no one had thought about that before. They had just gone on fighting. And because no one could come up with an answer, they carried on and conquered America.

## Revenge

The story "Revenge" highlights the risks of bullying for the aggressor, and contains an implicit request to modify behaviour in order to prevent a painful ending. The story is also suitable for dealing with conflict between siblings, partners, neighbours and work colleagues who "annoy each other".

TOPIC: Aggression, bullying, family, human resource management, relationship, responsibility, separation, team work, violence

INTERVENTION: Aversive suggestion, destabilisation through the prefigurement of negative consequences (metaphor, negative model)

Every morning when Mr Wagner arrived at work, the same large cage with the same white cockatoo would be standing on the desk of his secretary, Mrs Sievers. Mrs Sievers would talk and joke with the bird all day – one might even go so far as to say that she flirted with it. "Cockatoos need a lot of love," she used to say. Every time she left the room, Mr Wagner would harass the bird in some way. He would pull faces at it, blow in its face or poke a long ruler around in its cage. The cockatoo would respond by raising its crest, moving its head up and down as if it were scolding someone and flapping its wings, and Mr Wagner would not be able to stop himself from laughing. Mrs Sievers knew what he was up to, of course.

"You shouldn't tease the cockatoo. And please don't laugh at it," she said.

"That bird's too daft to understand anything!" replied Mr Wagner, and got back to work.

Eventually Mrs Sievers retired. "A real pity," said Mr Wagner – after all, they'd worked together for over twenty years. He had a very high opinion of Mrs Sievers, and somehow he even had a soft spot for the daft cockatoo.

Several years later, when Mr Wagner himself retired, he went to visit Mrs Sievers and her husband at their home. He rang the doorbell at seven on the dot, and Mrs Sievers let him in.

"Wait, the cockatoo!" she cried out as he opened the door from the hall into the living room – she had forgotten to put the bird back in its cage. "It's a miracle that it missed your eyes!" she said later, as she helped Mr Wagner to wipe the blood from his forehead and nose.

## That Day

The story "That Day" illustrates a method of unreal reframing, that is, inventing a fictitious new interpretation for real-life experiences and in the process emotionally neutralising these experiences or even casting them in a positive light. The intervention was inspired by the film *Life is Beautiful* (*La vita è bella*) by Roberto Benigni. The film tells the story of a father who make life in a concentration camp bearable for his son by telling him that it is a complicated game in which he can earn points for behaving correctly; if he manages to collect 1000 points, he will win the top prize of a tank. The young boy survives as a result of the intervention, which makes it possible for him to behave correctly and without fear. The procedure can be varied in many ways to make unbearable situations at work or home tolerable, or even pleasant and enjoyable.

TOPIC: Aggression, bullying, motivation, team work
INTERVENTION: Mental game, unreal reframing (example, positive model)

> That day I had so little desire to go and do my job at the hospital where I worked that I could barely find the motivation to do so at all. And so, in an effort to make things at least a little more bearable, I invented a new job description for myself.
>
> I decided that my real job was to spend time chatting with patients and to enjoy the beauty of the people and things around me. I would of course still do the things considered by some to be essential for someone in my profession, but this would be my secondary concern.
>
> That day I smiled happily at the people I met, and many of them smiled back.

### The Film

The story "The Film" can be used in similar contexts to the previous story.

TOPIC: Aggression, bullying, de-escalation, motivation, team work
INTERVENTION: Mental game (example, positive model), unreal reframing

> Imagine that your workplace is really the set of a new film, and everyone there is currently rehearsing their part. Will it be a cartoon, a comedy or an overblown historical romance? Look around you; some of your colleagues are already skilled at their roles, whereas others still need lots more practice. For the first time you realise why some of them seem to behave so strangely – they're not like that really, it's just the part they're playing. Maybe you can even identify the film's producer, director and make-up artist, and find some explanations for their previously puzzling behaviour.

### Social Noises

"Social Noises" can be used in similar contexts to the previous stories.

TOPIC: Aggression, bullying, de-escalation, motivation, team work
INTERVENTION: Anchoring, conditioning of waking behaviours, prioritisation, mental game, unreal reframing (example, positive model)

> Someone once asked me, "Do you have a story for workers who have to put up with members of the public insulting them and calling them names because they aren't allowed into a restricted area?"

I said, "Tell them about all the fascinating noises you can hear in nature. The snuffling of water buffalo at the river bank, for example, or the grunting of warthogs scratching themselves against trees, or the roaring of a waterfall, or the tremendous noise of an avalanche breaking free from the side of an immense mountain. The city is also a good place to find interesting sounds; traffic noise, building sites, the background jingle-jangle of music in department stores and the hum of chitchat in a pub garden. Ask the workers what sounds they are reminded of when they hear the ranting and raving of angry visitors. Spend some time talking to them about this similarity, and explain that the angry words are meaningless 'social noise' whose only purpose is to allow the speaker to communicate without taking on any obligations.

"Talk for a while about the social noises made by water buffalo and warthogs, and repeat the phrase 'social noise' often, emphasising it slightly. Whenever the workers are accosted by members of the public in future, they will think of water buffalo or traffic noise or a thundering avalanche – and they will think, 'social noise, social noise, social noise.'"

### The Secret Name

The story "The Secret Name" is suitable both for treating historical trauma and for working with ongoing and perhaps unavoidable trauma. It allows children and adults to protect their identity by introducing or uncovering a central part of their personality which is invulnerable to others. After telling the story, the therapist can hand over a stone and ask the listener to find his or her own secret name. In certain cases, the story can be modified so that the therapist plays the role of a shaman and gives the client a secret name, sowing the seeds of a new identity which liberates the client from the super-ego of a sect or other authority to which he or she was previously in thrall. It is important that the intervention in this modified form should only be used at the end of a course of therapy, and a high level of integrity and caution is required on the part of the therapist to ensure that he or she is only seen as a "guru" in formal terms and does not take the place of the individual who previously played this role. The story is contraindicated for patients with compulsive and personality disorders if they find it difficult to keep secrets.

TOPIC: Aggression, bullying, family, growing up, identity, names, parents, sects, sexual abuse, trauma, undercover investigators, violence, witness protection

INTERVENTION: Dissociation of parts of the personality, increasing complexity, metaphorical reframing, object as a metaphor, dissociation of connotated notions (metaphor, positive model / searching model)

When a Native American child is born, the name it is given by its parents is only temporary – it may change, or the child may be given other names as well. The child is also given a secret name by the tribe's medicine man, and this is his or her true name which only he or she knows. No one can misuse or abuse this name, which belongs to the child alone.

The Native American child is also given a stone by the shaman. If the medicine man dies before he has had a chance to tell the child his or her secret name, the young Native American child will take himself or herself off to a deserted location with the stone and stay there until the stone has revealed the true name through dreams or other revelations. Many of these stones are druses, or in other words rocks containing a cavity lined with gemstone crystals. Others contain gold, but all contain a healing magic and the power of the secret name.

### From the Crocodile's Mouth

The fable "From the Crocodile's Mouth" illustrates the dynamic of a double bind message and metaphorically describes the communicative traps into which not only zebras but all of us can fall when we respond to contradictory and simultaneous messages, and how every answer can be misunderstood.

TOPIC: Aggression, anxiety, borderline personality disorder, consultancy within an organisation, cutting, double bind, friends, love triangle, relationship, self-perception, sexual abuse, symbiosis, team coaching
INTERVENTION: Externalisation of ambivalence as a dialogue, inner team (metaphor, negative model / searching model)

"Good morning, my dear zebra!" The small bird who greeted his old friend the zebra in such a friendly fashion was sitting in Ali the crocodile's wide-open jaws and picking remnants of food out of his teeth. The zebra looked at him with a terrified expression, took a step backwards and then ran away.

"But zebra, you don't need to be afraid of me! We've always..." The bird looked at the crocodile. "What's up with him? Do you know?"

Ali shook his head. "No idea. Zebras are strange animals."

### How Do You Break a Spell?

Whereas the story about the crocodile focuses more on the natural dynamic of a contradictory message, the story "How Do You Break a Spell?" demonstrates a method for responding in kind with counter messages, or in other words for reflecting both sides of the contradictory ambivalence in a paradoxical answer. Anyone who finds answers to the original message or comes up with counter-questions which return (mirror) its bewildering contradictions by varying them rather than resolving them will rob the message of its power to ensnare.

TOPIC: Borderline personality disorder, bullying, double bind
INTERVENTION: Avoiding resistance, counter double bind, mirroring, promoting a searching attitude, trance induction through confusion (metaphor, searching model)

> Fedor the magician spoke again. "If a strange magician places you under a spell with a movement of his hands, you must free yourself by performing the same movement in reverse. If he throws an invisible rope around you, you must throw it back by performing his throw in reverse. If he throws two or three ropes around you, use all of his movements against him. Pretend you are his living double and be more like him than he is himself. Then there will be nothing that can bind you down, and the magician will be trapped by his own ropes."

### Table Tennis

The story "Table Tennis" illustrates an alternative counter double bind technique using a metaphorical approach.

TOPIC: Borderline personality disorder, bullying, double bind
INTERVENTION: Counter double bind, mirroring (metaphor, positive model)

> Someone once told me, "I often used to play table tennis with my older brother when we were children. He had the annoying habit of putting a spin on the ball so that it would fly off in all directions as soon as it hit my bat. Then I discovered that if I watched my brother's actions and the way in which the ball was turning, and put the same spin on the ball that he did, the ball would land wherever I wanted it to, and he would be left to deal with the spin which he had caused himself."

### The Cellar Spider I

The metaphor "The Cellar Spider I" makes it clear that underdogs can come out on top if they know how to make the most of their weapons. The story can be used as a warning for people who bully others, or to invite criticism of a dictatorship of the weak and encourage people to find ways of fighting and winning even if they believe themselves to be inferior.

TOPIC: Aggression, bullying, catatonic schizophrenia, double bind, violence
INTERVENTION: Aversive suggestion, expanding resources (metaphor, positive model / negative model), pattern interrupt by the client

I saw it on Sunday, underneath the sink in my apartment – one of those cellar spiders which have a tiny body but enormously long legs and look similar to daddy longlegs. It was in the process of wrapping something in the threads of its web, which on closer inspection proved to be one of the large, fat and hairy house spiders which scare some people so much. Then the day before yesterday I saw the small spider sitting on top of the large spider and feeding on it. How does such a tiny weak spider manage to kill such a large fast spider? It stays at a safe distance and throws thread after thread over the large spider, and the more the large spider tries to free itself, the more it gets stuck. The small spider only starts to feast on the large spider when the latter is unable to move.

### The Cellar Spider II

"The Cellar Spider II" uses a metaphorical approach to highlight opportunities for defence. It can also be used to encourage listeners to think about the causes and consequences of hyperactivity, mania and addictive behaviour.

TOPIC: Addiction, aggression, attention deficit disorder, bullying, hebephrenic schizophrenia, mania, work/life balance / workaholism
INTERVENTION: Pattern interrupt by the client, promoting a searching attitude (example / searching model)

Have you ever accidentally bumped into a cellar spider's web? If a cellar spider believes itself to be in danger, it starts to swing itself and its web backwards and forwards in such a rapid and sustained manner that for a long time it is impossible to see exactly where the spider is.

## Anxiety

This section examines ways of dealing with common and uncommon situations which cause anxiety, and methods for overcoming anxiety disorders. It goes without saying that anxiety is not an isolated phenomenon, and that its causes and effects are often interchangeable. A vicious circle often arises in which the mental and social consequences of experiencing anxiety reproduce or reinforce the various factors that trigger anxiety. My therapeutic work in this area is based on the following principles:

Anxiety is useful if it is focused on likely and avoidable current risks and if it heightens perception and results in more carefully planned action. If any one of these conditions is not met, however, reducing anxiety is a useful goal.

"Anxiety reaps what it fears." (Bernd Schumacher, seminar discussion, 2003.) Excessive worrying often results in the very thing which was the source of the worry, and a reduction in anxiety is therefore once again a useful goal.

Anxiety has its roots in past experiences. If unlikely events in the past mean that future risks are overestimated, it is important to overcome this fear of the past.

Anxiety is an illusion because it is based on worries about an unknown future.

Anxiety changes breathing patterns, and the reverse is also true – anyone who can change his or her breathing patterns will also change how anxious he or she feels.

Anxiety changes muscular tension, body position, movements, voice and heartbeat, and so anyone who changes any of these things will also change the level of anxiety he or she feels.

Bodily pain is proportional to perceived anxiety; anyone who can eliminate anxiety will also eliminate pain.

It is not the risk itself that worries people; people worry themselves.

Anxiety expresses itself in metaphorical images, and anyone who can alter these images will change his or her entire world – perception, thinking and acting – and at the same time change the way in which all living creatures respond to his or her behaviour.

Anxiety can be eliminated by imagining the subject, object or context of the anxiety in a modified form which is incompatible with anxiety.

Anyone who imagines anxiety as a person standing opposite and engages in dialogue with this person renders the anxiety powerless to infiltrate his or her body.

Anyone who imagines anxiety as a person, thing or structure in the room and then imagines how the person, thing or structure changes its shape and shrinks will find that the anxiety also changes and shrinks.

Anxiety-related problems are often inextricably linked with problematic aggression, compulsive thoughts, depression, grief and post-traumatic stress disorders, and many of the stories in the previous and following sections therefore also contain useful ideas in this respect.

## Dark Room

The story "Dark Room" highlights the fact that anxiety is a widespread human experience, and invites the listener to think about who and what can help to bring light into a life filled with darkness.

TOPIC: Anxiety, depression, falling asleep, grief, monsters, parents, sleep
INTERVENTION: Age regression, promoting positive expectations (example, positive model)

Do you still remember being a child and lying in bed in the dark? A dark that was so impenetrable that you were afraid of it. Perhaps you called for your parents, or perhaps you just stayed absolutely silent and pulled the quilt over your head and under your heels so that there was no way in at all. Anything might be lurking out there in the dark – a goblin, an animal or an evil person. I said "might", but one time there was definitely something moving around under the bed or in the wardrobe, I could just feel it!

Do you still remember how it felt when you called your parents and they came to see you? First you would hear your father's or your mother's footsteps, then the door would open and light would flood into the room. Perhaps you were dazzled by the light to begin with, but that wasn't a problem. The darkness had gone. Someone was there to look after you. The fear vanished, and all the night-time ghosts became powerless.

### How Do You Tame a Dragon?

The short story "How Do You Tame a Dragon?", which can be told to children and young people as an intervention for shyness or bullying at school, takes as its starting point the world of popular fantasy books, films, computer games and trading cards, and can be varied and embellished with characters or locations from the same genre. Once a child has immersed himself or herself in the story, he or she can be asked to remember how it felt to be a dragon tamer and to try and recreate this feeling when he or she is with people or in situations that were previously a source of anxiety. The story can be varied by omitting the suggestion to give the dragon commands and instead suggesting that a dragon tamer should simply behave as if there were no dragon or as if it presented no threat at all. Some threats only remain in existence if we perceive them as threats. For example, someone who does not suffer from a fear of falling is as unlikely to fall off the top of a skyscraper as he would be to fall off a book if he were to stand on one; Milton Erickson's story "Walking on Glare Ice" is a similar example (Rosen, 1982:110). The story can also be told as a computer game which takes place in the imagination and in which the aim is to collect mental power points while remaining at the same level of physical power, ensuring that the dragon cannot attack despite its superior physical power, and conquering it by treating it as an innocuous and inferior opponent. Killing the dragon is strictly forbidden and means that the game is over, since the tamed dragon is needed as a companion. Many metaphors can be framed similarly in a way that is appealing to children and young people. A listener who imagines that he or she is playing a computer game enters the same trance that he or she would be in while actually playing the game, or in other words a highly suggestible state. A final post-hypnotic suggestion could be added by noting that some children have even stopped being afraid of their real-life "dragons" after playing the game, since the dragons no longer have any power over them.

TOPIC: Aggression, anxiety, bullying, depression, self-confidence
INTERVENTION: Externalisation of a problem as a person, mental game, unreal
   reframing, visualisation (metaphor, positive model)

Fedor the magician once told me that if you want to tame a dragon, you
have to walk right up to him as though you were a master greeting his
pupils. Your steps must be confident, like those of the dragon lord when
he comes to claim homage from those who are younger and weaker than
him, and to take tributes from their stores of treasure. If you want to tame
a dragon, *you* must stand up straight and hold your head high. Look him
in the eyes! Your movements must resemble those of someone entirely
without fear, who is not afraid of the dragon's fiery and sulphurous
breath. Your walk must resemble that of someone whose skin cannot be
pierced by a dragon's claw and cannot be lacerated by a dragon's tooth,
and your voice should resemble that of someone who is used to issuing
commands. The dragon can only injure those who show their vulnerability when they approach him. Anyone who gives commands to the
dragon will not be injured by him.

### The Gang of Pigs

Children's imagined fears are sometimes impervious to explanations but
can be overcome by powerful counterimages. The logic that underpins fears
can be used to transform them from problems into solutions, as illustrated
by the story "The Gang of Pigs". (For more information on how problem
metaphors can be converted into solution metaphors, see the instructions on
transforming metaphors in Chapter 8, the story "Peer and Rasputin" and the
method for getting rid of ghosts in the story "The Persecuted II".)

TOPIC: Aggression, anxiety, bullying, monsters, self-confidence
INTERVENTION: Promoting age regression, unreal reframing (example,
   positive model)

"I'm scared of Peter. He always tells me, 'I'll get my big brother with his
gang of soldiers!'"
   Four-year-old Renate was very anxious about the threats she heard
from a kindergarten friend who had an older brother in the army.
   Her father asked, "Do you remember the big pigs at Uncle Arthur's
farm?"
   "Yes…" said Renate, her voice expressing her awe at the enormous pigs
which had left a deep impression on her.
   "The next time Peter tells you he's going to get his brother's gang of
soldiers, say to him, 'Then I'll get my Uncle Arthur's gang of pigs!'"
   "Good idea!" cried Renate.
   The gang of soldiers had already lost its hold over her.

## Fear of Moths

The case study "Fear of Moths" illustrates how the stressful feelings which are associated with a particular situation can be dissociated from the situation and replaced with feelings which are associated with a more pleasant situation. The story can be used for spiders and any other phobia triggers as well as for moths.

Three weeks after the encounter described below, the girl's father (a musician and neuroscientist in the field of hearing research) told me, "She still screams when she sees a moth, but she screams three octaves lower than she did before." Three months later, I visited the family again. "Look, there's a moth," said the mother to Constanze while we were chatting. The young girl, who was hoovering at the time, hoovered up the moth without any noticeable signs of alarm.

The procedure reverses a method used by Milton Erickson, who made pipe smoking unattractive for his pupil Jeff Zeig by giving him a lecture lasting more than an hour in which he described in painstaking detail how someone tried in every conceivable way to smoke a pipe but found all the possible options too "awkward". Erickson linked the term "awkward", which already held very negative connotations for Zeig, with a situation which had previously held positive connotations for him, whereas the above example demonstrates exactly the opposite. Zeig gave up smoking for good immediately after the conversation (Zeig, seminar discussion, 2007).

TOPIC: Anxiety, phobia (arachnophobia), trauma
INTERVENTION: Anchoring, conditioning of waking behaviours, paradox ("Don't think about hot chocolate!"), paradoxical intervention (example, positive model)

> Yesterday I visited some friends of mine.
> "Our daughter is afraid of moths," they told me. "Every time she sees a moth in the apartment she has a meltdown and makes a huge fuss. Is there anything you can do?"
> "I don't know," I said, and turned to the daughter, who was sitting at the table with us and drinking a mug of hot chocolate. "The next time you see a moth, make sure that you don't think about hot chocolate and that you don't think about not thinking about hot chocolate, and that you don't think about how the hot chocolate tastes right now and the way you feel when you drink hot chocolate, because if you think about hot chocolate and how you feel right now because you're drinking hot chocolate you might have hot chocolate feelings whenever you see a moth, accidentally and without meaning to. And what would happen if you felt as though you could almost taste and smell hot chocolate and as though you had hot chocolate feelings whenever you saw a moth? How would you cope?"
> "I wouldn't care."

"Watch out!" I said. "Even if you think you wouldn't care about having hot chocolate feelings whenever you saw a moth, you need to be careful that you don't end up not caring about the moths themselves, because it would be a shame if you didn't care about the moths so much that you got hot chocolate feelings whenever you saw them…"

The young girl saw a moth quarter of an hour later, and stayed calm and relaxed.

### Start of Term in the Staffroom

The situation described in the story "Start of Term in the Staffroom" makes it clear that people's widespread reluctance to talk about their problems can create the illusion that they are the only ones suffering. I have included the story as a reminder that people tend to underestimate themselves because they are unaware of how common their problems are.

TOPIC: Anxiety, motivation, responsibility, team work
INTERVENTION: Promoting openness, real reframing (example, positive model)

It was the first day of school after the summer holidays.

"Why do I always find the start of term so difficult?" a teacher asked herself as she entered the staffroom. "Everyone else seems to be happy that term is starting, and I'm the only one with this sense of crushing anxiety."

Then she had an idea, and asked a colleague, "How's it going?"

"Great!"

"And how's it *really* going?"

"How long do you have? I have so many problems I don't know where to start…"

## Compulsion

Instead of external and social compulsions, the following section deals with different forms of internal compulsions; compulsive perception (compulsive focusing of attention), compulsive thoughts, compulsive action and compulsive inaction, as well as everyday variations on these themes that are not covered by other sections. Compulsive behaviour is an everyday phenomenon rather than a rare occurrence; it happens every time that an individual attempts to act on paradoxical instructions such as "Be spontaneous for once!", "Just don't listen to them!" or "Stop worrying or you'll make it worse!"

Compulsive perceptions, compulsive action and compulsive inaction play a key role in many sexual disorders, anxiety disorders, sleep disorders, stammering, depression, pain and tinnitus, and many other relevant metaphors and model interventions can therefore be found in the chapters on these subjects.

### King of the Wood

Polycentric organisation is more effective than centralised organisation in many contexts. The fable "King of the Wood" is designed to encourage clients to relinquish conscious control and to trust in their unconscious (or alternatively in life, their community, nature, God). The wood can function as a metaphor for the way in which body and soul operate on an involuntary and unconscious basis, for example. The story can also be used to challenge controlling social systems.

TOPIC: Anxiety, compulsion (OCD), control, erectile dysfunction, falling asleep, parenting, sexuality, sleep
INTERVENTION: Increasing complexity, psychoeducation (metaphor, positive model)

> "There's too many of us," said the trees in the wood once upon a time. "We need someone to rule over us. We need someone to tell us where we should grow and how we should form our branches. We need someone to tell us when we should grow buds in spring and when we should change our leaves to bright colours in the autumn."
>
> And they elected an old oak as their king. Although trees grow very slowly, the king had a lot to do. He had to tell every tree where which branch should grow and when which leaf should be unfolded. He had to decide who should withdraw how much water from the soil, and he was even faced with the most challenging task of all – who should consume how many nutrients. After just a short time, the entire wood began to suffer from fungi and parasites; some trees dried out and others fell prey to root rot. The trees began to grumble and argue amongst themselves. The king accused his people of insubordination, the people accused the king of being incompetent and they all accused each other of being idiots and common rogues.
>
> On a beautiful July day, when the leaves were starting to fall, the king abdicated. All the trees were happy, and held a big feast. And from then on, things gradually improved for the trees.

### Tourette's

The story "Tourette's" illustrates how compulsive disorders can be reduced by using the symptom; the therapist exhibits the symptom and outdoes the client in doing so. In the case of Lisa, her manner of speech subsequently became more moderate, at least when she spoke to her father in the presence of her friends and acquaintances.

TOPIC: Compulsion (OCD), growing up, mirroring, scatological language, Tourette's syndrome
INTERVENTION: Utilisation of a symptom, utilisation of rapport (example, positive model)

> When Lisa was fifteen years old, every other word she said seemed to be an expletive or obscenity. Any encouragement to express herself more politely merely meant that her language become even more vulgar. Once Lisa asked her father rudely whether she could sleep over at a friend's house. Her friends were hanging around to hear his reply, and so he said calmly, "As far as I'm concerned you can get pissed out of your fucking head at the damn party."

### Grunting

The case study "Grunting" illustrates how the pattern of an unconscious action such as a tic can be interrupted by linking it to rules and (if necessary) setting additional homework of following the rules before the symptom occurs. Once the patient has learned the rules, the symptom can no longer occur unconsciously and is likely to disappear, since conscious production of the symptom will hold less attraction.

As for the girl mentioned in the case study, her tic reduced in frequency immediately. During the next few days she sometimes left the room at the start of a meal in order to "get out all the grunts". After a few relapses around two weeks later the parents started playing the game again, and the tic then disappeared entirely.

The method is based on the symptom prescription technique which is popular in the field of systemic therapy, and on methods developed by Milton Erickson. Erickson helped a young boy with a verbal tic who shouted out "eek" once a minute by asking him to make the sound twice a minute (and later three times and then four times a minute), and checking with a stopwatch to be sure that the frequency was exactly right. If not, he was sent to his room. This symptom too disappeared within just a few weeks (Short & Weinspach, 2007: 266).

TOPIC: Compulsion (OCD), tics, Tourette's syndrome, trichotillomania
INTERVENTION: Anchoring, conditioning of waking behaviours, homework, paradoxical intervention, symptom prescription, utilisation of the symptom (example, positive model)

> Yesterday I met some old friends at a wedding I was attending.

"Our eight-year-old daughter Marlene has developed a tic," they said. "She always makes this terrible grunting noise, and it's particularly bad when she's eating. Is there anything we can do?"

"Let's see," I said, and we discussed various ideas with each other.

Later, when we were in the playground, I told Marlene that I grunted every time I pressed my nose, and that her parents also grunted – with a different grunting noise – whenever they pressed their noses. I pressed her nose and heard her grunt. We discovered that she only grunted quietly when she pressed her own nose. We also discovered that pressing your nose lots of times helps to get rid of the grunts so that there are no grunts left for a while, and so we did this before dinner. She grunted once before eating, but noticed it immediately. We decided that each nose press needed a grunt, and that therefore each grunt needed a nose press. Whenever she grunted, she should therefore press herself on the nose straight away so that the number of nose presses was the same as the number of grunts. Ideally she should notice when a grunt was coming and press her nose first so that the grunt followed the nose press in the proper manner, and so she would have to learn to press her nose each time before she grunted. I told her how important this was. We had a lot of fun together, but I don't think Marlene will continue to grunt while eating for much longer.

## Dying at the Age of 26

The case study "Dying at the Age of 26" illustrates how compulsive ideas can be modelled in such a way as to eliminate what previously made them so worrying. This follows a cartoon approach; a problem symbol is visualised and metaphorically transformed without reference to any real-life contexts until it becomes a solution symbol. The result is reinforced by a final suggestive question which implies that the answer will be a solution. This procedure merely defuses the substance of the compulsive idea rather than challenging it or taking it away from the client. If the problem recurs at the age of 92, the patient can turn back the figures to 26 or double a figure so that she imagines dying at the age of 292 or 929... The method is also suitable for words imagined in writing, whose letters can be rotated, replaced and altered ("mad" can be changed to "sad", for example).

TOPIC: Compulsion (OCD)

INTERVENTION: Externalisation of a problem as writing, stabilisation through a suggestive question, unreal reframing, utilisation of the symptom, visualisation (example, positive model)

"I have a problem," a friend once said to me. "I've somehow got this idea into my head that I'm going to die at the age of 26. That's not all that long away. I know it's stupid, but I can't get rid of the idea, and it frightens me. What can I do about it?"

"Create a mental image of the number 26 and examine it very closely," I answered. "Now swap the figures around. What do you see?"

"The number 62," said my friend.

"Exactly. Now rotate the six by 180° and stand it on its head. What do you see now?"

"The number 92."

"So when do you expect to die?"

"At the age of 92."

"Is that ok?"

"Definitely," said my friend, who was free of the problem from then on.

### The Wrong Audience

The dialogue "The Wrong Audience" illustrates how we sometimes feel guilty regardless of whether someone has accused us of doing something wrong or would do so if they had all the relevant information at their disposal. Feelings of guilt towards others originate from feelings of self-reproach, which in turn are based on our own values rather than on those of the alleged victims. Apologies often resemble a monologue more than a dialogue, and it may be necessary to make forgiveness a more agreeable concept for the guilt-ridden party by alerting them to the difference between internal and external dialogue.

TOPIC:  Conscience, forgiveness
INTERVENTION:  Inner team, psychoeducation (example, positive model)

> A friend once had to cancel our arrangements because of an appointment, and kept on apologising for having done so. I reassured him every time that it didn't matter, but he wasn't convinced.
>
> I then said, "You're talking more to your guilty conscience than to me."
>
> "That's a good way of putting it," he answered. "I'll remember that."
>
> And I didn't hear any more apologies.

## Depression

Therapists working with individuals exhibiting depressive behaviours must take steps to ensure that they do not empathise with the client so much that they end up in the same state of hopelessness and lethargy which the client has experienced for so long. In the case of patients suffering from anxiety, compulsion, depression, suicidal tendencies or addictive behaviours, too much rapport can paralyse the therapeutic process because it progressively reduces the therapist's ability to think and act.

Storytelling is one way in which therapists can protect themselves and benefit their clients at the same time, since the therapy sessions will then appear to focus not on the paralysing problems, but on pleasant topics which are interesting in a positive sense and which – unlike conversations about problems – do not suck the energy out of the therapeutic dialogue.

### Wasted Time

The story "Wasted Time" highlights the paradoxical fact that worrying reproduces and reinforces the reasons for worrying in a vicious circle.

TOPIC: Depression
INTERVENTION: Aversive suggestion, paradoxical intervention (example, negative model)

> "I've made so many mistakes. I've wasted years of my life and have nothing to show for it," she sighed, and wasted the next few years saying exactly the same.

### Three Boxes

The story "Three Boxes" embodies a basic therapeutic principle, namely that problems must be separated and solutions must be linked. Whenever a client presents problems which appear to be linked, for example in the case of depression or psychosomatic involvement, it is recommended that the problems should be examined independently and separately as though they had nothing to do with each other in reality. In many cases the link (or inter-dependency) will vanish when it is challenged, even if it was plausible. Yet as soon as a solution is found for one or more of the problems, it is worth turning the question around and asking whether the solution could also be beneficial in another area and be transferred to another problem.

TOPIC: Depression, psychosomatic disorder
INTERVENTION: Increasing complexity, dissociation of connotated notions (example, positive model)

> "You must be mistaken," the man said to the other man. "You must keep your illness absolutely separate from your family problems and your family problems absolutely separate from your problems at work. These are two or rather three entirely different kettles of fish. Imagine putting these three things in three different boxes... Now close each of the three boxes and push them into three different corners of the room. Have you pushed them a long way apart? Good. Now we'll look at each box individually..."

And they discussed each problem separately. Whenever they found a solution, however, the first man said, "Might that also work for the other problem...?"

### The Filing Cabinet

If I meet someone who is dealing with so many different problems all at once that he or she feels overwhelmed, I sometimes ask him or her to imagine a filing cabinet and then to imagine opening the top drawer of the filing cabinet, placing the first problem in there, having one last look at it, labelling the drawer and closing it. I ask him or her to repeat the process with the other problems and the other drawers. The story "The Filing Cabinet" introduces an idea of separation which is similar to that embodied in the previous story, but differs in that time is more important than location. I occasionally add the following post-hypnotic instruction to the intervention: "Now you can keep the filing cabinet closed, and your problems will be there waiting for you if you want to tackle them one by one. The only thing you won't be able to do is to open all the drawers at once – you will only be able to open one at a time. If you want to deal with several problems at the same time, you must remove the contents of each drawer briefly and then put them back again afterwards. It's generally a good idea to leave things in the drawers where they belong, so that everything stays in order and you can spend your time on things that are more enjoyable and empowering."

TOPIC: Anxiety, depression, psychosomatic disorder
INTERVENTION: Dissociation of connotated notions (metaphor, positive model)

I used to have a filing cabinet in my office which had many different drawers. When I first started using my filing cabinet I thought that it was broken, because it was impossible to open two of its drawers at the same time. Pulling one drawer out meant that the others were locked shut – I could move them very slightly backwards and forwards, but they couldn't be opened until I had pushed the first drawer back into place; then I could pull out another drawer.

### Slides

The story "Slides" can also be used to separate out problems so that they can be dealt with individually and the interdependencies between the different sub-problems can be reduced.

TOPIC: Anxiety, depression, psychosomatic disorder
INTERVENTION: Dissociation of connotated notions, (metaphor, searching model)

A client once told her therapist a convoluted life story, in which all of the problems seemed to be mutually dependent and mutually reinforcing. The therapist took a number of OHP slides, placed them on top of each other and asked the woman to describe the pictures she could see on the slides and read out the writing.

"I can't," said the client. "I'd need to look at each one separately in order to do that."

The therapist placed the slides one by one in front of her, and she described the pictures and read out the writing.

Then the therapist said, "Now let's think about which of your problems belong on the same slide and which belong on different slides. Then we can get started with your course of therapy."

They discussed the different problems and the ways in which they over-lapped. When they came to start the course of therapy, they were already half finished.

### The Blade of Grass in the Crack

The story "The Blade of Grass in the Crack" can be told in many situations described by patients as hopeless. It illustrates a fundamental principle of systemic therapy, namely that it is important to identify anything which may be useful, no matter how innocuous, and multiply it until it becomes a force which can hold its own against the stresses which at first appeared unassail-able. The story can help clients who have resigned themselves to a situation – and their therapists – to adopt a searching attitude and identify solutions which previously appeared impossible.

TOPIC: Aggression, anxiety, Asperger syndrome/autism, compulsion (OCD), depression, freedom, penitentiary system, trauma, violence
INTERVENTION: Expanding resources , promoting a searching attitude, pro-moting positive expectations (metaphor, positive model)

The prisoner said, "Last night I dreamt that a blade of grass grew in a crack in our dungeon, just where the shaft of light which comes through the spy hole in the door hits our wall. It was watered by the mois-ture which drips from the dungeon roof and the walls. The roots grew stronger and forced the crack open a tiny amount, and a second blade of grass grew from these roots, right next to the first. Then we hung a belt on the door so that its silver buckle reflected a little light onto the second blade. This grew as well, and its powerful roots widened the crack a little more. We repeated this process again and again until the stone was surrounded by grass on all sides. When a year had passed, we pulled out the weeds, and the light shone through the cracks. We braced our-selves against the stone and pushed it outwards with all of our strength, inch by inch over the course of a day. Then we climbed out through the hole and were free."

"It's a shame there's no blades of grass growing in our dungeon," sighed his fellow prisoner.

The prisoner who had just related his dream stared at the wall for a long time. Then he asked, "And what do you think *that* is?"

### Numb Feet

In patients suffering from depression, certain forms of post-traumatic stress disorder and the shock phase of a grieving process (which may be a permanent condition in the case of pathological grieving), the unconscious avoids experiencing emotions and instead prefers to dissociate itself from all (or all currently relevant) feelings because the pain which would otherwise ensue would be overwhelming. In many cases such an attitude becomes entrenched, and remains in place even if the resources needed to deal with the critical events are available (additional family or therapeutic support, solutions to other problems or their disappearance). Leaving a state of mental numbness may mean that painful emotions resurface, and so it is sometimes important to provide the unconscious with the prospect of a better life after this painful phase in order to prepare the patient to move through the pain into a state where they are able to experience their emotions, for example by using the metaphor in the story "Numb Feet".

TOPIC: Addiction, convalescence, depression, grief, mobilisation, motivation, narcosis, operation, shock, trauma, withdrawal
INTERVENTION: Promoting positive expectations, sending the symptoms back into the past), systematic desensitisation (metaphor, positive model)

After walking through the snow for a long time on a cold winter's day, you sometimes get so cold that you can't feel your feet any more. Even after you come inside and into the warm, your feet remain numb at first. And the funny thing is that if you place them against a radiator to warm them up, that's exactly when they start to hurt – when they are out of the cold, instead of previously when they were buried in ice and snow. A fool might say, "If I don't thaw out my feet, then they won't hurt!" But anyone with a bit of common sense knows that the warm only hurts the cold feet for a short while. You just have to put up with the pain, and when it's over you'll feel pleasantly cosy and warm.

### Gramophone

The story "Gramophone" can be used in situations where psychological or physical symptoms need to be linked again with the events that triggered them and separated from the present which no longer needs them. This may be the case for patients suffering from post-traumatic stress disorder, but also for those suffering from phantom pain or post-operative pain without an organic explanation, as well as asthmatic disorders which occur for the first time or in greater severity in response to stressful events. The story is also useful in cases where traumatic events that occurred in previous generations overshadow an entire family's biography, since it allows a mental distinction to be made between the realms of the dead and the living (and therefore also between their competencies and responsibilities). Different performers can be chosen in order to allude to conflicts between particular countries, cultures, skin colours, religions etc., and separated out in line with the motto, "Every culture is responsible for itself, and you are only responsible for yourself." The "voices" of many different key figures from the past are interspersed in the story, together with the suggestion that they will fall silent and remain with the individuals to whom they belong.

TOPIC: Asthma, depression, family, grandparents, grief, intercultural conflict, pain, parents, phantom pain, trauma, war
INTERVENTION: Age regression, anchoring, interspersal technique, sending the symptoms back into the past, dissociation of connotated notions (example, positive model)

> I have a gramophone at home on which I play songs such as "Falling in Love Again" and "Lili Marlene". Marlene Dietrich sings them in such a wonderfully low register! Then I listen to the sandpapery voice of Louis Armstrong, and I can almost imagine that I'm meeting him in person. I listen to Caruso's vibrato echoing down the years, "O sole mio…" Their voices come to me out of the grooves of the record, without any electrical power, and they sound as though they are the real voices of the people themselves. When their voices sound through the horn of the gramophone, it is as though the singers were visiting the present day, and I were with them in the same room. Then the gramophone falls silent, and their voices return to the other world which is separate from ours, and which is where the former owners of these voices live.

### The Man Who Wins When He Loses

The story "The Man Who Wins When He Loses" illustrates a therapeutic approach to double binds in the form of a case study.

TOPIC: Depression, double bind, perfectionism, self-confidence
INTERVENTION: Counter double bind, inner team, mirroring, paradox ("What is wrong is right!"), provocation (example, positive model / negative model)

Some time ago a man came to ask me for some advice. He said, "I don't want you to be disappointed if you fail in your attempts to help me."

I answered, "I won't try to persuade you that you'll gain something from attending a course of therapy with me. If I try to prove to you that this is possible, and if you want to prove the opposite, you'll always succeed and I'll always fail. If you want to prove to me that you'll gain nothing from therapy, it would be a better idea for me to avoid wanting to achieve the opposite."

He said, "I've already been to see other counsellors. In my experience, the benefits last around three days, and then everything goes back to how it was before."

I replied, "If the voice of your experience tells you that, then all that your experience can tell you is that the benefits only last three days if that is what your experience says. The voice of your experience tells you that your experience makes things go badly for you. Maybe your experience could learn from this experience and take a break in order to allow other voices to speak, and say nothing for once and simply observe whether the other voices can achieve what it has previously failed to do. I'm sure your experience won't mind doing that, since it wants to help you."

He said, "I don't trust myself to do anything. I have zero self-confidence. I feel like I've done everything wrong. I'm too much of a perfectionist. I worry too much."

I answered, "You don't want to accept responsibility. Anyone who does something makes lots of little mistakes, but anyone who does nothing makes one single big mistake – doing nothing – but the mistake is hard to pin down. You disappoint people for fear of disappointing people, and people would be less disappointed if you did disappoint them."

He asked, "Do you think you can help me to know what I want?"

I answered, "I have some very clever tricks. You'll find out what you want, but you'll think it had nothing to do with me."

## Mania

As is the case for depressive disorders, the root cause of manic episodes may be avoidance of a stressful experience, with the unconscious following the strategy of creating the greatest possible emotional distance from a state in which biographical traumas may be experienced as painful. In a reversal of the approach described in the chapter on suicidal tendencies, the therapist can use the ambivalence seesaw technique by firstly copying the client's "manic" interpretation of the world and then very gradually introducing less euphoric, then neutral and finally slightly negative elements into this world view. He or she must be sure to keep these gradual steps towards a different perspective so small that the client moves along at the same pace, and if necessary tolerate steps backwards.

Another strategy involves telling stories which allegorise the positive aspects of mania but subtly and consistently sow the seeds of impending failure until it becomes unavoidable. The story must end with nothing more serious than a metaphorical black eye, however, in order to make the story comprehensible to a patient suffering from mania and avoid promoting a depressive episode through suggestion.

### The Desert

The short story entitled "The Desert" highlights the risk of extreme mood fluctuations and sudden changes of life plans, and of exhausting oneself or overstretching oneself by attempting to handle projects alone (at work or otherwise). The story can also be used to make it clear that the opposite of right is a different right, whereas the opposite of wrong is a different wrong, and that the opposite of a risk can be more hazardous than the risk itself. The story can be modified to describe someone who gets into difficulties in the mountains if the listener prefers Alpine landscapes.

TOPIC: Bipolar disorder, burnout syndrome, crisis, dream, goals, identity, loneliness, mania, responsibility, stress, survival, work/life balance
INTERVENTION: Metaphorical reframing (metaphor, positive model / negative model)

Top of his bucket list of dreams had been to experience the desert – the vast expanse of the Sahara. Now his dream had come true. He had travelled there by plane, coach and jeep, all the way to some tiny speck of a village somewhere on the edge of the Sahara which he had found on the map. And he knew that beyond this village was nothing – no roads, no settlements, no water, only sand, stones and rocks. He did not really know what had prompted him to travel there. Was it simply a longing from the depths of his soul? Or perhaps he had simply been surrounded for too long by too many people, too much commotion, too many voices who all wanted something from him – his colleagues at work, his neighbours, his family at home, all pulling him this way and that; can't you please... would you please... And now silence, nothing and no one around him.

He had longed for this for so many years, perhaps his whole life long. It is so quiet here than he can hear the sand and stones crunching under his feet with every step. He wants to drink in more of this vast expanse of solitude before night falls. The next rocky hill is not too far away in the distance, but the ascent is tiring – not because of the temperature, since the sun is already low in the sky and it has become remarkably cold, but because the sand slips out from under his feet whenever he takes a step forward, pulling him backwards. He finally reaches the summit of the hill, and looks forward into the desert and back at the village. The sun is starting to set in a red haze behind the village, and through the small windows of the huts he can clearly see the flickering of the fires which are already burning. Now he wants to leave this last piece of civilisation behind him. His heart longs for quiet, preferably away from everybody else. He makes his way down the valley towards the next hill. He wants to watch the red sunset once again from the top of this hill and see nothing but desert around him. The route there is not long, but it is exhausting because of the sand slipping out from under his feet and the boulders which he must climb around. Quickly it gets dark. When he reaches the top of the hill, the sun has disappeared. He stands there for a few minutes until his dream fades and he returns to reality. He is surrounded by pitch blackness – not the darkness he knows from home, to which one's eyes can get accustomed, but a darkness which makes it impossible to see his hand in front of his face. Returning to the village is now out of the question. His concern now is that it has become bitterly cold, and seems to be getting colder and colder. He would never have believed that it could be so cold in the desert. Standing there in the dark in his summer shirt, shorts and sandals, he feels completely helpless and is overcome by fear. He is afraid that he will not survive the night, that he will freeze to death, die alone and never be found. He thinks about his family, and his thoughts begin to go around in circles. What will they do when he doesn't come home? Will they search for him, and will they ever find out where he is? He wants to see them again so much. He sees three lights on the horizon, like stars rising in more or less the same place where the sun set before. He thinks to himself, "Stars don't rise in the west. Am I seeing things already? And these stars are moving sideways, almost as if they were electric torches..."

A few hours later, he is sitting around the fire in a hut with the three African men who were carrying the torches and a number of other villagers. A woman wearing a veil hands him a plate of roasted lamb and a cup of goat's milk. They communicate using their hands and feet, and he expresses his thanks to the villagers with signs and gestures.

"Inshallah," smiles a man, "...if Allah wills."

## Dream world, delusion and hallucination

Delusional ideas occur as a result of many different conditions, for example depressive and schizophrenic disorders, psychosis, substance abuse and dementia of different origins. As a basic principle, it is almost impossible to prove what is delusion and what is reality, and where the boundary lies between them. Sometimes people who think they are being watched and bugged have a problem of credibility rather than being delusional. It should also be remembered that a client's support network often regards things which are unlikely as delusional without having any hard evidence disproving the hypothesis that the client is simply providing an accurate description of the reality in which he or she finds himself or herself (either wholly or in part). Even if ideas can be positively identified as delusional, it is often helpful to accept the delusion as it is presented by the client in order to use its inherent logic to formulate exceptions or solutions.

It goes without saying that the role of storytelling is to expand the range of psychiatric and (if necessary) pharmacological options for the treatment of delusions rather than replacing them.

### Anna's Submarine

The case study "Anna's Submarine" makes it clear that a therapist can only lead someone out of a dream world if he or she also enters the dream world first. The path out of the dream world must also be attractive, and it must still be possible to return to the old patterns if necessary. The submarine intervention also involves the paradox that Anna is invited to leave her dream world while she is in her dream world, meaning that she can pursue both sides of the ambivalence with different parts of her personality; she can act in accordance with her previous pattern while at the same time trying a new pattern, although the old pattern will then not be quite the same as it was...

The course of therapy lasted two hours. In the two weeks after I told this story and the intervention "Mrs Brain", Anna's ability to concentrate and her interpersonal skills improved to the extent that she found school much easier and made friends with another girl for the first time in years. After four weeks, her mother reported that Anna had stopped pulling out her hair and chewing her fingernails, was participating more in lessons, was getting better marks and was continuing to play with her friend, and that Anna herself said that she was, "very happy".

TOPIC: Asperger syndrome / autism, attention deficit disorder (ADD/ADHD), developmental delay, mutism, nail biting, paranoid, hallucinatory or catatonic schizophrenia, psychosis, trichotillomania
INTERVENTION: Moving the focus of attention from the inner to the outer world, pacing and leading, paradox ("You'll wake up asleep!"), trance exduction (metaphor, positive model)

Anna dreams. She dreams while she's at school with the other Year Four pupils, and she continues dreaming when she comes home after school. She lives in her dreams to the extent that no one really knows whether she is talented or stupid, simple-minded or subtle, shy or inhibited, introverted or mentally disturbed. Anna has no friends, and seems content with her own company. Anna appears to be happy when she is dreaming, or perhaps she only dreams because of how unhappy she would be if she were not dreaming? Anna twists and tugs on her hair until it falls out. She chews her fingernails until they bleed. Is Anna ill, or just quirky? Which school should she attend, and what is the best way to help her? Her parents want answers to these questions, and so they bring her to therapy.

"I believe you live in a submarine," I say to Anna. She looks at me inquiringly.

"You dive down below the waves to a rainbow-like world of fish and coral and many other brightly coloured things which are unknown to the people living on the surface. Do you agree?"

"Yes," says Anna.

"It must be lovely down there. You can investigate the sea floor in peace, and no one can disturb you."

"That's right," says Anna.

"You can be a deep-sea researcher – someone who investigates the world of the deep on behalf of the people up on the surface. They find out everything there is to know about the animals and plants that live in the sea."

"That would be fun," says Anna.

"All submarines need a periscope, of course. That's a long tube with mirrors so that you can always see what's happening up top even when you're down below."

"And so I can watch the other people," says Anna.

"Exactly. And you'll also need a sonar system so that you don't crash into other submarines or ships while you're under water. The sonar system emits sound waves so that you know when others are coming too close, and when you should dive down deeper into the sea in order to avoid other submarines and ships."

"Do I have to go deeper?" asks Anna.

"Well, I'm sure you know that it's not a good idea for two submarines or a submarine and a ship to crash into each other. Both vessels can be damaged, even if the collision was a mistake. It's better to anticipate the accident and change course or dive down into the water in good time. In order to respond promptly, you need a microphone which picks up the signals of the other submarines and ships and a radio system so that you can talk to their crew even when you're under the water."

"Yes, that's a good idea. Then I won't collide with them again."

"Exactly. And of course every submarine has to come to the surface from time to time."

"Why?"

"For oxygen, and for food and drink. You need to come to the surface every now and again to take them on board."

"Yes, you're right."

"Research submarines also have to come to the surface regularly so that the researchers can talk to the people up top about what they should be investigating down below."

"Really?"

"Of course. The submarine's job is to find out what happens under the sea and to tell the people on land about it."

"Can submarines shoot at other people?"

"Yes, submarines have torpedoes, but they must only be used against enemy ships in an emergency. It's better to talk using the radio, or to come to the surface and use the megaphone; 'Hello, I heard your signals and came to the surface. What's up?' Submarine captains who are really good at their job spend a lot of time below the water and a lot of time above the water. They know the signals of the other ships so well that they always know when it's better to come to the surface and when it's better to dive down into the water. They also know when it's a good idea to be half up and half down, like a crocodile which keeps only its eyes, ears and nostrils above the water so that it can see everything happening above the water, but is still well camouflaged and can dive down quickly if necessary. Sometimes submarines also travel along just below the surface of the sea so that only their conning tower is poking out. This allows them to find out everything which is happening above the water, and to hear all the signals they need to hear and see everything they need to see, but to reach the bottom of the sea quickly if they ever need to dive down."

"Cool," says Anna. "I like that idea."

Like everyone else, submarine captains sometimes take a holiday and come on shore. They meet their friends, tell them about their voyages and hear about their friends' experiences. I once knew a submarine captain who liked to fly a hydroplane in his spare time, looking from above at what he normally saw from below – the land and the water, the ships, the submarines and everything else. And when he had seen everything, he landed again, or splashed down as hydroplane pilots say. He knew the world from every perspective, and he was very happy."

"Cool," said Anna. "I'd like to do that."

## Mrs Brain

The intervention "Mrs Brain" can be used to encourage children (and adults) to recondition themselves gradually with suggestive instructions in order to overcome recurrent problems. The method of autosuggestion introduced in the story can be transferred to many different solutions; a child can ask his or her brain to give him or her ideas of ways to make friends, to find the motivation to do homework, to control his or her impulses etc.

TOPIC: Asperger syndrome / autism, attention deficit disorder (ADD/ADHD), developmental delay, psychosis, schizophrenia, specific learning disability
INTERVENTION: Conditioning of waking behaviours, homework, invisible friends, rhetorical question, suggestive question, trance induction through questions, unreal reframing, yes set (example, positive model)

I'm sure you know that you have a brain and that it can think. But have you ever tried talking to your brain? No?

Then it's high time you started. What's your brain called? Is it a man or a woman?

Great... Now you can say to your brain, "Hello, Mrs Brain!" and it will undoubtedly answer, "Hello, dear Anna!" You can ask iTopic: "Dear Mrs Brain, could you make sure I always concentrate when my teacher is explaining the homework we need to do?" and Mrs Brain will answer, "Of course I can, dear Anna, you should have asked me before!"

"I see," you can reply, "but now I am asking you. Would you please make sure I'm always alert and listening hard when the teacher explains the homework, dear Mrs Brain?"

"Absolutely, dear Anna!"


### The Persecuted I

The case study "The Persecuted I" illustrates how the rules of a delusional idea can be used to achieve the gradual dismantling of the same idea. In order to achieve this goal, a distinction is made between the persecutors and the effects of their actions.

TOPIC: Bullying, erotomania, paranoid personality disorder, paranoid-hallucinatory schizophrenia, persecutory delusion, psychosis, sects, stalking, undercover investigators

INTERVENTION: Pacing and leading, utilisation of the symptom, yes set (example, positive model)

"I'm being systematically terrorised by a man I knew many years ago – he asked me out but I refused," the woman told me. "He used to work for the secret police and has a network of old friends who help him. My phone is being tapped. Objects in my apartment and my car are being moved around to unsettle me. Rumours about me getting married have been spread at each of the places I work. I can't relax any more."

"That doesn't sound very likely," I answered, "but it is possible. The secret police had ways of 'taking apart' a person by spreading rumours. And we know that certain secret services and sects sometimes try to induce delusional beliefs in people on a systematic basis. There was one case in which a man who had previously belonged to a sect was terrorised – the sect leaders arranged for him to be shadowed and for a black car with two men in sunglasses to be parked wherever he went. The man told his friends, his family and health professionals, until in the end everyone thought he had gone crazy, and even he was starting to worry about his sanity. Before long he was looking for black cars with men in sunglasses everywhere, even after the black cars had all disappeared. If there was a black car or a pair of black sunglasses in the vicinity, you can be sure that the man would spot them – even if they had nothing whatsoever to do with him. The sect had induced persecutory delusions in him."

"That's what's happened to me," said the woman.

"Maybe someone has indeed induced persecutory delusions in you," I continued. "I think that if someone had moved things in *my* apartment a few times, I would start to look to see if anything else had moved as soon as I entered the apartment, and then I'd ask myself, 'Was that really there before?' And sometimes I would think that things had moved simply because I couldn't remember where they had been before. I think I'd become paranoid."

"That's exactly what's happened to me," replied the woman. "I'm becoming paranoid."

"I think what we need to do is find out what is really paranoia and what is really interference in your private life. If we are right in what we think, after a certain period of time only a few small hints at interference would be necessary to keep the persecutory delusion alive, and perhaps ultimately none at all."

"I think that there is still some evidence of interference," said the women, "and at least at the start there must have been lots."

"I don't dispute that – I wasn't there! I just think that sometimes real persecution induces persecutory delusions, and I think that we can reduce your suffering if we find out how much of what you believe to be persecution is paranoia, because there is no evidence of real persecution. Perhaps 20 percent, perhaps 40 percent, perhaps even 80 percent or 95 percent of what you believe to be persecution is no longer caused by the persecutor, but by your fears. Are you happy to follow this line of investigation as far as it takes us?"

"Yes, I am."

### The Persecuted II

The case study "The Persecuted II" serves as a continuation of the previous story, and illustrates how delusions can be eliminated by using the logic inherent to them. The client is asked to discourage her persecutors by making them so bored that they give up, and at the same time to discourage the part of her personality responsible for the fear of persecution by removing the relevant stimuli.

In the second therapy session which followed the session described, the woman told me that her telephone was no longer being tapped; she had decided that this was the case because she could no longer hear any clicking noises on the line, and she believed it was a consequence of the Telekom tapping scandal, which was big news in the media at the time.

A more detailed version of the embedded case study "Getting Rid of Ghosts" was published in Hammel 2012b: 72.

TOPIC: Anxiety, bullying, erotomania, monsters, paranoid personality disorder, paranoid-hallucinatory schizophrenia, persecutory delusion, psychosis, sects, stalking, undercover investigators

INTERVENTION: Pacing and leading, series of stories, utilisation of the symptom, yes set (example, positive model)

"So these people who move things around in your apartment and spread rumours at your workplace that you're getting married – what is it that they want? Presumably to cause you mental distress?" I asked.

"I guess so," answered the woman.

"And since these people are tapping your phone and watching you, they must also see how you respond to being terrorised like this," I replied.

"That's right."

"So your persecutors would find these games a lot less fun if they no longer achieved anything," I pointed out. "What I'm going to tell you might not seem to have anything to do with your situation, but I believe that it does. Once upon a time I knew a small girl who was afraid of the ghosts in her house. Some of the grown-ups she knew thought that there really were ghosts. I didn't know quite what to think, so I said to the child, 'Are you having problems with ghosts in your house? I can help you with that – I know them and have quite a lot of experience in dealing with them. I used to meet them lots when I was a child, and I still do from time to time. I was terribly afraid of them when I was little, but then I found out something about them – they can't really do much at all, they just pretend that they can. All they want is to make you scared, and they find that great fun. If they can't make you scared, they get bored, and after they've been bored for a while they go away. You can even tease the ghosts by saying, "Good morning, dear ghost! How are you today? Did you sleep well? Will you eat some breakfast with us?" Then the ghost will be really annoyed. Perhaps it will try and scare you even more. But if you continue doing what I've suggested, the ghost will get bored to death and go and look for something else to do.'

"What do you think? Could you find a similar way of dealing with the people terrorising you?"

"I think I could," said the woman.

## Celibacy

The need to reinterpret the past can be an obstacle standing in the way of the therapeutic treatment of compulsive actions or delusional ideas which are of decisive importance for an individual's biography, either because they have been acted out over long periods of time with the involvement of the individual's family and the public or because they have entailed major sacrifices. Rewriting the past and standing by this new-found interpretation and structure, both in private and in public, is a huge undertaking, and it can be useful to highlight the price that must be paid – which often includes grieving for opportunities which have been wasted in the past – in order to help the client make the leap into a new life, earning well-deserved respect and admiration. The story "Celibacy" can be told together with a story about someone who only learns as an adult that he was adopted, and who has to reinterpret his past and overcome a crisis, but who eventually, after restructuring his biography, becomes happier than he would ever have been able to before. Similarly, a story can be told of someone who discovers that his partner has been cheating on him for some time, but who survives the crisis and finally gets his life back on track and finds happiness again.

TOPIC: Addiction, belief, compulsion (OCD), delusion, relationship, sects, self-perception, separation, undercover investigators

INTERVENTION: Metaphorical reframing (metaphor, searching model)

One morning, at some point in the future, a pope woke up from a strange dream. In his dream he had been giving a talk to thousands of priests when in a sudden flash of inspiration he had called out, "From this day forward, celibacy will be abolished. Priests may now marry again!" But the priests did not cheer and rejoice – they looked at him in silence.

Then he heard a voice behind him saying, "I've denied myself so many pleasures for so many years, and lived my life according to doctrine. Has it all been a waste of time?"

He turned around and looked in a mirror. Then he heard a choir of priests singing "Has it all been a waste of time?"

"Please say no, please say no!" in the form of a psalm and antiphon.

Later that morning, the priest met a cardinal and asked, "What would happen if I abolished celibacy?"

"You would have spent all your life doing and not doing many things, and it would all have been a waste. You would be surrounded by people who had done and not done the same. We would have to start our lives afresh, and a crisis would ensue. Think about what you are doing."

"Yes," said the priest, "it would be a truly courageous step."

## Me Too

Many people who otherwise appear thoroughly sensible report that they hear voices or see visions and kinaesthetic hallucinations at times, and almost all of these people have a close affinity with the spiritual aspects of life; it was probably this phenomenon which gave rise to the visions seen and voices heard by Biblical figures and subsequently by saints throughout the history of the Church, and which allows the shamans and mystics of other cultures to see auras, spirits and totem animals. Someone once said to me, "When I visited Indonesia, I realised that I'm not mad, I'm just living in the wrong culture." For the most part, hallucinations only result in delusions if the individual in question cannot distinguish his or her individual experiences from the experiences accessible to everyone, and develop socially acceptable behaviour on this basis. The quote-based story "Me Too" deals with hallucinatory experiences that are often regarded as schizophrenia but should be clinically distinguished from this disease.

TOPIC: Belief, hallucination (hearing voices), paranoid-hallucinatory schizophrenia
INTERVENTION: Imagined rapport, increasing complexity (example, searching model)

"I hear voices and see things which no one else sees, just like some of my patients," a consultant psychiatrist once told me. "I just don't tell my colleagues about it."

## Suicidal tendencies

Anyone who wants to stop someone committing suicide must be familiar with their values and utilise them for therapeutic purposes. There is very little point in contradicting the suicidal patient's claims that life is not worth living, since arguments along these lines often merely result in the client feeling even more isolated and misunderstood. The concept of the ambivalence seesaw, combined with the principles of pacing and leading, is more likely to allow progress to be made in a therapeutic setting; the therapist mentions how hopeless the client's life appears to be and continues talking in this vein for a short while, then introduces a tiny element of hope into what he or she is saying – so tiny that the client cannot contradict it – before continuing to speak again for a while about the hopelessness of life, and keeps on introducing aspects of hope into the conversation with very gradual increases in frequency and intensity. These positive perspectives are initially linked very closely (within the same sentence) with negative perspectives in order to avoid the client contradicting them. If the therapist can persuade the client to accept and take on the positive aspects of what he or she is saying, the focus of attention can be shifted more boldly from negative to positive thoughts. Until the very last, however, the therapist should retain a small element of negativity in the repertoire of his or her arguments in order to make it easier for the client to focus his or her attention on the positive aspects.

It goes without saying that effective prevention often requires not only therapeutic conversations, but also the involvement – with the client's consent – of other individuals and institutions in the therapeutic work (family members, doctors, psychiatric services, social institutions, self-help groups etc.).

### When You Meet Your Brother...

The thought experiment "When You Meet Your Brother" is an intervention which can be used for patients with suicidal tendencies. The patient's family structures and the values of both the patient and any predeceased family members are used as a basis for demonstrating that life is worth living. This prevents "copycat deaths" and utilises the patient's bond with these individuals by hypothesising what they would think about the planned suicide. The dialogue can alternatively be used with individuals who are (or feel) responsible for the death of another person.

The living person can ask questions or offer apologies, while the deceased person provides a fictitious (but often realistic) opinion on what is said. In my experience the deceased are kind-hearted, and the outcome of such a dialogue is almost always (with the possible exception of murders) that the deceased denies any guilt on the part of the individual who is still living, or forgives him or her. If an outcome of this kind cannot be achieved, the therapist should mediate between the two sides – one fictitious and one real – in order to ensure that each side has the best possible opinion of the other, for example using methods from systemic counselling, family constellation therapy, Gestalt therapy or ego state therapy. Interventions of this kind can also be used to travel to heaven or another meeting point to say farewell to an individual – or a pet – in cases where a final farewell was impossible before their death.

TOPIC: Abortion, conscience, copycat death, family, grief, murder, suicidal tendencies, war

INTERVENTION: Age progression, imagined rapport, inner team, preventive suggestion, thought experiment, trance induction through age progression, through questions, through alienation of the familiar, through confusion and through stereotype, utilisation of values and social structures (example, searching model)

> When you're on the other side, and have escaped this world – a world I can see you're eager to leave – and when, after arriving, you meet your mother and say, "Hello Mum, I'm here already! I decided to catch an earlier train, as you might say," what will she reply? What questions will she ask? And when you meet your brother, who died before you, how will he greet you? What will you tell him, and how will you answer him?

### A Single Request

The story "A Single Request" can be used in the same context as the previous story, and again utilises the patient's family structures and values to demonstrate that life is worth living. The intervention was developed in 2007 in conversation with a patient who had undergone a biopsy and had announced that if cancerous cells were found he would commit suicide. Half a week after this conversation, the patient said that he had thought about the request and decided against killing himself.

TOPIC:  Conscience, family, suicidal tendencies, trauma
INTERVENTION:  Imagined rapport, preventive suggestion, utilisation of values and social structures (example, negative model)

"You're free to end your life, and I won't try to stop you. I just have a single request, and there's something I need to tell you first. I once worked in the out-patient department of a hospital, and we saw lots of people who had tried to kill themselves, or in other words to do exactly what you're considering. We saw people who had slashed their wrists open, people who had poisoned themselves, people whose legs had been torn from their bodies, people whose stomachs had burst open and much more. Some of the people whose job it is to care for these people become mentally and physically ill themselves.

We also have to remember the police officers, the fire fighters, the paramedics, the motorway maintenance workers and the railway staff who have to clean up all the mess.

And then there's the mothers and fathers, the siblings, the children and the grandchildren, who can't understand why it has happened and often suffer for all the rest of their life as a result.

And so I have a single request – when you do end your life, do it in such a way that the sum total of unhappiness you cause for those around you is not more than you yourself have to suffer at this moment."

### The Dance of the Thorns and the Knives

"The Dance of the Thorns and the Knives" is an intervention which can help patients to stop cutting and accept responsibility. The story exaggerates the self-harming behaviour in keeping with the principle of a symptom prescription, and also treats it – albeit with a sense of affectionate irony – as something valuable, mirroring to the client the polyvalent nature of cutting as a courageous but self-degrading behaviour, as a cry for help but a rejection of one's surroundings, as a way of feeling alive and a way of damaging oneself, as self-dialogue and symbolic suicide. At the same time, cutting with knives is presented as an escalation of the previous lacerations with thorns and mentioned only in passing as something relatively inconsequential, thus utilising the ambivalence which exists between trivialising and dramatising the behaviour.

TOPIC: Cutting, double bind, growing up, Munchhausen's syndrome by proxy, Munchhausen's syndrome, self-harming behaviour

INTERVENTION: Ambiguity, aversive suggestion, increasing complexity, metaphorical reframing, paradoxical intervention, positive connotation, ritual, dissociation of connoted notions, symptom prescription, utilisation of the symptom (metaphor / example, positive model / negative model)

The native tribes of the Amazonas basin have some fascinating customs. For example, there are certain rituals which must be performed before a child can become an adult – the ethnologists who study these tribes refer to them as initiation rites. They are not simply tests of courage, but traditions which represent a doorway into a new stage of life, or the next rung on a ladder which they must climb up in order to reach a higher level. These rites are really quite impressive – the young people of one tribe dance for a whole night long, and while they dance they flog their backs with long, thorny vines. They drag the vines across their skin until it is hanging in shreds from their backs, and they dance together in pools of their blood.

After this dance comes a second dance, during which they use sharp knives to cut their arms and legs, and then rub each other's wounds – first with the blood running out of their veins, then with spit which they rub onto the wounds, and lastly with salt.

Then they keep on dancing, ever more wildly, before finally sinking exhausted into each other's arms and sleeping for a very long time. Their dreams are full of images showing them the way into their adult life, which will be different from the life they led before.

Once they have performed this ritual they are much stronger than they were before. They must complete several more initiation rites before entering new stages of life, but the ritual of the thorns and the knives is performed only once. After they have entered the adult world they leave the past behind them, because they are now in a new era which follows new rules.

## Loss and farewell

Grief is triggered by loss experiences. Grief responses – sometimes described in terms of phases through which the grieving individual passes, and sometimes described as the interplay between different psychological aspirations – are experienced not only after the death of a loved one, but also after a separation, the loss of an irreplaceable object, a job loss, the loss of health or the loss of something which was joyfully anticipated but never became reality. Major grief experiences can also be triggered by moving house or emigrating, since people's responses to all of these events are similar in every respect.

### Stand Up

The metaphorically framed rhetorical question in the story "Stand Up" suggests that the only way forward for someone who has been shipwrecked is into the future and a new life. The rest of the story plays out in the listener's head as he or she thinks about what must have happened beforehand and what will happen afterwards. It can also be used with patients who have undergone a serious illness or an operation in order to motivate them to go on living (or to engage with physiotherapy).

TOPIC: Caretaking, convalescence, crisis, grief, health, mobilisation, motivation, operation, relationship, separation, trauma
INTERVENTION: Metaphorical reframing, promoting a searching attitude, rhetorical question, suggestive question (metaphor, searching model)

What does the victim of a shipwreck do when he reaches dry land?

### On the Riverbed

The story "On the Riverbed" illustrates that being rescued is often a question of timing and waiting for the right moment – which is sometimes the very last second.

TOPIC: Crisis, grief, separation, success, survival, time management
INTERVENTION: Structuring of processes (metaphor, positive model)

A driving instructor was practising parking manoeuvres with his pupil in a car park next to a river. The learner driver put the car into reverse, put his foot down hard on the accelerator – and seconds later they were both on the riverbed.

"Stay calm!" said the instructor. "Leave the door closed, undo your seatbelt and wind the window down just a little so that the water trickles in."

The driver's compartment slowly filled up with water while the two of them waited on the riverbed.

When the water was up to their necks, the teacher said, "Now open the door and swim upwards!"

The rescue operation succeeded, and both teacher and pupil survived.

### Almost Too Late but not Too Early

The quote-based story "Almost Too Late and not Too Early" can be used in the same context as the previous story. Experiences of squeezing spots can also be used in certain situations as a metaphor for time management when solving problems …

TOPIC: Addiction, anxiety, grief, time management
INTERVENTION: Structuring of processes (metaphor, positive model)

> A lifeguard once told me, "If someone who is drowning is still panicking and flailing around, it's impossible to get them to dry land. You have to wait until they've calmed down, and then you can rescue them."

## Motorway Roadworks

The story "Motorway Roadworks" highlights the stressful and risky nature of the grief experience, but also the meaning behind it. If someone who made a vital contribution to an individual's identity is no longer available, the individual in question must reorganise his or her thoughts and feelings and to a certain extent reinvent himself or herself as a result. The unconscious often responds to crises of this kind in a way which appears incoherent and devoid of purpose to the conscious self, but which in fact pursues the useful goal of rebuilding an identity.

TOPIC: Crisis, grief, identity, separation, suicidal tendencies
INTERVENTION: Promoting a searching attitude, rhetorical question, trance induction through description of a trance situation (metaphor, searching model)

> How do you feel about motorway roadworks? I find it annoying when I need to get somewhere quickly on the motorway and then suddenly find myself in the middle of roadworks. I have to pay attention because the road layout has changed and the lanes are narrower, and the build-up of traffic means that it's even more important to keep your distance and avoid causing an accident. I was recently weaving my way through the road signs and lane markings at yet another set of motorway roadworks, and I wondered to myself, "What could possibly be the use of roadworks on motorways?"

## Surfing the Waves

The story "Surfing the Waves" conveys the message that grief comes in waves, and that the power of these waves can often be overwhelming. It is, however, possible to learn how to be carried along by the waves in order to avoid being knocked over by them most of the time, and sometimes even to gain strength from them – or at least to avoid losing any more strength than is absolutely necessary.

TOPIC: Cancer, chemotherapy, chronic disease, crisis, cyclic illness, economy, grief, growing up, relationship, time management

INTERVENTION: Structuring of processes (metaphor, positive model)

> When we were children we once went swimming on a beach with strong surf, where the waves rose two metres or more up into the air before thundering down onto the sand. We had to learn to be lifted up by the waves in order to avoid being knocked down by them. We had to wait until the crest of the wave was almost directly above us, because if we jumped too early, we would sink into the wave and have to hold our breath for a long time until the momentum of the wave had passed, but if we jumped too late we might not come up again at all – the wave would press us down onto the sand, and we would lie there unable to move until it had passed. Yet if we jumped at exactly the moment when the wave lifted us slightly upwards and we could harness its power for our jump, it would lift us high up onto its crest, move past our face with a small splash and then let us glide softly on the back of the wave down to the trough. Wave by wave, we gradually learned how best to control the power of the surf.

### Trying It Out

The case study "Trying It Out" is an intervention that helps patients overcome the fear of ageing and death.

Anyone who can actively shape the unavoidable in his or her thoughts and deeds will stop being a victim of fate.

TOPIC: Ageing, dying

INTERVENTION: Age progression, unreal reframing (example, positive model)

> "I'm looking forward to dying," she said and looked quite cheerful as she said it. "It's all prepared. I visited the undertaker with a few of my friends from the old people's home, and asked him, 'Can I look at the coffins?'
>
> "'Of course,' he said, and showed them to me.
>
> "'Can I try one out?' I asked, "just to check that it fits?'
>
> "The undertaker gave me a funny look.
>
> "'There's something pressing into my hip just here,' I said once I was in the coffin. 'Would it be possible to have some foam padding?'"

### I'll Come Again

The story "I'll Come Again" sets out instructions for communicating with people in comas or other states of reduced awareness. It is a good idea to base conversations of this kind on what the patient formerly loved and believed, and what was significant in his or her previous life. Establishing physical contact and speaking in the same rhythm as the patient's breathing promotes attention and rapport, and it is also useful to monitor his or her pulse, movements and breathing for responses to what has been said. Physical responses such as turning the head, wrinkling the forehead or moving the hands and eyes often bear a clear relation to the content of the conversation, and repetition of what has just been said will generally make it possible to ascertain whether the patient is indeed responding to the relevant words and themes. In my experience, ritual texts with familiar meanings are easier for coma patients to interpret than new content, and simple sentences and words and repeated sentences are also easier to understand. Abstract concepts and words like "not" are more difficult to understand than figurative concepts and may therefore be completely ignored by the patient, changing the whole meaning of the statement. Concepts associated with stressful connotations should be avoided, but it is also possible to embark on a process of systematic desensitisation by repeating the relevant terms in a calming voice and linking them to vivid descriptions of positive concepts. Calming and positively connoted concepts and ideas can also be interspersed into a conversation until the patient shows – by means of corresponding psycho-autonomic responses – that he or she has entered an anxiety-free and relaxed state. ("The Good Shepherd" is Psalm 23 of the Book of Psalms in the Bible).

TOPIC: Belief, body language, coma, death, delirium, narcosis, ritual, sedation, sleep, somnolence
INTERVENTION: Interspersal technique, prioritisation, systematic desensitisation, utilisation of values (example, positive model)

"Would you mind going to see Mrs Seiberth?" asked the nurse. "She was in a somnolent state when she was admitted yesterday, and I think the end is close."

I'd met Mrs Seiberth several times before and we'd got on well, but when I approached her bed this time she didn't respond to my greeting – she was in a coma, and her gaze was vacant. Every breath was accompanied by a coughing noise. I knew that Mrs Seiberth was a religious person, and I placed my hands on her arm and recited the Psalm of the Good Shepherd, slowly and calmly with long pauses timed to match the rhythm of her breath. Her breathing became calmer, and the coughing noise stopped.

When I reached the words "comfort me", however, she started to cough again. I repeated the words in a calm tone of voice until the coughing stopped, and then I carried on. When I reached the line "in the presence of my enemies," the same thing happened and I repeated this line too with a soft, calm voice until the coughing stopped and she was breathing calmly again. When I came to the line, "Only goodness and faithful love will pursue me all the days of my life," her breath became yet calmer, and I repeated it again and again until she was breathing quietly and serenely.

Then I came to the end of the psalm, and told Mrs Seiberth, "It's time for me to say goodbye." Mrs Seiberth coughed again, so I repeated, "I'll come again, I'll come again, I'll come again, I'll come again, I'll come again," until her breathing was quite calm again.

The next day I repeated the ritual, and this time her breath remained calm the whole time, with the coughing noise only returning when I said goodbye.

"I'll come again, I'll come again, I'll come again," I said, and her breathing became soft and smooth. On the third day, I arrived to see Mrs Seiberth a little later than usual.

I met her son at her bed, who told me, "She died an hour ago."

## The Legacy

One of the characteristic features of the suffering associated with grief is that we cannot receive from the deceased what we once valued or give anything back to them – at least not in the habitual sense. Grandparents who experience the loss of an adult child and subsequently become carers for their grandchildren in his or her place often find great comfort in doing so; similarly, self-help groups and initiatives often spring up out of a desire to help people in similar situations to process difficult bereavements, with the assistance provided to these people acting as a substitute for what the bereaved would like to give to the dead. The reciprocal relationship of giving and taking is continued despite the interruption of death, and a new meaning is ascribed to fate. The story "The Legacy" illustrates a basic legacy-related intervention which can be used in most grief situations and which makes it possible for those in the world of the living to express thanks to the deceased and if necessary to make reparations. It can also be used to prevent "copycat deaths" through disease, accident or suicide. The legacy intervention is based on the Hellinger balance of giving and taking (Weber, 1997: 22; Mücke, 2001: 102).

TOPIC: Biography, family, grief, identity, meaning
INTERVENTION: Positive connotation, preventive suggestion, real reframing, thought experiment, trance induction through questions and through stereotype, yes set (example, positive model)

You've told me lots of good things about your late brother, who must have been a wonderful person. I've learned that he was a good listener, that he was patient, that he was touchingly concerned about his family, that he had a brilliant sense of humour...

I have the impression that you have similar talents – perhaps he passed them on to you. I'm sure he's a big part of the reason why you are the way you are, and this was the gift he gave you – a kind of legacy which will allow you to help others in turn, particularly those who are also grieving for your brother. You can pass on all the wonderful things you received from your brother to the people he loved – to your children, to your pupils and to everyone you think would benefit from such a gift.

Do you think your brother would approve of you passing on to others the gifts he gave to you?

He would then be acting through you in a manner of speaking, and giving the same gifts to others thanks to your actions.

And you would be acting on his behalf by doing the good deeds that he used to do.

And you would also be giving him a gift as well, do you agree?

Whatever you do in his interest and on his behalf is a gift you are giving him out of gratitude. Am I right? That would mean that your brother could keep on giving his gifts to the world, and you could keep on giving your brother something in return for as long as you like.

# Chapter 5

# Promoting successful relationships

## Romantic relationships

The benefits offered by stories told during sessions of couples therapy are not simply multiplied by two because they are told to two people at once; the stories also affect the interactions between the pair, leading to an exponential increase in the benefits gained. Neither of the parties involved can continue behaving in the same way if the other party starts to behave differently, and if this different behaviour provokes a different response, the behaviour of the first party will undergo yet further change in turn, following the pattern of reciprocal resonance.

### At the First Fart

Falling in love may be a good start to a romantic relationship, but the success and duration of such a relationship does not depend on whether and how long the couple were initially "in love" with each other. The significance for a romantic relationship of falling in love is relativised in the story "At the First Fart"…

TOPIC: Faithfulness, romantic relationship
INTERVENTION: provocation, psychoeducation, reducing complexity (example, searching model)

> My mother, who has been happily married for many years, was talking to me about what makes a happy relationship. "Being head over heels in love is all well and good," she said, "but all of that goes out the window at the first fart…"

### Fact

The dialogue "Fact" asks when one should work on oneself and when one should come to terms with the truth about a romantic relationship. Anyone who makes a concerted effort to change irritating habits or be more demonstrative in his or her affection can achieve great things, but as a general rule the struggle of changing one's personality to please one's partner is not a worthwhile one. The risk is high that one partner will go to great efforts and make only moderate progress, while the other is left with the impression that these efforts to bring about change fall short. Anger, despondency, rage and hardship become part of everyday life when one half of a couple tries to change himself or herself to stop the other from leaving, and it is often better to learn new ways of dealing with the situation at hand without changing its basic features.

TOPIC:  Habit, identity, relationship
INTERVENTION:  Externalisation of ambivalence as a dialogue, provocation, psychoeducation, reducing complexity (example, searching model)

> The woman was incandescent with rage.
> "Can't you make any effort at all? Why does nothing ever change? Why do you do the same thing over and over again?"
> "That's just the way I am," answered the man.

### The Eagle and The Falconer

The description of the relationship between "The Eagle and The Falconer" is one way of examining relationship problems – in particular faithfulness and jealousy, monogamy, potential separation and the ambivalence which exists between the desire for freedom and emotional ties – from the perspective of a curious onlooker.

TOPIC:  Faithfulness, freedom, jealousy, relationship, separation
INTERVENTION:  Externalisation of ambivalence as two locations, visualisation (metaphor, positive model)

> High up on the Potzberg mountain is a birds of prey centre which puts on daily shows between spring and autumn, featuring eagles, falcons and vultures.
> Some of the people who watch the shows ask, "Isn't it cruel to keep these magnificent birds imprisoned here when they would rather be free?"
> In response, the falconer answers, "No one who hunts with an eagle can keep him captive – if the eagle decides not to come back from a flight, no one can stop him. An eagle only decides to come back if he thinks that he's better off living with humans than being free. Strictly speaking he's already free, because he can decide every day whether to stay or go – but the eagle loves his human and regards him as a partner, and not just a hunting partner, but a marriage partner, if we can speak of such things

in relation to birds; a partner in everything, from hunting and everyday life through to rearing chicks... Eagles are long-term monogamists, and become very jealous if they see other birds of prey together with their human, to the point that they will drive off their rivals. The eagle and his falconer are therefore married in a sense, but the eagle can get a divorce whenever he wants one. Now and again an eagle does fly away and never returns, but this is a rare occurrence. In some cases a human must also leave an eagle because he is at risk from the magnificent creature, but this too is rare. If neither of these exceptional situations occur, the eagle and the falconer will stick together through good times and bad alike..."

### A Lovely Christmas

Situations in which the story "A Lovely Christmas" can be used include those where there is a possibility that a couple might be happier if they developed their own new customs instead of sticking to family traditions and beliefs passed down through the generations. The story can also be used in cases where one partner has a closer relationship with his or her parents than with his or her new partner (in-law conflicts) and where parents or a partner's grown children attempt to take control of parenting decisions.

TOPIC:  Emigration, family, growing up, identity, intercultural conflict, moving house, relationship

INTERVENTION: Externalisation of ambivalence as two locations, pattern interrupt by the client, ritual, visualisation (example, positive model)

> They had already been living together for a few years, and their life together was generally very harmonious – except when Christmas came around each year. She came from a well-to-do Hamburg family, whereas he came from a well-to-do Heidelberg family. Until they moved in together, she had spent a lovely Christmas each year with her parents in Hamburg, and he had spent a lovely Christmas each year with his parents in Heidelberg. Now they lived in Darmstadt. The first year after moving in together, they celebrated a miserable Heidelberg Christmas there. The second year after moving in together, they tried a Hamburg Christmas, but that was also miserable. The third year they tried a joint Heidelberg and Hamburg Christmas, and that was the worst of all. After thinking for a while about what to do this year, they decided on a Darmstadt Christmas, and they had a lovely time.

### Shiny or Matt

The metaphor "Shiny or Matt" highlights the fact that what we regard as beautiful often changes over the course of a relationship, and that although beauty is in the eye of the beholder, what the beholder sees may also change.

TOPIC:  Relationship
INTERVENTION:  Metaphorical reframing (metaphor, searching model)

> When I got married many years ago, my wife and I bought each other gold rings. We could choose between polished rings or matt rings, and we choose a shiny, polished pair of rings. Friends of ours got married at around the same time as us, and they chose matt rings. After several years had passed, we held our rings next to each other and compared them. We saw that there was no longer any difference between the pairs of rings – the shiny rings had acquired a matt finish, and the matt rings had become shinier. They had come to resemble each other completely.

## Ugly and Beautiful

The story "Ugly and Beautiful" can be told in similar contexts as the previous story.

TOPIC:  Relationship, sexuality
INTERVENTION:  Increasing complexity (example, positive model)

> I've known people who found each other drop-dead gorgeous when they first met, but who claimed after they had been together for several years that even though they still loved each other, they no longer noticed what the other person looked like because they had grown so used to seeing each other. I also once knew a man who had gone out with a model, and who said, "I got used to her beauty after a few years, and what counted then was her character." I've even known people who found each other unattractive when they first met and still learned to love each other. The woman told me, "After I fell in love with my boyfriend, he stopped being ugly and turned into the most handsome man in the world, and that's how he's stayed for me."

## Temptation

The dialogue about "Temptation" can be transferred to many different situations, including faithfulness within a relationship and addiction issues. "Out of sight, out of mind," says the proverb, and placing a temptation (and anything closely associated with it) firmly out of sight helps a great deal in getting the offending object or other negative thoughts out of mind – cigarettes can be stored in the loft or cakes in the freezer, for example. It is interesting to note that people often avoid taking similar action, even if it would be possible with a minimum of effort and they claim to wish to be rid of the temptation. (On suggestive therapy for obesity, cf. Kohen & Olness 2011: 199.)

TOPIC:  Addiction, alcohol, attention, bulimia, eating disorder, faithfulness, obesity, relationship, sexuality

INTERVENTION: Avoiding a trigger, externalisation of ambivalence as a dialogue, reducing complexity (metaphor, positive model)

> Mr Gundolf said, "I can't look at a piece of cake without wanting to eat it."
> I asked, "Does that bother you?"
> "Yes."
> "Then don't look at the cake."

## Jellyfish I

The metaphorical story "Jellyfish I" serves as a model for understanding aggression by a member of one's close family or by a partner or former partner, potentially caused by his or her need for physical and psychological integrity. It provides a metaphorical illustration of the fact that other people can quite legitimately have different protection-related requirements and protective mechanisms as a result of their different personalities, biographies and lifestyles. The metaphor can also be used to increase understanding of patterns of behaviour relating to separation or (perhaps long-past) trauma which are experienced as exaggerated. The story contains a therapeutic double bind, since it expresses the beauty and vulnerability of the creatures in positive terms, but at the same time describes the client or a friend or relation as a jellyfish, thus pacing and reframing accusations or self-accusations which have been expressed. The story respects the listener's need to justify his or her own aggressive behaviour as necessary defence, under the condition that the person excusing the behaviour in this way accepts the comparison to a jellyfish. The emphasis on describing the jellyfish in positive terms makes it hard for the conscious mind to reject the comparison, but no one wants to behave in a way which is reminiscent of a jellyfish, however much they love jellyfish.

TOPIC: Aggression, double bind, growing up, jealousy, premenstrual syndrome, relationship, separation, sexual abuse, trauma
INTERVENTION: Aversive suggestion, counter double bind, metaphorical reframing (metaphor, negative model / positive model)

> I think that jellyfish are beautiful creatures, whose movements are fascinating to watch. But why do they sting? Why do they hurt you as soon as you touch them? Other animals only bite when they are attacked... The body of a jellyfish is formed from a jelly-like substance, and they are so delicate that a single rough touch can injure them and a blow – even an accidental blow from a well-meaning human – can kill them.
> In my opinion, jellyfish are just as scared of a human's touch as humans are of being touched by a jellyfish. The jellyfish has no other way of escaping the encounter it fears so much, but people have many different

options both before and after the event. They can check whether there are any jellyfish warnings, and decide whether or not to risk going for a swim and whether to be particularly careful. If they do get stung after all, they can wash the sore area with vinegar and keep out of the sun, or apply lotion which mitigates the effects of the poison.

## Jellyfish II

"Jellyfish II" encourages the listener to think about his or her choice of partner, sexual compatibility and the right way to deal with aggression between family members. The metaphor can also be used if the listener is involved in a bullying situation or is faced with choosing a new job or other social environment. The story refocuses attention from the destructive behaviour towards sexuality, thus prompting the listener to let off steam by using his or her energy for desire and creativity instead of aggression. Connotations of sexual experiences (associated with jellylike substances and the movements of the jellyfish in the water) also appear in the story.

TOPIC: Aggression, bullying, jealousy, relationship, sexuality, team work
INTERVENTION: Counter double bind, promoting a searching attitude, shifting the focus of attention from a deficit to a resource, utilisation of connotations (metaphor, searching model)

How do jellyfish reproduce, and why don't they sting each other in the process?

## The Emergency Alarm Button

"The Emergency Alarm Button" is a procedure for helping people who want to reduce their propensity for violence or their tendency to use violence in the heat of the moment. As fort the couple in the case example, the man did not attend any further therapy sessions, but his wife came to see me again twice. In a telephone conversation three months later, she told me that no further problems had occurred, and the marriage had become a happy one again.

TOPIC: Aggression, family, impulse control, intercultural conflict, relationship, violence
INTERVENTION: Metaphorical reframing (metaphor, positive model)

"Can you really hypnotise people?" asked the man. "Maybe you could just hypnotise me and get rid of my problem!"

He laughed. His wife had brought him to therapy, and he had no real interest in attending.

"Which problem is that?" I asked.

"He hit me," answered the woman sitting next to him. "While I was holding our son."

"It felt like someone had pressed my emergency alarm button," he said. "It was an automatic reaction. I didn't mean to do it."

"I don't need to hypnotise you," I replied. "You can do it yourself. Have you seen those red fire alarm points they have in hospitals and public buildings, with a layer of glass covering up the alarm?"

"Of course," said the man. "Why do they have the glass there?"

"So that no one presses the alarm by accident."

"What if it was a wafer-thin layer of glass, like the glass slides used to view specimens on a microscope?"

"That might break if someone leaned against it."

"What about bulletproof glass?"

"That would be too thick."

"Think about how thick your layer of glass needs to be to ensure that your wife cannot break it. Take a good look at this layer of glass and place it in front of your emergency alarm button."

## Past the Expiry Date

The metaphorical story "Past the Expiry Date" can be told to someone who remains in a romantic or professional relationship even though he or she no longer values it.

TOPIC:  Bullying, compulsion (OCD / hoarding), double bind, economy, faith-fulness, human resource management, neglect, quality, relationship, separation

INTERVENTION:  Externalisation of ambivalence as a dialogue, psychoeducation (metaphor, negative model / searching model)

> I find it impossible to get rid of left-over food, because I was taught that, "Food should never be thrown away!" – at least not as long as it looks edible. And so I keep food which I don't fancy eating in the fridge so that it doesn't go off. I keep it for one, two or three weeks, or perhaps even a month, and then when it shows the first signs of mould, I throw it away with an almost clear conscience because it can no longer be eaten.
>
> "Why don't you just throw it straight in the bin?" a friend asked me recently. "You're not suddenly going to start wanting to eat something if you don't like the look of it from the start."
>
> "Who knows?" I asked.

## Love

The title of the story "Love" conceals an intervention for those who are worried about being "left on the shelf" or have resigned themselves to remaining single after a long spell of loneliness. The story champions the idea of enjoying romantic relationships – and life itself – at any age.

TOPIC: Ageing, relationship
INTERVENTION: Age progression, promoting a searching attitude, promoting positive expectations (example, positive model)

> I was travelling in the same train carriage as them. My diary was stuffed full of meetings, whereas they were two people in love who had all the time in the world. She looked into his eyes and smiled. He smiled back. "If you hadn't talked to me when I was sitting on the park bench that day, I'd still be sat on my own in the home with all the other old dears."

## Family

The traditional family constellation with two parents and several children is no longer the dominant model which it used to be, and there has been a rise in the number of single-parent families, parents with 50/50 shared residence, blended families with long-term or short-term arrangements of partners and siblings, and of course families with fostered or adopted children.

Children growing up in non-traditional family structures often come to therapy with the same problems as children from traditional families, but the adults involved often suspect or claim that these problems are caused by the issues which the family has had to overcome (e.g. divorce). Given that it is impossible to prove whether or not the root cause of a teenager's lack of punctuality and sloppiness is the fact that he misses his father and would prefer to be living with both his parents (which is probably the excuse he uses), it is more productive to challenge the plausibility of similar arguments and instead to discuss who can do what in the given situation to improve the family's life together – perhaps under the condition that the other party makes a different contribution which is negotiated in conversation between the two sides.

In certain situations, problems are caused not by conflict but by a child's lack of self-confidence and his or her anxiety about people and the uncertainties of life.

Anxiety can sometimes be increased rather than reduced by talking about it, and in any case often follows its own logic and is impervious to rational arguments. It is therefore a good idea to incorporate "I"-reinforcing therapeutic interventions into therapy unobtrusively by telling stories.

### The Schneiders

The story "The Schneiders" demonstrates a procedure which can be used to build cohesion in families, for example among siblings.

TOPIC: Aggression, de-escalation, family, growing up
INTERVENTION: Anchoring, conditioning of waking behaviours, framework
suggestion (example, positive model)

"We are the Schneiders. We stick together." That was what she said to her children when she was telling them to share their toys.

"We are the Schneiders. We stick together." That was what she said to them when they argued.

"We are the Schneiders. We stick together." That was what she said to them when she helped them out of a tricky situation.

"We are the Schneiders. We stick together." That was what she said to them when she asked them to help her.

"We are the Schneiders. We stick together." The children heard their mother say these words many hundreds of times, and they reflected the truth not only while they were growing up, but also when they were adults – they were the Schneiders. They stuck together.

### The Eagle Chick

The metaphor in the story "The Eagle Chick" is designed for children in care, but is also suitable for children from traditional families who may suffer from the widespread latent fear of losing their parents. The reference to a very slight injury to the eagle is a useful way of mentioning the listener's injuries without reinforcing them, and of suggesting by implication their rapid healing.

TOPIC: Adoption, blended family, family, grief, growing up, parents, self-confidence, separation, siblings
INTERVENTION: Metaphorical reframing, promoting positive expectations
(metaphor, positive model)

I can no longer remember exactly where this story happened, but I think it must have been in a village in the Balkans, in the former Yugoslavia. What I do remember is that an eagle chick had fallen out of his nest. When the family found him, he was full of beans, flapping his wings and opening his beak wide, and he did not appear to be injured except for a little blood in one spot. The parents hesitated and looked around. There were no mother or father eagles to be seen anywhere, and if they left the chick to its own devices it would die. What should they do? The children urged their parents to help the chick, and so eventually they took him home with them. After arriving home, they put the chick in a cage which had previously housed a pair of cockatiels, and the parents then spoke to a hunter who told them what they should do. They cleared out a room in the basement for the eagle chick and placed an old car tyre on a wooden box in the centre of the room, lining it with scraps of fabric and old clothes, and then they put the large chick inside. They gave him scraps of meat to eat and water to drink. The children had fun cawing like they had heard eagles cawing in their eyries, and the young eagle cawed back, providing hours of entertainment for everyone. The eagle grew and thrived, and his plumage began to change, with the feathers becoming smooth and dark brown.

One day the hunter came to visit. He looked at the eagle and said, "You're a big boy now!" And then he said to the family, "It's time to take him outside."

He gave the father a leather glove with a long cuff and placed the eagle on his arm, and then they went for a walk together. The bird looked around, curious and eager to explore. The children thought it was funny next day at breakfast when their father said that his arm muscles still ached. The hunter's visits became more frequent, and their walks became longer and longer. One day they saw other birds of prey in the sky, and the eagle saw them too. He gave loud cries and beat his powerful wings so violently that the father had to take care to avoid being hit.

The next few walks they took were more like hikes, and finally they walked up to the top of the rocky outcrop at whose base the eagle had been found. They looked to the ground, and saw a large eagle and two somewhat smaller eagles circling in the air further down. The young eagles were still clumsy, flapping their wings more frequently and sometimes seeming to lose their balance for a moment when they were hit by a strong gust of wind.

The eagle watching from the top appeared to be deep in concentration, stretching his neck out and standing still as a statue on the father's arm. As though he was trying to remember and understand... Then he once again flapped his wings violently, cawed and let out a cry like only an eagle can. When the bird had calmed down, the father gripped his body with his left arm and held him tight, then moved his right arm out from under the bird's talons and gripped his legs so that the claws were dangling in the air. The irritated bird pecked with his beak at the father's hand which held his legs – not badly enough to hurt him, but badly enough to make him jump. The next move had to happen very quickly. The father gently spun backwards in a circle, and then threw the bird downwards with all his force. The eagle was clearly surprised, and gave a muffled cry. He wobbled and staggered in the air, and appeared to fall for a while, but finally he caught himself and moved through the air with clumsy flaps of his wings. After a while he settled down on a rocky ledge to recover. For a while they watched him, and then they all went home. Over the next few days they walked up to the rocky outcrop another few times, and were happy to see four eagles circling in the sky. They seemed to have recognised each other. When autumn came the eagles left, and they didn't spot any circling there in winter either. Once, when the snow was at its deepest and the frost at its coldest, they looked out of the back window of their house and saw their eagle sitting there. They gave him a piece of dried sausage which he wolfed down greedily, and over the next few days he returned a few times. Then the snow thawed, and the eagle's visits stopped.

Eighteen months later, an aunt who lived in a distant village wrote to say that a pair of eagles was nesting and raising young chicks in the area for the first time ever. The family went on a trip there, officially to visit the aunt, but in reality to see the birds. When they came in sight of the eyrie, one of the eagles there flapped his wings violently and gave a loud cry. Was that their eagle?

### Zero-Problem Therapy

The case study "Zero-Problem Therapy" illustrates firstly that solutions are found by focusing on solutions instead of on problems, and secondly that the "ordeal" technique can be a useful tool if it is applied directly to the thera-peutic conversation. The idea of the ordeal is to make involuntary processes, that is, those controlled by the unconscious mind, unattractive for this latter by associating the relevant behaviour with a punishment that is guaranteed to happen. An ordeal is therefore based on an agreement that there will be additional unpleasant consequences in the event that the problem is not solved, with the aim of making the solution a much more attractive option for the unconscious mind. In this story, an agreement is reached that the anticipated unpleasant events will only occur if the solution cannot succeed without them.

TOPIC: Aggression, de-escalation, growing up, violence
INTERVENTION: Ordeal (example, positive model), reward and punishment

> Two boys of eight and ten who were attending therapy had bickered and fought every day for as long as they could remember. Their parents were also present and listening to the session.
>
> I asked the boys why they were there, and they avoided answering. When I suggested that they didn't like talking about their problems, they agreed with me, and so I explained to them, "Me too. People always want to talk to me about their problems, but I don't like talking about problems at all. I'd much rather talk about solutions and what it would be like if all the problems had gone away. How does this sound – as long as we can keep on thinking up solutions, we won't talk about problems. We'll only talk about them if we run out of ideas for things which might help."
>
> The boys agreed, and I asked them what they might do to get along better with each other. They had lots of imaginative ideas, and cooperated with each other to find ways of arguing less. They came up with ways of making up with each other after an argument and even of stopping

arguments before they happened, and they developed methods of foreseeing arguments and leaving the room before they happened. I made them promise to try out all the ideas and to do more of what worked, and it turned out to be a very productive conversation.

### When Someone Says "Stefan Hammel"

The following story illustrates how an agreed pattern interrupt can be used to avoid recurring and therefore predictable disputes. The course of therapy lasted two hours.

TOPIC: Aggression, de-escalation, growing up, siblings, violence
INTERVENTION: Pattern interrupt by the client (example, positive model)

> When I met again with the boys who argued constantly, they told me, "We only had three or four arguments this week – it used to be three or four times a day!"
>
> "How did you manage it?" I asked, and they answered, "We agreed that every time one of us thinks an argument might happen, he must say 'Stefan Hammel!' and then we must both go straight to our rooms for ten minutes. If we can't go to our rooms, like when we're in the car or in a canoe, we both have to be silent for five minutes before we can talk to each other again."

### Pest

The story "Pest" demonstrates an intervention for preventing antisocial behaviour in gifted children who are bored and insufficiently challenged, and for developing their talents. The case study also illustrates how a network of stories can be built up, all targeted towards the same solution.

TOPIC: Aggression, attention deficit disorder (ADD / ADHD), family, gifted-ness, growing up
INTERVENTION: Age progression, homework, real reframing, series of stories, utilisation of the symptom (example, positive model)

> A mother brought her nine-year-old son to therapy because he was pestering her and his three-year-old brother all day long. The boy said that he was very good at pestering people, and that he was doing it because he was bored. His report card from school was full of As and Bs, although he moaned about his teacher because she was too strict. He never did any homework at home – every time he finished the work which had been set in a lesson, the teacher would tell him, "Do your homework," and there'd be none left to do by the end of the school day.

I explained to the boy that his habit of pestering his family was nothing more than an understandable desire to learn more about people and their behaviour. Then I told him, "My niece is only fourteen, but she already carries out psychological experiments. She carried out an experiment in the bathroom to find out whether the members of her family were more likely to pick a roll of toilet paper which was closer but had a crumpled end, or one with a neat end which was further away. When I asked her whether she was planning any more experiments, she said, 'I've discovered that if I imagine I'm seventeen years old and can run the way I can run in my imagination, I get ignored by the boys who normally annoy me on purpose.' She investigates how people treat her differently if she is dressed differently, and she observes what happens if she has a pretend argument with a friend and then both of them explain to the teacher who comes over to settle the quarrel that they're having a great time, with a broad smile on their faces."

I told the boy that if he carried out lots of experiments like these, he could make a fortune selling things at car sales as a teenager or become an outstanding teacher or therapist as an adult. I told him about all the experiments I could remember carrying out which had heightened my perception of non-verbal behaviours, and then I instructed him to get started right away with the task of researching the behaviour of his fellow human beings, to write down all his findings and to report them to me.

I said, "There's just one condition. You must not pester or harm anyone during these experiments."

The boy said, "Do you know what I'm going to do first? I'm going to find out whether my brother copies me if I do a forward roll."

### The Winter Rose

"The Winter Rose" is a suggestive story aimed in particular at girls growing up in conditions which are challenging in terms of space, social environment or family structure. Alternatively, a child can be asked to name his or her favourite animal, and the story can be turned into one about a zoo owner or breeder who succeeds in finding a way to raise this animal in particularly difficult conditions despite all the doom-mongering of his critics, so that it grows up healthy and happy, is admired by many and later becomes the mother or father of wonderful young animals. The story can also be used to boost the morale of patients during long hospital stays, for example while undergoing chemotherapy.

TOPIC: Adoption, attractiveness, blended family, cancer, chemotherapy, children's home, chronic disease, family, grief, growing up, immune system, loneliness, moving house, poverty, self-confidence

INTERVENTION: Metaphorical reframing, promoting positive expectations (metaphor, positive model)

I have some very large terracotta pots on my balcony, and I decided that I'd like to plant roses in them.

"You can't grow roses in pots – they'll die," said my father.

"That's a shame," I said, but I couldn't get the idea out of my head, and so I visited a plant nursery.

"You can't grow roses in pots, at any rate not outdoors," said the sales assistant. "They'll freeze to death in winter because the whole root ball is surrounded by frost."

"Can't you bring them inside over the winter?" I asked.

"They don't like being moved around," said the sales assistant. "Take it from me, you can't grow roses outdoors in pots."

Then one of the gardeners who worked at the nursery entered the showroom. "Of course you can," he said. "There's a special variety of rose which doesn't mind frost at all. It looks a lot like a beautiful wild rose, and it isn't damaged by the weather at all. It can also be grown in a small space, even in a large terracotta pot on a balcony. It matures well, and its scent is exquisite. It's a very resilient plant, and you can take it with you whenever you move house – and if you ever move to a house with a large garden, you can of course replant it in the ground."

### The Replanted Tree

The story "The Replanted Tree" is designed in particular for children finding it hard to come to terms with a new living situation after a house move or adoption, or after their parents have divorced and the family has been restructured. Once again, it is a good idea to refer to a minor injury in the story in order to incorporate the problem which the listener is facing and its predicted improvement without lending too much gravity to the story (and by analogy to the way in which the patient handles the associated situation in his or her life). The story can also be used for patients who are forced – for age-related or health-related reasons – to move out of their own house in order to go and live with family or in a home, or adults with disabilities who are forced to move away from their families and into sheltered accommodation.

TOPIC: Adoption, ageing, attractiveness, blended family, children's home, foster care, grief, growing up, moving house, self-confidence

INTERVENTION: Metaphorical reframing, promoting positive expectations (metaphor, positive model)

One day a gardener was working in his garden when he found a small tree right in the middle of some shady undergrowth. "A shadbush!" he cried. "How on earth did that get here?" He would never have suspected that such a beautiful and valuable tree could be found in such a dark location. Perhaps the wind or a bird had carried its seeds there?

The gardener thought carefully about what he should do next. He knew that it is sometimes difficult to move a plant to a different location, but he also knew that his shadbush would never grow into a large, strong and beautiful tree if it stayed here in the shade. So he decided to replant it in a different location, where it would get enough sun and wind to thrive and flourish. He took his spade and dug out a broad ring of soil around the trunk of the tree before digging a hole in the ground where he wanted the tree to grow and placing the shadbush there, root ball and all. He then filled the hole back up with soil, added exactly the right amount of fertiliser, and gave the plant a good watering.

When he looked at his tree the next day, he was dismayed to see that all the leaves on it were drooping. He thought to himself that the tree's roots had probably extended a long way under the ground before it had been dug up, and that it must have lost some of its tiniest hair-like roots. The tree would need to conserve its energy to heal these injuries, but it should be able to regrow its roots, and so the gardener decided to give his tree the best possible care and simply be patient. He waited and gave the tree all the time it needed, and soon the leaves had indeed regained their former strength. After a few months the tree was a fine specimen, and after a few years it had grown into a large and strong tree.

## Parenting and detachment from the parental home

Growing up involves detaching oneself from one's parents in a series of many small steps, some of which are as hard for the parents as they are for the child. Stories are a particularly helpful therapeutic medium in such situations since they can be used to address both grown-ups and children at the same time. The use of stories for children and adolescents in detachment or crisis situations is discussed in Hammel, 2010.

Some of the following stories are aimed more at parents and some more at children. Most of them champion the child's right to develop freely and gain independence from his or her parents by forming independent opinions and becoming self-confident. Some encourage parents and children to take the next step, and others alert parents to behaviour of their own which might be hindering the development of their child. One of the stories highlights the fact that parents are entitled to use force against their children if necessary...

### Love of Cats

The aphorism in the story "Love of Cats" reminds the listener that love involves seeing the world from the perspective of whomever you love, and in order to do so it is necessary to spend time carefully and respectfully observing his or her individual thoughts and lifestyle. It is useful to distinguish between what the other party actually wants and what I might want if I were him or her. When direct questioning is impossible (in the case of young children, individuals with a mental disability, coma patients, people suffering from aphasia or people who speak a different language, for example), careful observation of non-verbal reactions is generally helpful.

TOPIC:  Friends, parenting, parents, relationship
INTERVENTION:  Promoting a searching attitude, psychoeducation, suggestive
    question (example / metaphor, negative model / searching model)

> A friend once asked me, "If cat owners only want the best for their pets, why can you buy venison-flavoured cat food and yet you can't buy mouse-flavoured cat food?"

## Pulling the Goat Home

The story "Pulling the Goat Home" reminds the listener that parents should not necessarily expect their children to be willing to be parented, and that an element of force is often unavoidable. The goal in such cases should then be to find the most humane way of applying this force. Pulling a goat on a cart is much more effective than trying to convince it with words to move in the right direction, but also more ethically acceptable and effective than beating it with a stick or pulling it along by its horns.

TOPIC:  Family, freedom, growing up, parenting, parents
INTERVENTION:  Pattern interrupt by the client, reducing complexity (meta-
    phor, positive model)

> It was a time of grinding poverty, shortly after the war. My father-in-law said, "Buy yourselves a goat, then you'll always have cheese, milk and butter." Shortly afterwards we walked to the market which was held three villages away and bought a goat. Unfortunately the goat didn't want to come home with us, so we bought a cart as well. We lifted the goat onto the cart, strapped it down, pulled it home and sold the cart.

## Blocked-Up Ears

The story "Blocked-Up Ears" highlights the importance of preparatory suggestions for the following therapeutic work. This includes not only shaping positive expectations, but also using various individual therapeutic techniques which introduce new ways of seeing and behaving. The metaphor can be used in supervision and parent coaching or as psychoeducation for clients.

TOPIC:  Growing up, motivation, parenting, parents, school

INTERVENTION: Destabilisation, finding resources, framework suggestion, interspersal technique, metaphorical reframing, pre-hypnotic suggestion, promoting positive expectations, psychoeducation, seeding (example, positive model)

"We put a few drops of olive oil into our patients' ears around half an hour before we syringe out the wax," explained the doctor's assistant. "It softens up the wax so it's easier to get out."

"I do exactly the same when I want to work together with a client to solve a problem," I answered.

### The Shoelace Debate

The story "The Shoelace Debate" illustrates how unsolicited advice (whether direct or indirect) can provoke resistance, and how other interventions are often more effective.

TOPIC: Growing up, human resource management, overprotectiveness
INTERVENTION: Externalisation of ambivalence as a dialogue, psychoeducation (example, searching model)

"Your shoelaces are trailing on the ground," my father said to me yesterday as we were strolling around the garden.

"Yes," I replied.

"You look ridiculous," he said.

"Ah well," I answered.

"You might trip over them," he said.

"I might do many things…" I pondered.

He carried on nagging for a long time, before finally concluding, "Giving children advice is a good way of making sure they won't do what you want them to do – in fact they'll generally do the opposite. My mother would often remind me that my favourite TV show was on soon. I knew that it would start before long and I wanted to watch it, but my mother's reminders annoyed me so much that I didn't watch it at all. My father rarely gave us advice. He was a wise man."

We looked into the pond and thought of my father's father while gazing at the reflections of the sky and the clouds in the water.

### The Little Cat

The fable "The Little Cat" is an intervention which promotes children's independence and prevents parental overprotectiveness. It is intended to ease the transition from kindergarten to primary school

TOPIC: Growing up, kindergarten, overprotectiveness, school, self-confidence
INTERVENTION: Age progression, externalisation of ambivalence as two
   locations (metaphor, positive model)

The little cat sat all alone high up in a tree.

The baker came by, spotted the creature and cried out, "That poor little cat, she's climbed all that way up and is too scared to come down!" Then the baker said to the priest who happened to be passing by, "Father, we must help that poor little cat!"

The mayor was also passing by, and came to see what was happening.

"Mr Mayor," said the baker and the priest. "Please help us to get that poor little cat down!"

"Yes," said the mayor. "Of course we must help that poor little cat. I'll call the fire brigade!"

The fire engine came up with sirens howling, and the firefighters jumped out. They placed their ladder against the branch on which the cat was sitting, and one of them climbed up. "You poor little cat!" he said as he came closer to her.

The cat looked at the firefighter in surprise, before getting to her feet, scurrying down the tree trunk and jumping easily and nimbly to the ground.

"People really are very strange," thought the cat, and walked over to the school playground where she climbed the next tree with astonishing agility. "What can they all be doing over there?" she wondered, as she watched all the people who had collected around the first tree.

### The Schoolchildren's Fairy

The story "The Schoolchildren's Fairy" can be used in the same contexts as "The Little Cat". Both stories were first published in Hammel, 2007. This one is based on an intervention by Milton Erickson, who sent a six-year-old girl reported to be a kleptomaniac and pathological liar a letter from the "six-year-old-growing-up fairy". The letter said that the fairy saw everything the girl did and heard everything she said, and that she was her growing-up fairy. The girl then invited the fairy to her seventh birthday party, but the fairy refused and said that the fairy for seven-year-olds was now responsible for her (Rosen, 1982: 241).

TOPIC: Growing up, kindergarten, school
INTERVENTION: Age progression, promoting a learning attitude, promoting a
   searching attitude (metaphor, positive model / searching model)

The kindergarten children's fairy is beautiful, but her big sister, the schoolchildren's fairy, is even more beautiful and magical. The schoolchildren's fairy makes children dream about numbers and letters, and teaches them clever thoughts and fun games to play in the playground. When the kindergarten children's fairy grows up, she wants to become a schoolchildren's fairy too, and she hopes that this will happen as soon as possible. Then a younger fairy can take over her job and become a kindergarten children's fairy.

### *A Girl Like Robin Hood*

The story "A Girl Like Robin Hood" demonstrates how problem anamnesis is possible using barely perceptible voice signals, how symptoms which are experienced negatively often have positive intentions and how a symptom can be cured by setting homework for the friends and family of the index client.

Physical gestures are similar to changes in the voice in that they provide information on the root causes of a problem. Certain ways in which an individual rubs his or her eyes with a finger or fist are a very reliable indication that the unconscious wants to cry or is remembering a time when the individual cried, and are triggered by a slight itch in the eyes, which is sometimes described by the individual in question as the cause of the movement. Regular observation of an individual's movements in the context of what is currently being discussed proves that this is no coincidence, however. A distinction should be made between gestures that point to an unconscious desire to cry, and different ways of rubbing the eyes which are triggered when people talk about tiredness and sleep. Patients who are talking about or alluding to an illness frequently display the behaviour they displayed while suffering from this illness. For example, when allergy patients think about allergies they often start before long to cough, to scratch their skin and to tug at their nose and in general to give non-verbal demonstrations of all the symptoms of their illness. If a client is revisiting a traumatic period of his or her life during a therapeutic conversation, he or she will sometimes cough in a way that sounds asthmatic or reminiscent of vomiting, and some of these patients do in fact suffer from asthma which may have been triggered or made worse by the relevant events.

TOPIC: Body language, delusion of poverty, emigration, family, growing up, intercultural conflict, moving house, poverty, theft

INTERVENTION: Anamnesis questions, anamnesis through bodily signals and changes to the voice, homework, positive connotation, real reframing (example, positive model)

Whei-Ing was 14 years old, and her mother had brought her to therapy because she had been shoplifting again. She told me that she ran a Chinese restaurant, that Whei-Ing's father ran a shop selling Asian food and that the daughter often helped her mother out in the restaurant. I asked Whei-Ing whether she got any pocket money. She said that she got enough, and her mother explained that she could have more if she wanted, but that she had never asked for more. When Whei-Ing used the word "money", her voice broke a little, as though she had lost her voice temporarily.

I interrupted her to ask, "What do you think about when you hear the word 'money'? Tell me the first words which come into your head."

She listed a few words, and her voice broke again a little when she said "grief".

"What do you think about when you hear the word 'grief'?"

"Poverty," she answered, and her voice sounded different again.

"And what do you think about when you hear the word 'poverty'?"

"My mother is always talking about how poor we are. And my father sends all the money we could save or spend to his mother and siblings in China." Then she started crying.

"No one could argue with the fact that you have a good reason for shoplifting," I said to Whei-Ing. "You're doing it out of love, to protect your mother. But whether you mean to or not, you're making your mother unhappy and harming yourself. You might have an excellent reason to shoplift, but shoplifting is not the answer. I'd like you to stop, out of love for your mother."

Then I said to Whei-Ing's mother, "You should be proud that the members of your family love and support each other so much. Stop talking about how poor you are, and before we meet again I'd like you to go shopping with your daughter and spend some money on something unnecessary but beautiful."

She did not appear to understand what I was asking her to do, and I had to repeat my instructions several times.

"That will be very difficult for me," she finally answered, squirming and giggling. "I've never done anything like that before in my whole life."

"That will be your homework," I answered.

Next week the mother and daughter told me that the father had paid for them to visit Hong Kong on holiday.

"You should treat yourselves to a mini-Hong Kong every week," I said.

Soon they told me that they had gone shopping and to the cinema together. Even though they expected him to say no, they had asked the father to come along as well, and to their surprise he had gone to the cinema for the first time ever with them and bought the family popcorn – also for the first time ever.

"The course of therapy is complete," I told them.

Later I received postcards from WheiIng and her mother which they had sent from Hong Kong and Shanghai.

## Managing Without Them

The aphorisms in the story "Managing Without Them" can be used during conversations with parents to promote the detachment of parents (and if necessary grandparents) from children, or in conversations with children to promote detachment from parents. The story can also be used in conversations with people working in the helping professions, since there is a risk that the emotional benefits to helpers from their altruistic work are so great that they avoid setting their charges free (thereby accepting that they can no longer provide help), while their charges tolerate this as a result of various advantages they derive from the situation or simply because it is convenient.

TOPIC:  Goals, growing up, parents, self-confidence
INTERVENTION: Framework suggestion, provocation, reducing complexity
       (example, positive model)

> "The job of parents is to make sure that their children can manage without them," said one mother.
> "Children are only given to us on loan," said one father.

## On the Threshold

Children and young people want to grow up and to be seen as being almost grown up already. There are few things more humiliating than being regarded and treated as younger than you are, and few things offer more prestige than being treated seriously like a grown up. The story "On the Threshold" highlights the challenge involved in achieving a balance in this respect; an insecure young girl may find it empowering if she is perceived by grown-ups as attractive, but at the same time it is important to avoid the feelings of humiliation which are easily provoked as a result of her insecurity.

TOPIC:  Attractiveness, growing up, self-confidence
INTERVENTION: Positive connotation, promoting positive expectations
       (example, positive model)

> "Your freckles are beautiful," said the man.
> The girl shook her head violently. "No, they're not!"
> It was clear that she felt ashamed of her freckles each and every day of her life. The man thought carefully about what to do next. He didn't want the conversation to end there, but what should he say?
> "I always wanted a girlfriend with freckles," he replied. "Then I found one without freckles, and decided that not having freckles was ok too."
> Then he changed the subject. Had he overstepped the line? He didn't want to offend her, or – God forbid! – cause any misunderstandings. But

the girl was beaming with pride. She didn't want to be a child any more, and she understood that he had seen the beautiful woman inside her.

## Middle-aged and elderly people

This chapter is devoted to a range of therapeutic approaches that can be used for older family members and their relatives who find themselves in a challenging situation, for example because of disability, misfortune, accusations or differences in attitude between family members. It also contains ideas for dealing with issues that increase in importance from mid-life onwards.

### A Desire for Life

The story "A Desire for Life" highlights the fact that strong family relationships play a vital role in an individual's health and his or her will to go on living. People tend to want either to live in a tribe or not to live at all, and the majority of suicides and attempted suicides are a result of isolation and loneliness. Similarly, some people only survive an illness because of the presence of loving relatives.

TOPIC: Death, depression, family, goals, health, loneliness, pain, relationship
INTERVENTION: Increasing complexity, psychoeducation (example, positive model)

> I meet patients at the hospital where I work who want to die even though they are relatively healthy, who hope that they will not wake up after an operation or who ask me to kill them.
>
> I meet other patients who are trying with all their strength to conquer their illness even though the doctors have told them that this is impossible, or patients trying to extend their lives by just a few weeks even though they are in terrible pain and have no hope of recovery.
>
> Again and again I meet desperately unhappy people who are almost healthy, and people who are full of the joys of life and yet are close to death. The difference between them is that those in the first group have no one caring for them, whereas those in the second group have partners, children, grandchildren and friends who care for them with love and affection. A desire for life is a desire to live for someone else.

### Time Adjustment

The case study "Time Adjustment" demonstrates an intervention for adjusting one's perception of time when interacting with people who live life at a slower pace, in order to respond in a patient and relaxed manner.

TOPIC:  Ageing, slowness
INTERVENTION:  Time distortion (example, positive model)

> Today I was chatting to an old man who spoke very slowly. He kept on pausing while he searched for the right word, and many of his sentences were left unfinished. The man couldn't help it, but I could feel myself becoming impatient and even angry at the slow pace of the conversation. So I imagined a dial which I could turn to adjust how quickly or slowly I perceived time; within less than a minute, the man seemed to be talking at an entirely normal pace, and since he was no longer too slow, all my impatience vanished.

### Behind the Wardrobe!

The story "Behind the Wardrobe!" reminds us that older people may sometimes act in a way that appears strange not because of memory loss, but because of the stigmatisation, social isolation and personal frustration suffered by many – particularly dementia patients – as they get older. Many of the "crazy" aspects of a person's life actually make perfect sense when viewed in the context of the associations he or she makes between the information available to him. Dementia patients are not always and not exclusively "crazy", and their illness may perhaps also draw out latent craziness in the members of his or her family or support system.

TOPIC:  Ageing, aggression, de-escalation, dementia, family
INTERVENTION:  Real reframing (example, positive model)

> "Behind the wardrobe!" our grandfather would bellow every time something irritated him.
> "He's suffering from dementia," our parents would say to any friends who were visiting, excusing his behaviour.
> "Behind the wardrobe! Behind the wardrobe!" our grandfather would then roar even louder. Us children were used to the fact that grandfather was a bit strange.
> When he died not long afterwards, we helped to empty out his rooms, and the wardrobe was also taken apart. On the wall behind it was written in large black letters; "Fuck off!"

### The Difference

A person who imagines himself or herself to be at an earlier stage of life involuntary assumes the facial expressions associated with younger people, and anyone who imagines himself or herself to be very old or identifies with older people will again assume the matching facial expressions. In many cases, the age a person imagines himself or herself to be can be estimated from his or her countenance. Given that an individual's neutral facial expression reflects his or her prevailing mood in previous years, it is noticeable that children who are mainly surrounded by older children or adults often appear older than they are, whereas those surrounded by younger children often appear younger. The same applies to habitual facial expressions; anyone who often wrinkles his or her brow in worry or concentration will in the long run find that these wrinkles become part of his or her neutral facial expression. Individuals who take an objective and distanced approach to their job will have a countenance that reflects this fact, and the same is also true for those who regularly offer empathy to suffering individuals. The way we identify with people, moods and values determines how we look. The story "The Difference" encourages the listener to ask his or her unconscious to identify with attitudes, people and times in a way that will eventually be reflected in his or her facial expressions. Most people will intuitively select low-stress and symptom-free points of iden-tification, which also promote physical, psychological and social wellbeing. It is also possible to suggest that stressful identifications should be regularly interrupted. (See the story "The Worry Catapult".) Suggestions of these kind should preferably be given to the unconscious on an experimental basis to start with, together with an instruction to do more of the same if the new pattern proves useful or otherwise to return to the previous physical behaviour.

TOPIC:  Ageing, cosmetic concerns

INTERVENTION: Age progression, age regression, anchoring, promoting a searching attitude (example, searching model)

> "Are you really her identical twin?" asked the man in disbelief. "How come you look so much younger?"
>
> "I'm not sure," she answered, "but my sister works in an old people's home and I'm a paediatric nurse."

## Friends

How are friendships made? The answer to this question has a lot to do with the discovery of commonalities such as shared patterns of behaviour, shared ways of thinking and seeing the world and shared interests. Two people may become friends if they discover that their past or future feature the same unusual events. What matters most is that the friends' respective interests are handled in a socially acceptable way, that both sides believe a balance has been achieved in terms of giving and taking and that conflicts are resolved in such a way as to prevent any lasting harm or feelings of ill will on either side.

### Gregor the Dragon

"Gregor the Dragon" encourages children to be aware of the harm caused by their own violence, to use their power carefully, to accept themselves as lovable, to discover their talents, to win back former friends and to find new ones. This story was developed to help a young boy who regularly scratched other children and drew blood. It was first published in Hammel, 2008.

TOPIC: Aggression, attention deficit disorder (ADD / ADHD), bullying, children's home, de-escalation, friends, kindergarten, loneliness, school, violence

INTERVENTION: Promoting a searching attitude, promoting positive expectations, psychoeducation (metaphor, positive model)

Gregor the dragon huffed and puffed away to himself, feeling sad and angry. He had been looking for someone to play with all day long, but no one wanted to play with him. He had asked the fox whether he would like to play, but the fox had replied, "No way! You'll only burn our skin and hair again with your fiery breath."

The badger, the hare and the bear had said the same when he had asked them. And yet he had not meant to burn their fur – it had just happened. At least most of the time. As Gregor the dragon sat there and brooded, a tear rolled down his cheek and fell with a small plop to the ground. The owl Laila, who – like all owls – had excellent hearing and was very wise, was sitting high up in the tree.

"What kind of a plop was that?" she asked herself. "It sounded like the noise a dragon's tear would make." And she peered out to see, since it's not every day that you see a dragon crying.

"Why are you crying, dragon?" she asked.

"None of the animals want to play with me. They say it's because I burned their fur. But I didn't mean to," answered Gregor.

"What should I do?" Laila scratched her head.

"You want to do them good instead of doing them harm, but it will take a long time until they believe that. It will take the whole day and perhaps even the whole night, and maybe even longer until they can trust you again. Why don't you start with me?" said the owl, flying down and landing on Gregor's shoulder. "Tell me some stories about dragons!"

And so Gregor began to tell the owl stories about dragons, and there were so many exciting stories that it took a very long time for him to tell them all… The forest creatures heard him in the distance, and their curiosity forced them to come a little closer and then yet closer still in order to catch every word of the dragon's enthralling stories. The dragon's voice grew quieter and calmer, and the other creatures came even closer. Night fell, and the temperature with it. The owl nuzzled into the dragon's neck, which was lovely and warm thanks to the dragon fire smouldering within.

Many hours went by, and when the sun came up next morning, it bathed in its rays a group of animals huddled closely around the dragon, enjoying the warmth which he radiated. And Gregor was still telling dragon stories.

## What Use Are Friends?

The dialogue "What Use Are Friends?" makes it clear that stable friendships and individual interests play a vital role in overcoming serious crises within a family; the same applies to crises within a relationship, regardless of whether the two halves of a couple decided to stay together or separate. Isolation from the rest of the world is sometimes also encountered in the case of single parents and their children, or carers and their charges. The first priority in a course of therapy for a couple who have isolated themselves from the rest of the world should be to ask about their previous friendships and interests, and how these could be re-established.

TOPIC: Caretaking, friends, grief, loneliness, relationship, separation
INTERVENTION: Promoting a searching attitude (example, positive model)

I was chatting to Mr Gundolf about a woman who had stopped seeing all of her friends to please her husband, and then found herself wondering whether she still loved him.

"The woman will only survive a divorce if she has a group of friends to support her," said Mr Gundolf.

"The same is true if she decides to stay," I said.

## The Cardboard Box Dressing

The isolation of an individual, a couple or a group of people from the rest of society can lead to serious psychological and social damage, and a certain degree of openness is required before healing can happen. The symptoms caused by isolation often isolate the victim yet further, but social and psychological succour can be provided by considerate friends and helpers who open up the way to a better life. The story "The Cardboard Box Dressing" contains an implied request to take the plunge into a new openness which will hopefully bring healing.

TOPIC: Addiction, aggression, compulsion (OCD), psychosomatic disorder, sects, sexual abuse, suicidal tendencies, violence
INTERVENTION: Promoting openness, pattern interrupt by the therapist (metaphor, positive model)

The graze on his thigh kept on becoming inflamed. "No wonder," he thought to himself. "My trousers are rubbing on it." He put a dressing on the wound, but even though the trousers were no longer rubbing on it, the skin was still inflamed. "It's because no air can get to it," explained a friend. But what was he supposed to do, walk around in his underwear?

He applied another dressing, but this time he placed a small cardboard box underneath it, with the open side pointing inwards towards his thigh. Now air could get to the wound, but nothing was rubbing against it. The inflammation subsided on the very same day.

# Chapter 6

# Promoting development

## Development and maturity

Many stories about development can be used to promote both the development of children and the professional and personal development of adults if they are introduced into the conversation appropriately. Similarly, the topic of success is relevant both to those wishing to achieve an elite position and those wishing to escape various forms of self-abandonment and neglect. Many stories are as helpful for successful businesspeople as they are for people whose lives seem utterly devoid of success. The concepts of young and old, rich and poor are all relative, and the only deciding factor is that the story is introduced appropriately, if necessary framing it as a madcap idea from a completely different sphere of life.

### *Different*

Anyone who is "different" to the other people in his or her life will find that there is always a price to pay as well as rewards to be reaped. A patient suffering in this respect can be asked whom he or she would rather resemble or be if this were possible, and what would be gained and lost from such a swap. It often becomes clear that the individual is different for a good reason, and that there is a value in remaining so.

TOPIC: Asperger syndrome / autism, attention deficit disorder (ADD / ADHD), disability, giftedness, goals, homosexuality, identity, transsexuality
INTERVENTION: Externalisation of ambivalence as a dialogue, trance induction through confusion (example, positive model / searching model)

> "I'm different to all the others."
> "Do you want the others to be different?"
> "If the others were different, I'd want to be the same, but as they're all the same, I'd rather be different."

## Finished

Being "Finished" is a question of the punctuation applied to the flow of life events. Both projects and human beings are often regarded as finished when they are not yet complete, and it is often more helpful to think of their "completion" as simply another stage in their development. The aphorism (or fable) comments on the confusion between looking back and looking forward which sometimes occurs in connection with a long-anticipated event.

A longer version of the story can be found in Hammel, 2012b: 97.

TOPIC: Growing up, learning, perfectionism, relationship, success
INTERVENTION: Promoting a learning attitude, promoting a searching attitude (metaphor, searching model)

"Finished!" said the egg after it had been laid.

## You'll Manage It

The story "You'll Manage It" can be used to counteract negative suggestions which may be self-fulfilling, and to build positive expectations.

TOPIC: Anxiety, Asperger syndrome / autism, attention deficit disorder (ADD / ADHD), compulsion (OCD), friends, growing up, school, trauma
INTERVENTION: Destabilisation through antitheses, promoting positive expectations, stabilisation through the prefigurement of success (example, positive model)

On 19 June 1974, Stefan's class teacher was writing reports. In his report she wrote, "Stefan's achievements are satisfactory, but he would achieve much more if he did not suffer from such severe behavioural problems. He is tense and unfocused, has no self-confidence and often appears to be terrified. He must find a more orderly way of working."

On 16 June 2008, Stefan was talking to eight children in a psychiatric outpatients' clinic. "When I was your age," he said, "I had hardly any friends. The other children teased me and laughed at me. The teacher wrote in my report, 'He will fail because of his inability to apply himself and to behave himself.' She was wrong – I made a success out of my life. You'll manage it too."

## The Three Principles

The following case study illustrates how a therapist can help a client to apply the "three principles" to cure themselves of depression, anxiety and a lack of self-confidence.

TOPIC: Depression, hebephrenic schizophrenia, learning, motivation, self-confidence, success

INTERVENTION: Inner team, paradox ("I am not here!"), positive connotation, promoting positive expectations, reversing the focus of attention, trance induction through confusion, through dissociation and through the suggestion of trance characteristics (knowing everything or nothing, being everything or nothing and being capable of everything or nothing), utilisation of the symptom and of values (example, positive model)

"My life is governed by three simple principles," she said. "'I know nothing,' 'I am nothing,' and 'I'm capable of nothing.'"

"Those are three useful principles," I replied. "And you have three useful inner voices who make sure that you remember them. But everyone knows that people spend most of their time talking about themselves. Whatever Hans says about Fritz says more about Hans than about Fritz. That's also true in this case; if an inner voice says, 'I know nothing,' it only means that that particular inner voice knows nothing. If an inner voice says, 'I am nothing,' it only means that that particular voice is nothing. If an inner voice says, 'I am capable of nothing,' it only means that that particular voice is capable of nothing. I'd stop worrying about it if I were you – the voices will soon disappear."

## Children's Shoes

The story "Children's Shoes" illustrates how the vision of a reality creates that very reality. Imagining a different reality and identity (acting as if something were the case) tends to result in the manifestation of whatever social construct has been imagined.

TOPIC: Learning, reality, self-confidence

INTERVENTION: pretended achievement ("act as if" intervention), destabilisation of beliefs, externalisation of ambivalence as a dialogue, promoting a learning attitude, promoting a searching attitude (metaphor, searching model)

"I've only just started learning what to do," said the apprentice. "How can I pretend to know everything already?"

"Buy children's shoes which are one size larger," replied his instructor.

## Invisible Friends

"Invisible Friends" are valuable companions. The story demonstrates the basic interventions of unreal reframing and the use of imagined rapport.

TOPIC: Learning, motivation, neglect, order (tidiness), quality, self-confidence, success, work organisation

INTERVENTION: Imagined rapport, invisible friends, promoting a learning attitude, promoting positive expectations, unreal reframing (example, positive model)

You can learn a lot from children. For example, many children have invisible friends. What use are they?

Have you ever noticed that you clean the house more effectively if your invisible companions – R2D2, Superman or the seven dwarves – go ahead of you and show you what to do? Their enthusiasm is infectious! Or have you ever noticed that tax returns are easier to complete and much more fun if five clones of your accountant presort the necessary documents, give you tips and tell you that you're better at the job than most other people? If you'd like to take advice from Sigmund Freud, Albert Einstein and John Rockefeller during challenging times, simply give the three gentlemen a voice and listen to their words out loud – first making sure that no one else is in the house with you who will think that you have gone mad, of course!

### The Genie

The story of "The Genie" can be used to promote responsibility, commitment and detachment from the parental home; it can also be used in situations where dreams have been voiced but have not yet found real-life expression.

TOPIC: Attention deficit disorder (ADD / ADHD), compulsion (OCD / hoarding), dream, goals, growing up, mania, neglect, responsibility, success

INTERVENTION: Aversive suggestion, destabilisation through the prefigurement of negative consequences, provocation (metaphor, negative model)

A young man once went for a walk along a beach. While he was walking along he saw part of an oddly old-fashioned lamp sticking out of the sand. "Perhaps it contains hidden treasure!" he thought, before digging out the lamp and carefully opening its lid. Out came a genie who said, "I have been trapped in this lamp for many hundreds of years, and now you have freed me. I grant you one wish!"

The young man was as amazed as he was delighted. "Brilliant! I'd like a big castle where I can live."

The genie answered, "I am master over the spirit world, but unfortunately not over the earthly elements. Otherwise it would have been hard to trap me in a lamp."

The young man nodded his understanding. "But if you can bring me the building materials required for your project, I can use them to build you an exquisite castle with no effort at all."

"How long will it take?" asked the man, who wanted his castle straight away. "As long as you take to bring me the materials, and not a second longer."

So the young man set off in search of materials – first gold and marble, but they were hard to come by and he would have had to work long hours and save lots of money. Then he looked for stone and wooden beams, but they were heavy to carry, and would have required a great deal of toil and sweat. Finally the young man returned to the beach, where he found flotsam, shells, sand and seaweed.

"Build me a castle from these," said the man.

"As you wish," answered the genie, and in the blink of an eye a large and beautiful castle built from flotsam, seaweed, shells and sand stood in front of the man. The genie vanished, and the man surveyed his castle while the tide slowly rose...

### Of Following and Leading

The intervention "Of Following and Leading" is useful in situations where it is difficult for individuals to establish and maintain rapport with others, for example if they suffer from autism, social anxiety, compulsive disorders and certain sexual disorders. It can be told to patients who would like to learn to be more loving towards their partner or who wish to regain their partner's trust in the face of impending separation. It is also suitable as an observation task for highly gifted children in order to challenge them on a cognitive and emotional level, to improve their social skills or to distract them from aggressive or depressive behavioural patterns.

TOPIC: Asperger syndrome / autism, attention deficit disorder (ADD / ADHD), compulsion (OCD), giftedness, loneliness, relationship, sexuality
INTERVENTION: Pacing and leading, pattern interrupt by the client, psychoeducation, utilisation of rapport (example, positive model)

While I was explaining the fundamental principles of hypnotherapy to a sixteen-year-old boy with autism, I said, "A group of researchers have discovered something quite astonishing. When someone is panicking and breathing very quickly, and you breathe just as quickly and then gradually slow down your breathing so that his breathing changes along with yours, he will become calmer and experience less pain. When a person is bent over and groaning with anxiety and you bend over and groan along with him, and then becoming gradually more relaxed, so gradually that he changes his behaviour at the same time, his fears will be dispersed.

"When a person is irritated and talks hesitantly and with an unfriendly tone of voice, and you use the same tone of voice and manner of speaking and then gradually change your speech in such a way that he copies you, he will become more friendly.

"This principle is referred to as 'following and leading', and it applies in every conceivable situation. You can use it to good effect in many different circumstances, but you have to be very careful that the other people involved do not think you are mocking them, and you should therefore carry out your experiments very discreetly.

"This group of researchers have also found out something else. If you closely observe someone whose state of mind and mood is different to yours, and copy his demeanour as closely as possible, you'll experience something of his state of mind and mood, and feel how it must feel to be in his shoes.

"This technique makes it possible to learn many interesting things about other people and the way they communicate unconsciously. In particular, it teaches you to see things from other people's points of view while at the same time encouraging them to see your point of view, strengthening the bonds between you."

## Learning

This section presents storytelling interventions which can be used to support learning and improve exam performance. Further factors which play a role in this area are covered in the following sections; for example, the section on anxiety contains stories that can be used in situations involving fear of exams, and the section on parenting and detachment contains stories that are useful in situations involving learning by children.

### Exam Revision

The story "Exam Revision" outlines one way in which students can mentally prepare themselves for the task of revision. In order to learn effectively, it is often useful to start by asking questions and to provide the unconscious with an overview of the unknown territory so that it can create an internal map into which the answers to these questions can later be slotted. It is also useful to distinguish between central and peripheral content before tackling the main task of revision.

TOPIC: Economy, exam revision, learning, motivation, success, time management, work organisation
INTERVENTION: Promoting a learning attitude, structuring of processes (example, positive model)

A man once had only five months to revise for an important exam, even though he knew that most other students spent twelve or eighteen months revising for it, and even then many failed and had to resit. How could he do all the necessary work in such a short time?

He gathered together the books he needed to study, and started off by reading the indexes at the end of the books again and again over several days. He wondered to himself what all the technical and foreign terms could mean, thought up explanations for them and asked himself which chapters would feature them most frequently. Then he examined the tables of contents, learned them off by heart and thought about how the books were structured. After that he read all the sections of the books printed in bold or italics, and the introductions and summaries for each chapter. He tried to work out where the key messages, explanations and supplementary information could be found in each book. Finally he returned to the indexes. After spending a few days like this he began to revise in the conventional fashion, and passed the exam at his first attempt.

## A Sacred Agreement

"A Sacred Agreement" can be concluded in situations where resolutions have previously been broken and the individual concerned – for example an addict – has lost credibility with himself or herself. The story can also be told in a modified form to alcoholics who damage their self-credibility through various forms of appeasement. Similarly, the story can be told to anorexic patients who deceive themselves when negotiating contracts with themselves about losing and gaining weight.

TOPIC: Addiction, compulsion (OCD), exam revision, learning, motivation, success, time management, work organisation
INTERVENTION: Promoting a learning attitude, psychoeducation, reward and punishment (example, positive model)

A young man who was revising for an exam kept on repeating to himself statements such as the following: "If you manage 100 pages by six o'clock tonight, you can take the evening off." After achieving his goal by five o'clock, he worked for another hour and increased his total to 120 pages. And because he was making such good progress that day, he worked for another hour until seven o'clock, and managed 130 pages in total. A few weeks later he noticed that his revision was becoming sluggish and half-hearted. His pace of work had slowed down, and he was no longer achieving successful days like the one described above.

He talked to an acquaintance about the problem, who replied, "It's hardly surprising. When you make an agreement with yourself, you have to treat yourself like a trusting child or your very best friend. You have to do whatever you promise, otherwise the inner voice or person you have deceived will refuse to cooperate in future, just like a friend will refuse to cooperate at some point if you keep on deceiving and cheating him.

If for some reason you can't keep a particular agreement with yourself, you must apologise to your inner friend. And if you want to change an agreement of this kind permanently, you must ask the friend or child in you for his opinion, and respect his answer. If in doubt, leave everything as it was. Anyone who cannot believe in himself is a poor wretch. An agreement you make with yourself should be a sacred agreement!"

## Mental Block

In the case of patients with a situational speech impediment or other "blocks" in relation to specific actions, it is a good idea to identify the trigger as accurately as possible and to find out in which cases the block does not apply. If the speech impediment only occurs in rare situations such as certain types of exam, all that needs to be done is to construct a slightly different course of events which does not feature the blocking trigger. The following case study illustrates this approach.

TOPIC: Exam revision, fear of exams, learning, motivation, success, work organisation

INTERVENTION: Anamnesis questions, avoiding the trigger (example, positive model)

A student once said to me, "I have to take an oral exam for Greek during which I have to read a text out loud and then translate it into English. The translating bit isn't a problem, but I have a complete mental block about reading things out loud in Greek."

I replied, "I'm sure I've heard you reading out Greek vocabulary, and your pronunciation sounded great to me."

She answered, "Yes, I suppose my pronunciation is ok."

I asked, "Can you learn a Greek sentence off by heart once you've read it?"

She said yes.

"When you're in the exam, read a sentence, close your eyes, say it off by heart, read the next sentence, close your eyes and say that one off by heart..."

She took my advice and passed the exam with flying colours.

## The Price of Success

The story "The Price of Success" illustrates a way of freeing oneself from the mental blocks which may arise if an inner voice categorically prohibits failure and thus makes it impossible to take potentially worthwhile risks. The story asks the listener to come to terms with the idea of failure through the realisation that it can be regarded as honourable; the price of success is always the possibility of failure.

TOPIC: Anxiety, economy, fear of exams, relationship, separation, success
INTERVENTION: Psychoeducation, reversing the focus of attention (example, positive model)

> When Mr Gundolf was asked for the secret of his success, he answered, "Before every new venture I weighed up the price of failure. I agreed with myself that this was the price I would pay if it came to it, without beating myself up. Then I weighed up the price of success and got started."

## Wishes, will and vision

"The wish is father to the thought" is a phrase sometimes used to express the fact that certain wishes never come true, but wishes are also father to the thoughts that result in deeds and manifest social and material realities. This proves that not all wishes are a waste of time, but it is vital to take the first, second and subsequent steps towards achieving the relevant goal in order to avoid visions getting stuck at the wishing stage. Belief in the realisation of a vision (or at least its potential realisation) is just as important as the willingness to pay the associated price. Living one's dreams and making them reality might sound good, but it also means confronting the part of reality which has not yet been altered by the transformative power of our vision.

### The Route Through the Mountain

The fable "The Route Through the Mountain" can be used to help the listener to search for or realise his or her vision. It implies the existence of great and as-yet-untapped opportunities, and encourages the exploration of new avenues of thought. Although disguised as a fable, in structural terms it is the biography of an inventor or explorer. Actually, a group of migrating swallows regularly flew through the St Gotthard Tunnel for several years. (Fables with a similar theme can be found in Bach, 1991 and Bambaren, 1994.)

TOPIC: Human resource management, learning, motivation, responsibility, success, team work, vision
INTERVENTION: Promoting a learning attitude, promoting positive expectations, promoting a searching attitude (metaphor, positive model / searching model)

> "What's that?" a young swallow asked her mother. It was the first time she had joined the flock in its annual migration over the Alps.

"Those are the rolling boxes which carry people around," answered her mother.

"But why are they coming out of the mountain here? This morning, when we were on the other side, they went into the mountain. Is it the same boxes which go in over there and come out over here?"

"I suppose so," answered her mother absent-mindedly.

"Couldn't we do that too?" continued the young swallow. "It's cold and windy up here, and the route over the mountain must be much longer than the route which the boxes take."

"No swallow has ever flown through a mountain."

"Really?" asked the young swallow. She was already elsewhere in her thoughts, and these thoughts caused her eyes to light up.

## Catching Up

The biographical story "Catching Up" can be told in a wide variety of situations where people think they are too late, have missed out on too much or have wasted the opportunities given to them.

TOPIC:  Success, time management, vision
INTERVENTION:  Promoting a learning attitude (example, positive model)

> I'd overslept, and we had a maths test in our first lesson of the day. When I finally arrived in the classroom I was handed the test paper – I had wasted a whole quarter of an hour, one-third of the time available. For a moment I almost gave the whole thing up for a bad job, but then I focused on doing my absolute best. After 20 minutes, the teacher looked over my shoulder at my test paper.
>
> "Strange," she said, "the pupil who arrived last has finished first."

## Dung Beetle

The story "Dung Beetle" can be told to highlight what can be achieved through the listener's will power, and to support him or her in the pursuit of his or her goals. The story can also be used to remind clients not to underestimate what another person can achieve through will power. The implication that the listener or the listener's partner is a "dung beetle" has aggressive overtones, which is useful for building rapport if the client's irritation, dissatisfaction or self-aggression are contributing factors, or in culture where insults delivered with a wink of the eye are a form of tenderness. Alternatively, reference can simply be made to a "black beetle".

TOPIC:  Growing up, motivation, success, vision

INTERVENTION: Promoting positive expectations, stabilisation of behaviour through the prefiguration of success (metaphor, positive model)

When we were children we sometimes went for walks with our parents, and while we were walking our father would often place a shimmering blue-black dung beetle in our hands.

"Close your hands around it once, and see how long it stays there," he would say.

We would do as he asked, and the beetle would soon get to work. With irresistible force it would push, scrabble and press our fingers apart with its legs and body, making relentless progress towards the light. Before long it had escaped from our hands.

### Heaven on Earth

"Heaven on Earth" is a story for idealists, perfectionists and those seeking happiness. The search for perfection is doomed to failure, but does not need to be in vain...

TOPIC: Belief, dream, family, goals, growing up, identity, loneliness, moving house, perfectionism, quality, relationship, responsibility
INTERVENTION: Promoting a searching attitude, reducing complexity (metaphor, positive model / searching model)

A man and a woman were once eating breakfast together.

"My dear," said the man, "I have something important to say to you. Today I'm going to set out on a journey. I'm going to search for heaven on earth."

The woman choked on her coffee. "Don't be ridiculous – you can't mean that. Have you lost your mind?"

"Last night I had a dream," said the man. "I was somewhere that looked like our village, but it was all quite different."

"How was it different?" asked the woman.

"It was a wonderful place. I found it after walking for a long way. When I approached, I noticed that there was no sign with the name of the village, but a radiantly beautiful angel was standing at the first house.

"I asked him, 'What is this village called?'

"He answered, 'I'll show you round if you like. This is heaven on earth.'

"I was shocked. I'd imagined heaven on earth to be larger, and quite different – a palace in the clouds, or a city with towers and golden cupolas. But this village looked almost exactly like our own, and I was almost a little disappointed by heaven on earth. The angel looked at me as though he was waiting for an answer, and I started to find him a bit creepy.

"'Show me around?' I asked. 'I think I can find my own way around.'

"'I think it's better if I show you,' said the angel mischievously, and so off we went. We came across people who were talking to each other and laughing. 'Like in our village,' I thought, but it seemed to me that something here was different. And as we walked through the village, I felt myself becoming ever more favourably inclined towards the angel and the people who lived there.

"I asked the angel, 'What does heaven on earth have which my village does not?'

"He answered, 'Heaven on earth can never be the place you are looking towards – it can only be the place you are looking from. Didn't you know?'

"I was silent, and for an instant I thought I saw a smile on his face.

"'Go and search for heaven on earth,' said the angel. He remained for a second longer, and then he disappeared, together with the people and the village. I was awake and lying in bed."

After the man finished recounting his dream, the woman took a sip of her coffee and was silent.

"My dear," said the man again, "I was given instructions by an angel. I have to set off and search for heaven on earth."

Nothing the wife did or said could change his mind, and on that very same day he said farewell to his wife, his family and his neighbours. Then he set off to search for the heaven he had seen in his dream.

He travelled through many countries. He went to Africa, but heaven did not look like Africa. He went to Siberia, but heaven did not look like Siberia. He went to China, but heaven did not look like China. And he went to America, but heaven did not look like America either, and he did not find heaven on earth. He was often welcomed warmly, and occasionally people asked him to stay – and sometimes he even thought that the angel was close by again, but it was never quite the same as it had been in the dream. He never found the heaven he was searching for, and so after a long time he returned home.

"Can you forgive me for staying away for so long?" he asked his wife. "I didn't find heaven on earth, but I've missed you so much."

She took him in her arms. "And I missed all of you as well!" he called over to the other members of his family and the neighbours who were approaching from all directions. "I've learned how much I can miss you."

"So you didn't find heaven on earth anywhere," repeated his wife. "What did heaven look in your dream? Which village did it look like?"

"Oh God," said the man.

### Marks Out of Ten

The story "Marks Out of Ten" can be told in similar contexts as the previous story.

TOPIC: Belief, family, goals, growing up, identity, loneliness, perfectionism, quality, relationship, responsibility, vision

INTERVENTION: Promoting a searching attitude, promoting positive expectations (example, searching model)

> Mr Gundolf said, "My search for a life that deserves ten out of ten has left me with a life that deserves four out of ten."
>
> I replied. "If you start searching now for a life that deserves six out of ten, you might find one that deserves eight out of ten."

### The Consultation

The story "The Consultation" illustrates the problems that can arise as a result of consistently focusing on deficits. It is suitable for highlighting depressive patterns of behaviour and double bind strategies in a therapeutic context.

TOPIC: Depression, double bind, dream, perfectionism, reality

INTERVENTION: Clarifying goals, promoting a searching attitude (metaphor, negative model)

> An elderly lady once entered a bookshop.
> "Good morning. I'd like to buy a Bible."
> "Of course, ma'am. We have a wide range of editions. Here's a very attractive leather-bound edition with gilt edging and illustrations..."
> "Oh no, that one is much too big. I need one which fits in my handbag!"
> "I see. Here's a pocket-sized edition which I'm sure you'll like..."
> "Are you joking? How on earth am I supposed to read these tiny letters? I'd need a magnifying glass! I need something with a much larger font."
> "I see. I'm sure you'll like this edition – it has a large font, and yet it's still small enough for your handbag..."
> "But that's only the New Testament. I want the whole Bible, not just a small part of it!"
> "A complete Bible which is pocket-sized but printed in a large font...? I'm afraid we don't stock anything suitable, ma'am."
> "Then I'd like to order one."
> "I'm afraid that won't be possible, because such a book is impossible to find. You see..."
> "I don't see anything. All I see is that you are incapable of doing your job. I'll come back again when your colleague is on duty, he talks a lot more sense!"

## Economy, order, efficiency and quality

What is economy? What is order? What is efficiency? What is quality? Entire degree courses are devoted to these questions, and the answers are controversial and multi-faceted, extending far into the realms of philosophy and mathematics. For the purpose of counselling and therapy, it is easier to express the problems and possible solutions associated with these questions in the form of metaphors. Although this may not provide clear definitions, the associated images can help bring about the desired transformations in ways of thinking and behaving.

### *Of Artists and Strategists*

The dialogue "Of Artists and Strategists" relates to the delicate balance between the investment of time and money in either "art" (literature, education etc.) or "strategy" (marketing, business management etc.). Even if one-sided priorities appear justified (by the quality of the output or the commercial success of the business), they ultimately lead to either financial losses or unhappiness at work.

TOPIC: Economy, perfectionism, quality, success
INTERVENTION: Externalisation of ambivalence as a dialogue (example, positive model)

> I was talking with a colleague about the meaning of professional success.
> "There are two types of people on the market – those who strive for perfection and those who strive for career success," she said.
> She could also have called them artists and strategists. We agreed that the members of these two groups are often jealous of each other – the artists produce the better results, while the strategists have nicer cars. Those focused on career success worry that their work is overvalued and that they will be found out, while the perfectionists worry that their work is undervalued and that no one will find out about them.
> "There's no point worrying about other people," I said to my colleague. "We should concentrate on being an artist and a strategist at the same time."
> And it turns out that this is the secret to enjoying one's job.

### *The Potential of Weeds*

"The Potential of Weeds" is a fable about principles. Every principle applies only in the context from which it originates, and a change in circumstances makes it necessary to review the principles which previously applied. Principles which dictate how to think and act in a particular situation may impede development if they are carried over to different situations.

TOPIC:  Belief, economy, growing up, identity, learning, perfectionism, quality, success, work organisation

INTERVENTION:  Externalisation of ambivalence as a dialogue, visualisation (metaphor, negative model)

> They were silent for a long time. Then the little dandelion asked his much larger neighbour, "What are you doing?"
>
> "I'm growing my taproot."
>
> "That's what I'm doing too. But I've made no progress for days. My root has hit a stone."
>
> "Just do what the couch grass does and grow your root around the stone. Grow more roots if necessary," said the big dandelion.
>
> "I can't do that," said the small dandelion. "A taproot is a taproot."
>
> And he never grew any larger.

## Dirty Children

The story "Dirty Children" also serves as a metaphor for a flexible approach to principles and rituals in the broadest sense of these terms. It can be applied to any "pure doctrine" in the fields of religion, ethics, aesthetics, science, therapy or economics.

TOPIC:  Anxiety, belief, compulsion (OCD), conscience, delusion of poisoning, eating disorder, hypochondria, immune system, parenting, perfectionism, washing compulsion

INTERVENTION:  Externalisation of ambivalence as a dialogue, reducing complexity (metaphor, positive model)

> "Children nowadays are all so clean," the old man said. "I remember that when I was young, the dirtiest children in our village were the healthiest."
>
> "And were you one of the dirty ones or one of the clean ones?" asked someone who was listening.
>
> The old man grinned and said; "We would come in from playing with our hands covered in sand and mud, grab an apple and bite into it without washing our hands – and nothing bad happened to us."

## Day's March

The story "Day's March" can be used not only in therapeutic contexts but also in coaching and mental training, where clients sometimes ask their therapist to help them deliver outstanding performances in one area of life (for example their career) even though other areas (health, family relationships, ethical standards) are being dangerously neglected. The story speaks out in favour of moderate stress in these weaker areas of life. The "inner troop" needs to look after all of its members and to achieve a balance between challenge and self-protection.

TOPIC:  Burnout syndrome, family, consultancy within an organisation, goals, health, relationship, success, team work, work/life balance,
INTERVENTION: protecting resources, inner team (example / metaphor, positive model)

> "I was an officer in the army for many years," he said. "There were many times when I had to lead my soldiers on a long day's march. I always made sure that the weakest members of my troop were well prepared but not overstretched, and that the strongest were challenged but also learned to watch out for those less strong than themselves. This approach – focusing on the troop as a whole rather than the individuals within it – was not only more humane but also produced better results."

### Balance

Partners should be equals. The aphorism in the story "Balance" illustrates an imbalance which can only be resolved if both partners stop the game and – if a mutual agreement can be reached – play something else.

TOPIC:  Consultancy within an organisation, human resource management, prioritisation, relationship, team work
INTERVENTION: Reducing complexity (metaphor, negative model / searching model)

> "Playing seesaw with you is boring," the ant said to the elephant.

### Target Practice

The story "Target Practice" highlights the paradoxical fact that an outstanding performance can sometimes result in structural and status-related changes, which are contrary to the interests of the individual in question; the reward for good work is more work. Those who work quickly or productively are therefore often unpopular with the rest of their team, and anyone who speeds up their rate of work to avoid dismissal or chase a promotion may find that this has the (otherwise avoidable) consequence of a colleague being dismissed and his or her tasks being added to the original workload.

TOPIC:  Burnout syndrome, borderline personality disorder, cutting, civil disobedience, double bind, motivation, Munchhausen's syndrome, Munchhausen's syndrome by proxy, protecting resources, self-harming behaviour, simulant, success, suicidal tendencies, war, work

INTERVENTION: Externalisation of ambivalence as two persons, paradox ("failure is success"), provocation (example / metaphor, positive model / negative model)

"One of the things they made us do when we trained as soldiers during the war was target practice. Some of our comrades shot a bull's eye as often as possible – they were sent to the front, and most of them died. Other comrades deliberately missed, and they survived the war."

### Exemplary

The story "Exemplary" can be used in the same contexts.

TOPIC: burnout syndrome, civil disobedience, motivation, protecting resources, work, success
INTERVENTION: Paradox ("Failure is success!"), provocation (example / metaphor, positive model / negative model)

After ten years of conscientiously exercising his duties, the mayor of a village in the Rheinish Palatinate in the eighteenth century wrote to the French occupying forces asking for permission to retire from his post. The authority reviewed his application and responded as follows:

"Honoured Sir, you have performed your duties with such dedication over the years that we refuse your application for retirement."

### Bad English

"Bad English" is a paradigmatic story which encourages the listener to learn from mistakes and to tolerate a deterioration in quality if it results in long-term learning within an organisation and among its members.

TOPIC: Learning, perfectionism, quality
INTERVENTION: Externalisation of ambivalence as two persons, promoting a learning attitude, stabilisation of behaviour through the prefiguration of success (example, positive model)

When I was growing up, my parents took us to America to visit relatives. My elder sister wanted to speak English correctly, and so didn't say a word. I just wanted people to understand me, and so I gestured with my hands and feet and made countless mistakes. My relatives were impressed, my parents were proud and I suspect my sister was envious. I learned English by speaking bad English.

## *Speed*

Like every other variable, "speed" is relative, or in other words depends on the context in which it is examined. The fable-like aphorism in the following story relativises statements which compare and assign value by deconstructing versions of reality, in order to reconstruct other versions (reframing).

TOPIC: Ageing, developmental delay, disability, economy, growing up, learning, slowness, specific learning disability, success, time management, work organisation

INTERVENTION: Externalisation of ambivalence as two patterns of movement, metaphorical reframing (metaphor, search model)

"Well done," said the tree when the snails overtook him.

## *The Door*

The story "The Door" can be used in most contexts where someone is trying to solve a problem in such a strained, hectic or panicky way that he or she may lose sight of obvious solutions. If necessary, a discussion can be held on what should be done if the door gets stuck, the key is in the room or the door is not really locked but merely bolted from inside. Special door knobs and handles with a device which prevents them being unlocked by children or dogs can additionally be mentioned.

TOPIC: Aggression, belief, compulsion (OCD), de-escalation, mania, reality, success, violence

INTERVENTION: Pattern interrupt by the therapist, reducing complexity (metaphor, positive model / negative model)

"Let me out! Let me out!" He pounded against the door with both fists and kicked it with his feet. The door did not budge by even a millimetre. He searched for a solid object in the room – a hammer or an axe – but there was nothing of any use. He screamed and sobbed, but no one opened the door. He appealed to God, prayed and cursed, but God did not respond and the door remained closed. Finally, he fell asleep from exhaustion. He tossed and turned, dreaming restless dreams in which miracles occurred and the impossible came true. In the middle of the night he woke up, got out of bed, walked over to the door, pressed down the handle and pulled the door towards him. The door opened, and he looked outside.

## Progress

The fable "Progress" can also be used in widely differing contexts; for example, if household tasks have been neglected somewhat owing to a busy period at work or a general inability to cope with life, it is often better to restore the house to its previous order simply by trying to ensure that the house looks a little better every evening than it did in that morning, even if the progress made in this way is very slow. Attempts to increase the rate of work often achieve the very opposite of what is intended. Similarly, certain chronic diseases (both physical and psychological) can be more easily overcome or kept under control if expectations of recovery are minimised; symptoms are allowed, provided they gradually occur less frequently and for shorter periods. Sometimes it is a good idea to imagine the route that must be followed when healing from an illness as essentially resembling an upward-sloping zigzag path (in this case, the contract which the patient would conclude with himself or herself would be as follows; as long as I get a little bit better every week, every month or every year, I'll be making adequate progress). The same applies to the task of ongoing weight loss or gain, and addicts can sometimes gradually reduce their consumption of the addictive substance in this way (or the frequency of major relapses); this is however dependent on a high degree of self-motivation, truthfulness and self-control, which is by no means always a given. This procedure can sometimes also be used to treat alcoholism without complete abstinence, depending on the patient's personality and his or her social environment.

TOPIC: Addiction, Asperger syndrome / autism, attention deficit disorder (ADD / ADHD), burnout syndrome, cancer, chemotherapy, chronic disease, compulsion (OCD / hoarding), debt, eating disorder, learning, motivation, neglect, obesity, specific learning disability, success, withdrawal, work organisation, order (tidiness), work/life balance,

INTERVENTION: Externalisation of ambivalence as two patterns of movement (metaphor, positive model)

A salmon was travelling along the annual salmon run, further and further upstream. He had leapt up rapids and jumped over enormous boulders – and even used all of his power and skill to ascend waterfalls.

"Not long now," said the salmon to himself at last. "I remember being here before – I passed it on my first evening on the journey down. I'm much larger and stronger now, and I'll have reached my destination in just a few hours."

The salmon redoubled his efforts, wanting to make faster progress. But as he did so, the current also seemed to become stronger. The path down the river had seemed easy, but the way back seemed pure torture. Sometimes he was too tired to swim, often he lacked the concentration to jump properly, occasionally he had to swim around the rods and creels of the salmon fishers and once he even had to avoid the paw of a hungry bear. Again and again he stopped to regather his strength, but the river kept on flowing to the sea. By the evening the salmon noticed that he had not made any progress – if anything, he had gone backwards. Sad and disappointed, he found a protected spot between two boulders on the bank.

He thought to himself, "It must be possible to reach my destination – others before me have managed it. But how?"

Then the clever fish had an idea. "I'm not going to try and get there as quickly as possible any more; I just want to make progress. All I will ask of myself is to get a little bit closer to my goal every evening than I was in the morning, and if I do that day after day I'll eventually reach my destination. As long as I've made some progress by every evening, it won't matter how short a distance I've travelled – even if it's only half an inch."

The salmon plucked up his courage and started again. Some days he barely made any progress at all, but mostly he travelled much further than he expected – and if he didn't, he remembered his resolution and was content with what he had managed.

After a few weeks, he reached his destination; a lake near the source of the river. He looked around, and found that only a few other salmon had reached the lake before him – most were still trying to reach their destination in the shortest possible time.

### The Goal Behind the Goal

A karate master who breaks a brick with his bare hands imagines to himself that the brick is further away than where he actually sees it. It is a good idea for runners to set themselves a personal goal that lies behind the finish line, so that they pass the finish at the fastest possible speed. The story "The Goal Behind the Goal" demonstrates that success sometimes requires imagining that a goal will be achieved at a time or in a place that differs from the real time and place.

TOPIC: Bulimia, competitive sport, gastroenteritis, learning, motivation, success, time management, vision, vomiting

INTERVENTION: Paradoxical intervention, structuring of processes, time distortion, unreal reframing (example, positive model)

One morning I woke up with an upset stomach. I felt sick, and I knew that I probably would be sick at some point. As long as I lay in bed, I was more or less ok. But when I decided to go to the bathroom, I had to run because a wave of sickness was approaching ever more rapidly, and the faster I ran, the faster it came. I was racing against the sickness, and the sickness won. An hour later the same thing happened. In order to prevent a repetition of last time, I imagined that the toilet was ten metres further away than it was in reality, and I walked with deliberate slowness. I arrived in plenty of time.

## Playing I

"Playing" is a series of metaphors that illustrate the conditions necessary for learning, effectiveness, success and quality. Anyone who learns how to play a musical instrument enhances many other physical and mental processes at the same time, and anything that proves useful in this area can be transferred to other spheres of learning, working and life in general. The first metaphor concerns resource protection during activities that take only a little effort, but are repeated many times over the course of a day. The story can also be used to express the idea that a verbal (and potentially physical) conflict can sometimes be de-escalated with little effort through silence alone.

TOPIC: Aggression, learning, protecting resources, success, work organisation
INTERVENTION: Reducing complexity (metaphor, positive model)

> A saxophone teacher once asked his pupil, "How much force do you need to apply to close the key? Use this much force and no more. And, what do you think: How much pressure do you need to blow a note? Use this much pressure and no more.".

## Playing II

The second metaphor in the series highlights the fact that it is a mistake to ascribe perceived phenomena only to the person in question or the surrounding system (the other person, situation, instrument or piece); reality is made up of interactions between the internal world and the external world.

TOPIC: Motivation, reality, responsibility
INTERVENTION: Promoting a searching attitude (metaphor, searching model)

> The resonance in the saxophone creates the second half of the note, but the resonance in the musician playing the saxophone creates the first half.

## Playing III

The third metaphor in the series highlights the problem that a higher quality of work is often confused with an increase in the rate of work, a quantitative increase in output or an increase in the amount of stress which is experienced and (in some cases) reported to others.

TOPIC: Quality, slowness, time management, work organisation
INTERVENTION: Increasing complexity (metaphor, positive model)

> If you play a piece of music quickly, you can hide all your mistakes – any note which is played too long or not long enough, or which is misplayed or out of tune is immediately replaced by another. That's why it's harder to play a piece slowly than it is to play it quickly, and why anyone who can play slowly is truly talented.

### Playing IV

The fourth metaphor in the series highlights the problem that the unconscious mind often only suggests solutions to the conscious mind after a delay, making it seem as though no progress is being made. Once changes have been made, the context for the initial problem has often disappeared and is ignored.

TOPIC: Motivation, quality, work organisation
INTERVENTION: Promoting positive expectations, psychoeducation (metaphor, searching model)

> "Sometimes I feel like my playing hasn't improved at all for weeks, even though I've spent many long hours practicing on my instrument. And yet other times I seem to make progress quickly," said a pupil to his music teacher.
> "You can't have the one without the other," replied his teacher.

### The Camel

"The Camel" is a fairy tale that deals with the issue of managing meagre or vulnerable resources. One context in which it could be used is as follows; many people who are unable to meet requirements (imposed either by themselves or by others) immediately "correct" their mistake verbally by excusing themselves and expressing their resolutions and promises to do better next time. This verbal and symbolic self-exculpation reduces the suffering caused by the situation to such an extent that in the long run nothing changes, and this procedure may be repeated any number of times. In order to interrupt this pattern, the guilty party must keep their resolutions and apologies secret until they can demonstrate concrete changes in their place. Good resolutions should be kept hidden away until they have multiplied and brought forth offspring!

TOPIC: Economy, protecting resources, success
INTERVENTION: Aversive suggestion (metaphor, negative model)

> There was once a sheikh who had two sons. When he was on his deathbed, he called both of them to him and said, "As you well know, these are

challenging times. Famine and inflation have destroyed everything I once possessed, and my entire herd of camels has been reduced to these two camel mares. Take one animal each and use them wisely, and you will be able to build a life for yourselves."

The sheikh died soon afterwards. The older son sold his camel mare and bought a hut with the money he had made. He mended the roof, cleaned the hut, bought furniture and then set off in search of a well-paid job.

The younger son bartered with a camel breeder, "Let your best male camel mate with my camel mare, this year and for the next six years. You will have the camel's first foal in return."

The man agreed, and after a few years the younger son had a fine herd. He occasionally sold some of his camels, but never more than the number of new camels being born.

After five years he bought a house, after seven years he got married, and after eight years he employed a stable boy – his elder brother.

### The New Word

The fable "The New Word" highlights the relativity and subjectivity of terms such as "economical"; the context and the goals being pursued determine what is economical, efficient, competent, innovative or professional. Even in the same context and if the same goals are being pursued, there may be alternative courses of action that are equally economical (or professional, or competent). The strategy which works best from a particular point of view can only be reliably identified on a statistical rather than an individual basis.

TOPIC: Economy, reality

INTERVENTION: Clarifying goals, promoting a searching attitude, reducing complexity (metaphor, searching model)

A squirrel once poked an ear out of his drey to listen to two business people having a conversation directly in front of the tree in which he lived. While he was eavesdropping, he heard a word he had never come across before in his life. Squirrels are well known for their inquisitiveness, and so the animal bade his wife and children farewell and set off on a journey to learn what this new word meant. Soon he met a spider.

"The spider might know!" thought the squirrel, and asked, "Spider, what does economy mean?"

"Economy means that you wait in silence and alone until your prey comes along, and then you act very quickly."

The squirrel did not quite understand the spider, but did not dare to ask any more questions. He continued on his way, and soon he met a lioness.

"The lioness might know!" he thought, and asked, "Lioness, what does economy mean?"

"Economy means that you hunt in a pack, and every lioness does what is needed for a successful hunt."

The squirrel did not quite understand the lioness, but continued on his way and soon came across a hummingbird.

"The hummingbird might know!" he thought, and asked, "Hummingbird, what does economy mean?"

"Economy means that I move my wings so quickly that I can hover in the air easily while I'm sucking nectar out of the flowers."

The squirrel did not quite understand, but continued on his way and soon met an elephant.

"The elephant might know!" he thought, and asked, "Elephant, what does economy mean?"

"Economy means that I knock over a few trees with my trunk so that the rest of me can pass through the forest more easily."

The squirrel was puzzled by this answer, but continued on his way, and soon he met a sloth.

"The sloth might know!" thought the squirrel, and asked, "Sloth, what does economy mean?"

"Not wasting any energy," replied the sloth.

Then the squirrel's gaze fell on an ancient old tree.

"The tree might know!" he thought, and asked, "Tree, what does economy mean?"

"Economy means growing very tall, up to where the sunlight is."

The squirrel did not understand the tree, and he was looking at the ground, deep in thought, when he noticed a fern.

"The fern might know!" he thought, and asked, "Fern, what does economy mean?"

"Becoming a beautiful plant even though you only receive a little sunlight," answered the fern.

The squirrel did not really understand what the fern meant.

"Have you found out what economy means?" his wife asked him when he returned home.

He answered, "I think that economy means living in a drey."


### The King Is Coming

"The King Is Coming" illustrates a strategy for improving work motivation and performance by imagining the real workplace in a new context and with new rules, which are not only more entertaining than the real rules but also deliver a better result.

TOPIC: Competitive sport, growing up, motivation, order (tidiness), success, time management, work organisation

INTERVENTION: Mental game (example, positive model), unreal reframing

"The king is coming! The king is coming! The king is coming!" She was expected to have tidied the apartment, cleaned the kitchen and got dinner on the table every day by the time her mother returned home from work. She would play "The king is coming!" while doing so, and welcome her mother into a spotlessly clean and tidy apartment, tired out from playing and with a smile on her face.

## Grandma's Cooking

"Grandma's Cooking" reminds the listener that the goal of therapy can be to make good things better as well as to solve problems.

TOPIC: Learning, quality, success
INTERVENTION: Optimising resources, promoting a learning attitude (example / metaphor, positive model)

"Your cooking always tastes nicer than Mum's cooking."
"Once upon a time I used to say exactly the same thing to my own grandma. She would answer, 'That's because grandmas spend a long time learning how to make good things even better.'"

## The Bin Monster

"The Bin Monster" illustrates a method of prompting the unconscious mind to improve the quality of counselling, therapy and self-coaching. The papier-mâché monster, which helps to prevent undesirable side effects of hypnotic suggestions and unwanted thoughts, images and dreams in general, can be seen at www.stefanhammel.de/blog/2007/05/01/89.

TOPIC: Dream, learning, success, trauma
INTERVENTION: Mental game, object as metaphor, dissociation of connotated notions, unreal reframing (example / metaphor, positive model)

"It's a bin!" explained Luise as she handed me the papier-mâché monster with gaping jaws.
From then on, Fred the bin monster sat in my counselling room and waited to be fed. Fred was initially happy to eat office waste, but gradually – perhaps because he had absorbed the psychological waste of so many conversations – he acquired a taste for all the things which were not needed by my clients and which they wanted to leave behind in my counselling room.
I began to introduce my clients to Fred, and over time he munched his way through the therapist's clumsy words and clients' oppressive

thoughts, as well as painful memories and unwelcome habits. One client even sent Fred her depressive thoughts when she was at home.

Eventually Fred also started eating anything that bothered me, and I allowed him to swallow all my bad dreams at night.

### Returning the Key

The story "Returning the Key" illustrates how an agreement involving a penalty of some sort (ordeal) can help to prevent involuntary mistakes, since the unconscious mind views them as too risky. As for the mistake mentioned, I never made this one again.

TOPIC: Memory
INTERVENTION: Reward and punishment, ordeal (example, positive model)

"You took my key with you, and I didn't realise I was locked out until I was standing right in front of the door!" my colleague berated me. "Please never do that again!"

"If I do, I'll drive the 160 km to bring you back the key, right away and in the middle of the night if necessary," I replied.

"You don't need to do that," she answered. "If you tell me in advance, I can bring the spare key."

"I'll do it anyway," I said. "If I know that that's what I've got to do, I won't forget in the first place."

# PART TWO

# The methods

# Chapter 7

# Identifying therapeutic stories

## Using intuition

There are many different ways of finding therapeutic stories; it is possible to search for them consciously, or to enter a trance with positive expectations and allow them simply to come to you.

One criterion for gauging the usefulness of a story is the presence of a climactic turning point, and almost all stories with such a turning point (as well as some without) can be used for therapeutic purposes. The element of surprise introduced by the turning point generally involves a reinterpretation ("reframing") of what has been heard up until that point so that it is now seen from a fresh perspective, increasing the number of ways in which the world can be interpreted and in which the listener can behave. If the story in question can be applied to the client's life, the unspoken implication is that the reinterpretation suggested by the climactic turning point can also be applied to his or her life. The patient will understand the story (either consciously or unconsciously) as an invitation to examine similar solutions to his or her own problems.

Many "therapeutic" stories can be discovered by examining the climactic turning point of a story and then searching for analogous structures in other spheres of life, for example in therapeutic and medical contexts. If we accept that the presence of a turning point in a story provides an indication that it might be useful, a reader searching for suitable stories need only agree an internal signal (an anchor) with himself or herself as a reminder to examine every such turning point to ascertain where and how (rather than whether) the story can be used.

Conversely, a therapist can find therapeutic stories by remaining open to the dream-like images suggested by his or her mind during counselling sessions, and agreeing with himself or herself that these images should be recorded on an "internal photo" or "internal film". Many metaphors that provide a figurative description of the relevant situation and imply solutions can be found in this way; although these internal images are often initially problem-based rather than solution-focused, several ways for a therapist to transform images of this kind from problem metaphors into solution metaphors are described in detail in the section on problem and solution metaphors.

Instead of recording the images that occur spontaneously in his or her mind, the counsellor can also carry out a systematic search for metaphors, for example in the fields of nature, medicine, technology, economics or historical research. Anyone who adopts a playful approach to the search for spheres of life with existing or potential structures resembling a current problem will soon notice how many solutions have been invented by nature, science, the body, society or an author, and these solutions can often be applied to one's own life or the life of the person seeking advice.

The art of therapeutic storytelling is therefore less about finding stories which are "therapeutic" per se, and more about identifying situations that match existing stories and stories that match existing situations through the innate human skill of associative and metaphorical dreaming, and if necessary adapting the stories to the therapeutic context. This happens on a daily (and nightly) basis in our dreams and in unconscious verbal and nonverbal communication, but for therapeutic purposes it is vital for these involuntary metaphorical bridges to be consciously identified, remembered and if necessary written down. It is a good idea to train oneself to be on the alert for metaphorical and paradigmatic stories during therapeutic and everyday conversations, and to learn to be consciously aware of the internal daydreams that act as a constant commentary on what is being discussed.

## Using written sources

A treasure trove of insightful anecdotes, paradigmatic stories and metaphors suitable for use as therapeutic stories can be found in the books of wisdom and oral traditions of various cultures and religions. Jesus' parables in the first three Gospels are just as useful for therapeutic purposes as the Old Testament stories, and rabbinical anecdotes and Oriental and Chinese wisdom tales are just as valuable as the fables of Aesop, Jean de la Fontaine and James Thurber.

Endless inspiration can be found in the stories told by therapists of recent generations, for example the therapeutic stories of Paul Watzlawick and Milton Erickson.

Memorable "calendar stories" (of the type found in old almanacs) or newspaper stories, as well as biographies and biographical tales, provide further sources of inspiration. Valuable material can be found in anecdotes told by musicians or politicians, or in cartoons, jokes and newspaper or magazine articles.

Any story with a climactic turning point or a tantalisingly open ending, or which contains an example serving as a model or a deterrent, can help clients to move on from problem-induced paralysis and prompt them to search for solutions.

## Using oral sources

It is not only jokes, anecdotes and literary stories that include climactic turning points, but also many stories told in more everyday contexts, for example experiences shared between colleagues, friends and acquaintances. All of the strategies tested out by people in challenging situations and found useful can be helpful solutions, and even failed strategies can serve as an example of "how not to do it", or in other words a negative model. Many of the stories in this book are based on experiences recounted orally between friends, as indicated in the footnotes. Dialogues, proverbs and trenchant individual thoughts can, however, also be transformed into memorable stories if they are divided up between two individuals in a question/answer format, inventing a context if necessary.

It is useful to reiterate the fact that every story – including those told orally – serves a therapeutic purpose, and that the task of the therapist is to identify this purpose. Many oral stories are like uncut diamonds; they look rough, unremarkable and not very different from the rocks surrounding them, although they do have a certain glint. When the diamond is cut, however, everything that hides its clarity and beauty is removed, and a story's linguistic rhythm, sentence structure and choice of words can also be polished in order to reveal the diamond hidden inside it. The difference between good stories and diamonds is that anyone capable of recognising a story can discover new ones every day.

## Using one's own life as a source

Every experience that allows an individual to develop on a personal level is likely to serve as a valuable example for others and a metaphor for similar solutions in other spheres of life. Experiences associated with an increase in patterns of seeing and behaving are particularly valuable; by way of contrast, generalisations expressed with absolute statements such as "all", "always" or "never" are seldom helpful, since they tend to restrict potential ways of thinking and behaving rather than expand them. For example, conclusions starting, "Never again will I..." reduce existing opportunities for action and are therefore of questionable benefit. It is often better to present new perspectives in such a way that they supplement existing points of view rather than replacing them, ensuring that the new patterns of behaviour act as additional options that will increasingly supplant the old patterns of behaviour if they prove useful, but allowing the client (who is asked to test out different options and to keep what is beneficial) to decide what is useful.

The specific counselling context and the therapist's own views on the disclosure of personal information will determine whether a recounted story is referred to as one that he or she has personally experienced. Some may prefer to ascribe their own experiences to a protagonist such as "my friend

Peter", "a colleague", "a girl of your age" or an imaginary figure, although in my experience there is generally no reason why a therapist should not reveal that the events being discussed originate from his or her own past. Examples of stories I have experienced myself and which are told in the first or third person include "Exam Revision", "Catching Up" and "Bad English".

This approach increases the authenticity and congruence of what is being discussed, and rapport is often heightened if it emerges during storytelling that the client and therapist share certain life experiences. The imbalance of power between the therapist and client can also be reduced in this way, allowing a conversation between equals. If the therapist recounts earlier crises and problems that are similar to those experienced by the client but have been successfully overcome, this suggests that the client will likewise overcome his or her problems; "I faced similar problems to you, and look what became of me!" Messages such as these can be particularly helpful for children in crisis situations, cf. the story "You'll Manage It".

As well as biographical experiences, case studies about a therapist's previous clients also represent a rich vein of stories which can be mined for counselling purposes. Examples include "The Bladder Alarm Clock" and "The Man Who Wins When He Loses".

## Using films and other media as sources

Films represent a treasure trove of stories that can be used for therapeutic purposes; once a therapist is familiar with his or her client's favourite films, the films themselves or the genre as a whole can be used as a source of examples and metaphors, opening up the path to possible solutions. A film can serve as the basis for a discussion on the risks of a particular course of action and possible false turnings, as well as on the price and value of a certain goal, in each case applied to the patient's life. Like books and computer games, films automatically have a hypnotic effect; they induce guided dreams and therefore speak to the unconscious mind directly while circumventing conscious thought. The memory of a trance experience (i.e. watching a film) also induces a trance, which means that the discussion of a film automatically creates a hypnotic trance, which can be instrumental in bringing about change. Searching processes that produce results that can be applied by the unconscious mind to the listener's own life are activated not only by the films and books themselves, but also by an individual's memories of them, and this effect can be used proactively in a counselling context. For example, typical situations from TV programmes can be used as a starting point for therapeutic conversations; some therapists have even started allowing teenagers to show clips from their favourite videos during therapy sessions as a discussion starter (Carmen Beilfuss, conference presentation, 2003).

Partners attending couples counselling can be asked to look for films that suggest solutions to their problem, and systemic questions starting, "If someone were to make a film of your life…" have a similar effect. Finally, current real-life experiences can be reframed as a "film" in order to allow a certain distancing from the events and provide opportunities for changed perspectives and new responses. This procedure is illustrated by the story "The Film".

Teenagers can also be asked to write an advertisement for themselves, or to invent an imaginary computer game which can be used to practise their new mental skills. Examples of imaginary computer games include "The Recovery Game" and "Life as a Game".

Conversely, computer games which exist in reality can be discussed in order to identify the skills needed to succeed at playing them, and how these skills can be transferred from the virtual world into the world of real encounters. In both cases, it is useful to tell players that they can transfer the skills acquired in the game into everyday real life by imagining that a particular everyday situation is simply part of the game, until they have "upgraded" their confidence in themselves and their skills and opportunities.

I once received an email from a teenager who had been suffering from severe depression for the past two months, containing a link to a video and the words, "I've found someone just like me." His depression was now lifting, and it was obvious that the song lyrics, music and images had moved him deeply. The music video showed a malfunctioning robot searching in a state of helplessness and confusion not only for someone to fix him, but also for other robots just like him and for some way of becoming acceptable to others despite his inefficiency and defectiveness. The rusty old robot (which can clearly be seen to be a costume worn by a human) can be understood as a metaphor for a person seeking friendship and identity, acceptance and self-acceptance. The video clip in question was filmed by the German pop group "Wir sind Helden" for the song "Kaputt".

## Using other sources of communication

Problems are bound up with communication; they originate from dialogue with the surrounding world and from internal dialogue with oneself. Anyone with a "problem" perceives a difference between the current state of affairs (or his or her interpretation of it) and the desired state of affairs; or, to put it another way, "Anyone experiencing a problem is refusing to accept some aspect of reality." (Ron Reid Wilson, seminar discussion, 2007).

All problems that are experienced follow similar recurring structures, and any story that talks about finding a solution to a problem or failing to do so can be metaphorically applied to other types of problem, in the same way that all stories about successful and unsuccessful communication can be transferred to other areas of communication – not only communication between individuals, but also complex forms of communication in areas such as finance, trade, jurisdiction and research. For example, the story "Africa" uses communication between researchers and cartographers as a metaphor for the internal communication that takes place within the brain when constructing reality.

If we also include the non-verbal exchange of information between pack animals or between different species of animal (cf. the fable "From the Crocodile's Mouth") as well as the exchange of information within groups, within an entire nation and between nations, we can find many more examples of successful and unsuccessful communication. Further inspiration can be found in forms of communication between people and animals (cf. the stories "The Bulls Are Coming" and "The Little Cat"), and plants too have forms of communication for controlling their own organic processes and fending off animal and plant enemies as well as fungi, bacteria and viruses; these defence strategies can also be used for problem-solving purposes (cf. the fables "The Potential of Weeds" and "King of the Wood"). If we regard our conversations with ourselves as communication between different parts of our personality (cf. the story "Dinner for One"), and the dialogue between different organs and parts of our body (cf. the story "Keep All Cells Alive") as another form of communication, this opens up another group of metaphors for successful and unsuccessful communication, and further examples emerge if we include technical communication, particularly in the fields of electronics, computers and the Internet (cf. the story "The Recovery Game"). All these areas serve as a rich source of metaphors for ways of solving problems through communication with others or with oneself.

# Chapter 8

# Developing therapeutic stories through dialogue

## Developing stories through systemic questions

Questions are an extremely useful tool when developing stories together with clients. In the context of systemic therapy work, questions are often asked to construct a positive vision, clarifying the client's goals and identifying what steps might need to be taken to get there. For example, the therapist might ask, "Imagine we had a time machine and we could go forward in time five years to a period when this problem no longer existed and you were managing everything really well – what would have happened between now and then, and what would have been the first step you took to achieve it?" Similarly, the film-based intervention referred to above ("If someone were to make a film of your life…") involves dialogic storytelling on the basis of systemic questions.

Systemic questions have other important features from a hypnotherapeutic perspective; for the most part they are by no means neutral but instead contain implications, and not only expand the available information but also introduce new ideas discreetly. The alternatives and paths of action offered and the focusing of attention on resources or exceptions etc. mean that they represent indirect suggestions pointing towards a solution (cf. Erickson & Rossi, 1979: 31). As a general rule these implications are accepted by clients and only rarely questioned, and they therefore help to construct a new edifice of ideas (leading to new actions) out of the client's own conceptual building blocks, in a continuous behind-the-scenes process of pacing and leading in which the therapist follows along with the client's experience and at intervals incorporates a new element into his or her thoughts, which – if it is accepted – will result in solution-focused change.

A story can also be constructed on the basis of a series of questions. The relevant questions can be structured suggestively as a yes set, in which questions are initially asked to which a positive answer is expected, and the later questions in the series – which will generally receive a positive answer in the same way as the earlier questions – can serve to unburden the client. (For further information on the concept of a yes set, cf. Erickson & Rossi, 1979: 32.) An example of this procedure is as follows:

Individuals grieving the death of a loved one often feel guilty for his or her death, even if this is hard for outsiders to understand, and in many cases a thought experiment can help these individuals. The therapist can ask the grieving client, "Imagine we could speak to your mother right know and tell her how you feel, what would she reply? Would she reproach you? Would she forgive you?" If the answer is in the affirmative (which is usually the case), the conversation can continue, "Would this answer help you? Would you believe what your mother said?" and also, "If you're sure that this is what your mother would think, can you believe it even though we haven't really spoken to her?"

Questions are furthermore always trance-enhancing, because the client must direct his or her attention inwards and ignore the triggers of the external world in order to answer them. (For further information on trance induction through questions, cf. Erickson & Rossi, 1979: 28.) This effect is particularly reinforced by:

• Questions that require introspection ("Which part of you…")
• Questions that involve scoring or ranking ("Using percentages, how would you score… and how would you score…")
• Questions about sensory experiences ("If you imagine a fragrant meadow…")
• Questions to the past or future (age regression or age progression)
• Questions about situations which involve an altered state of attention (trance induction through trance memory)
• Circular questions in the narrower sense (trance induction through confusion or overtaxing)
• Series of questions, in particular involving repetition of the start of the sentence (trance induction through stereotype).

Questions can furthermore be used within a metaphor in order to develop therapeutically useful internal images. The rhetorical question in the story "Stand Up" demonstrates how depressive and debilitating life stories can be given a positive slant if they are thought through to their logical conclusion (cf. the story "Stand Up".) In storytelling terms, metaphorical negative models are changed into positive models in the client's thoughts by means of leading questions.

## Changing problem metaphors into solution metaphors

A simple and effective way for a therapist to start telling therapeutic stories is to begin with the stories which clients tell themselves, thus ensuring the highest possible relevance to the client's concerns and mirroring as closely as possible his or her way of thinking. In the same way that we dream on a nightly (and daily) basis, figures of speech – examples and metaphors – can be found in almost all of the sentences we utter.

Many of these figures of speech are metaphors, and the metaphors used involuntarily by clients provide direct access to the world of dreams from which they originate. Almost all of these metaphors tend to describe unresolved problems or solutions to problems, and a distinction can therefore be made between solution metaphors and problem metaphors. The relatively small number of solution metaphors can be reinforced and expanded by the therapist, preferably in dialogue with the client. If the client uses the saying "who dares wins", the therapist can ask the client what he or she might win and what it might be appropriate to dare, as well as about opportunities and risks and the resulting strategies for winning. If a client talks about the "light at the end of the tunnel", the therapist can ask the client to estimate his or her walking pace and the distance that remains until the end of the tunnel, and discuss together how long it will take to get outside and what level of effort will be involved. Most of the metaphors used by clients are however problem metaphors; they talk about the "thin ice" on which they are walking, the "thread" by which their relationship is hanging, and the experiences that "ruffle their feathers".

A useful therapeutic procedure is to convert a problem metaphor into a solution metaphor, which the client will involuntarily reintegrate into his or her interpretation of reality since it originates from the metaphorical language of his or her own dreams. The modified metaphor thus opens up a new way of seeing reality, without undermining basic assumptions or likes and dislikes. The internal map of the client's values and beliefs is not replaced, but merely redrawn from a solution-focused perspective during the therapeutic conversation.

In order to transform a problem metaphor into a solution metaphor, the therapist should firstly imagine the metaphor as vividly as possible and as a visual reality, including acoustic and kinaesthetic aspects if appropriate. There are then a number of different approaches that can be followed, as described below.

### Rules approach: following a metaphor's rules

The rules underlying a metaphor are taken seriously by the therapist and followed through to their logical conclusion. Every figure of speech refers to and implies certain rules; for example, the image of a pecking order implies that there is a hierarchy among chickens, and the image of a ceasefire implies that there can be intermediate states between war and peace that are appropriate in a given situation. Almost all metaphors refer to meaningful experiences, and anyone who restructures a problem metaphor into a solution metaphor using the rules approach merely amplifies the rules that apply to the experiences described until solutions emerge that are valid according to these rules. In many cases it is sufficient to think the metaphors through to their logical conclusion.

If a client states that in certain situations he or she always "starts to sweat", the therapist can follow the rules of sweating through to their logical conclusion and reply, "Sweating can be a good thing if it cools you down on a hot day." He or she can then hold a monologue on the fascinating ability of warm-blooded animals to keep their body temperature constant, and also ask, "Do you enjoy simply being in a hot environment, or would you rather work up a sweat through exercise?" He or she can also point out that sweating is often a good way for the body to get rid of toxins when it is fighting illness, and talk for a while about the purging effects of lime blossom tea, and ask the client what he or she would most like to purge if it were possible to mentally "sweat things out". Regardless of what "start to sweat" might mean in the client's life, and even if the therapist does not know what it means to the client, this approach will reframe the symptom as something pleasant and useful, and the client's unconscious mind will search for similarly structured (isomorphic) solutions among the strategies available to him or her.

If the client can still demonstrate the symptomatic behaviour after a conversation similar to the above (which is by no means always the case), and if he or she still finds it problematic (which would be unusual), further consideration can be given to methods of dealing with sweating and its consequences, still following the rules approach. For example, the client might propose wearing fewer layers, applying deodorant, having a shower or similar ideas. Without saying so, the therapist implies to the client's unconscious mind that these responses should be applied (in metaphorical terms) to the situations in which he or she "starts to sweat"; the client has been led to a solution-based attitude allowing him or her to handle the situation very differently, and there is nothing more that needs to be done by the therapist.

If the therapist nevertheless wishes to go further, he or she can ask, "How will your mental outfit be different next time you find yourself in this situation? What might a shower for the mind look like? Or a psychological deodorant? What do you think it might smell like?" In cognitive terms these questions appear to be meaningless, but they prompt the unconscious mind to search in the world of dreams for solutions to the problem which gave rise to the metaphor.

One alternative to considering the positive implications of the client's metaphor is to think about what would happen in its absence. In order to do so, the therapist can present the client with a negative model of the metaphor he or she initially used, as follows;

"Sweating is generally regarded as the evolutionary trump card of certain mammals. Some people think the dinosaurs died out because most of them were cold-blooded and were unable to regulate their temperature." The above might have nothing whatsoever to do with the client's situation, but it will suggest the following to his or her unconscious mind; "Don't look for alternatives which are not available to you! Be modern and adaptable! If you don't want to be a dinosaur, be yourself and use the opportunities at your disposal!"

Whimsical digressions of this kind are generally well received by clients if they are presented in an entertaining manner and promote a searching attitude; as mentioned above, however, it is important to introduce and conclude such stories – which may be structurally and substantively different to anything the client has previously encountered – in such a way that he or she accepts them. After a conceptual detour of this kind, the therapist can return to the client's problem, apologising for his or her lack of self-discipline – or he or she can move on to another metaphor which relates more obviously to the client's questions.

A variant on the procedure of transforming problem metaphors into solution metaphors is the reframing approach, which involves adopting another perspective (based on a different place, time or person) and ascribing positive connotations to it. If a client says, "My husband told me I look like a whore when I wear a leather mini-skirt," the answer might be, "Perhaps that's because you turn him on."

Use of the rules approach to describe a situation in which a negative model leads to disaster can be described as a paradoxical approach. A client who says, "It would be like locking the stable door after the horse had bolted," could be told the following story:

"A long long time ago, a horse did bolt out of its stable in a village near here. A child saw it happen, ran to his mother and told her, 'The horse has bolted out of the stable!' 'Oh dear,' said the mother, and looked in the stable. The horse was indeed gone, so she went into the house and told the father. He went and looked in the stable, and agreed that the horse was really gone. He asked his parents what should be done, and they said he should call the vet. He called the vet, and he arrived and said that it was a job for the police. They called the police, and the police arrived and said it was no longer a job for them, since the horse had already been killed by a truck on the main road..."

### Exception approach: finding the exception to a metaphor

The rules that underlie metaphors can therefore be elucidated before transforming the metaphors themselves – which have been anchored for many years in the client's unconscious mind – and returning these transformed metaphors to the client as bearers of psychological health. Alternatively, the therapist and the client can work together to come up with plausible exceptions and modifications, which can be reintegrated into the patient's interpretation of the world together with the relevant metaphors.

If a patient says that he or she "missed the connection" or that "that train is long gone", the therapist can mention an interview he or she read with a woman who narrowly escaped the Eschede derailment because she missed the train, or tell a story about a man who missed a train but met the love of his life when waiting for the following one.

The disadvantage of the exception approach compared to the rules approach is that it is often less plausible; nevertheless, it is a reliable tool that can be used when clients employ extremely destructive metaphors. It is probably a bad idea to remind someone who refers to a challenging meeting with a boss and his colleagues as "meeting the firing squad" of the positive aspects of being executed at gunpoint; instead, the many different options offered by the exception approach can be used. From mock executions and jail breaks to last-minute pardons – even the looming enactment of a death penalty offers scope for exceptions, and the same applies for most other destructive metaphors.

When using the exception approach, it is important to prevent the patient from contradicting the exception with statements such as "that doesn't apply in my case". It is a good idea to ensure that an exception-based story is as plausible as possible, to deliver it in a self-assured manner, to ask the client how he or she thinks the story might have a "happy ending", and if necessary to avoid leaving time for "yes, but" objections.

### Cartoon approach: the flexible design of metaphors

A very effective way of designing metaphors involves recognising that a metaphor is in oneself rather than oneself being in the metaphor, and that a metaphor resembles an animated produced in one's head. I might previously have regarded my workplace as a gilded cage, but now that I know that this is simply a film inside my head, I understand that the cage is in me rather than the other way around. Once a client realises that metaphors of this kind are images created in his or her brain which can also be changed by the brain, he or she can make any changes he wishes and will generally also accept them. As the director of the film, he can decide whether to open the door of the cage, to saw through the bars or to bend them apart.

If a client regards a planned change as impossible, this means that his or her unconscious mind has decided against it because a solution of this kind is inappropriate. It might be that the client cannot imagine how a prison guard or owner of the cage comes to open its door, with the implication that his or her unconscious mind wishes to bring about a solution actively through its own efforts rather than to wait for other people. The same individual will however probably be able to imagine discovering a hidden key and opening the cage himself or herself, for example.

Introducing a film approach by referring to a cartoon is a good idea because literally everything is possible in cartoons, meaning that no restrictions are imposed on the potential solutions. Other genres can nevertheless be used if the therapist knows that these are particularly well suited to the client's individual preferences.

### Variations on the theme

These techniques can be implemented creatively with children (and with adults who are open to the idea) using paints, playdough, poetry, puppets, pantomime and other techniques. After the therapist has made verbal reference to the metaphor used by the client and interpreted it literally, he or she can ask the client to express it creatively, or create a picture or sculpture according to the client's instructions. For example, he or she might write out an imaginary package insert for medication and ask, "What symptoms could this behaviour – which you say is poisoning your daily life – be used to treat if the dosage were appropriately low? Would it be a conventional drug or a homeopathic remedy? Would it desensitise the patient, or act as an antibiotic? Would it be a sedative or a stimulant? For whom might it be useful in suitable doses, and what would be the indicated dose in specific cases?" Similarly, the therapist could draw on a flip chart a chemical plant for the manufacture of toxic behaviour, adding in routes to customers and asking why these customers might buy the relevant behaviour and keep the chemical plant in business despite complaints from the people who lived nearby. The therapist and client could then discuss whether it would be useful and feasible to impose a strict ban on the poisonous behaviour, and how environmental regulations might otherwise be applied to the production and use of this substance.

## Developing stories together with children

Telling stories is a particularly good way of engaging in dialogue with children; "Yes, and who do you think the sad eagle met there? ... That's right – a magician... And what did the magician tell the eagle to do so that his wings would heal as soon as possible? ... And what did the magician tell the eagle to do to stop the other eagles from picking on him? ... And if the magician could somehow see into the future and found out that the eagle later made lots of new friends, how do you think the eagle would have found these friends? How does the story continue, from the magician's idea to finding the new friends? What do you think happened in between?"

One of the good things about therapy sessions involving children is that they generally have very low demands in terms of the narrative completeness of an invented story. The therapist and the child can make up stories together to their hearts' content by engaging in dialogue; the only prerequisite for work of this kind is that everything that is told and played must have some kind of parallel to the child's situation and transform a problem into a solution in his or her imagination.

For example, the therapist and a child can play together with stuffed animals experiencing similar problems – as well as an animal who represents the child and an animal who represents the child's opponent, the therapist can also introduce friendly animals who help each other. The animals might represent family members or feelings, a symptom and freedom from that symptom or any conceivable source of strength and resources that can be used by the child and his family. What is most important is that the therapist allows plenty of space for the child's own ideas so that the child can play out various solutions with the animals (provided that the good side always wins, of course).

The simplest of methods can be used to invent effective stories during therapy sessions with children; for example, a shy girl can be told how knights at knight school used to learn to put on their suits of armour and use their weapons, and how a brave damsel once disguised herself and learned everything that the knights learned, and after a short period amazed everyone by proving herself to be much better at attacking and defending than any of the other knights. The therapist might talk about three brave mice who encounter problems every afternoon which are similar to those which the child experienced in school that morning, and who show the fox, the wolf and the bear how brave a mouse can really be.

In order to keep the dialogue going, and in some cases to gain extra thinking time, children can be asked questions such as the following; "After the small dragon had burned so many children by accident with his hot breath, no one wanted to play with him any more. But then the sad little dragon met someone who knew just what he should do – who do you think it was?"

I once put this question to a child who was busy blowing bubbles, and she answered, "A great big bubble!" Regardless of how illogical the answer may seem, the story can still continue: "That's right! The bubble said to the dragon, 'Listen, little dragon! I have an idea. It will soon be winter, and all the animals will be cold. Anyone who can burn people can also warm them up. Do you think you can manage to warm people up and find more friends?' What do you think the dragon answered? Did the dragon manage to warm up the other animals?"

Other family members who are present can naturally also be involved in the process; "Why don't we ask Mummy? Or maybe Daddy?" If a story is developed jointly in this way, further episodes of the story will often be told by the family at home.

Since the solutions that emerge during conversations of this kind have been jointly identified by the child, he or she will (consciously or unconsciously) transfer them to his or her everyday life and put them into practice. Stories of this kind generally deliver visible results with startling speed, generally by the following therapy session.

# Chapter 9

# Inventing therapeutic stories

## Types of therapeutic stories

### Paradigmatic and metaphorical stories

Therapeutic stories can be divided into rough genres on the basis of a distinction between metaphorical stories and paradigmatic stories, using the following criterion; metaphors involve the transfer of many elements from a different context into the patient's own life, whereas a paradigmatic story only requires changes to be made to a few elements, for example the protagonist or the time and place of the events, before it reflects the patient's current situation.

Metaphors tend to correspond to the situation in which they are told in structural terms and to differ from it in substantive terms, since they originate from a different context.

The story "The Dung Beetle" contains a metaphor; if the dung beetle is understood to be a person and his release from the child's hand interpreted as an escape from any challenging situation, the metaphor can be transferred to the listener's current problems. The similarities between the story and reality apply at a structural rather than a substantive level.

Paradigmatic stories tend to resemble the listener's current situation in both structural and substantial terms. There is no question of transferring situations from one sphere of life into another; instead, the listener merely needs to replace individual characters or locations to make the story applicable to his or her own life.

The story "The Schneiders" is a paradigmatic story, since only a few small details (possibly only the surname) would need to be changed to apply it to the listener's own circumstances.

In both genres, a distinction can be made between dynamic stories with active protagonists (as with the metaphor in the story "The Eagle Chick" and the example in the story "The Power of Thoughts"), and static descriptions and tales (as with the metaphor in the story "Africa").

There is no fixed boundary between metaphors and paradigmatic stories, and often the same story can be told once as a paradigmatic story for direct application to the patient's life, and again as a metaphor for application to a different sphere of life. This implies that it is not merely the form of a story that determines whether it is paradigmatic or metaphorical, but also the purpose for which it is used. Certain stories occupy an intermediate position since they can be very easily transferred to a different situation, for example cases where the relationship between a pet owner and his or her pet or between two animals serves as an illustration of similar behaviour between two people. Metonyms – which take one aspect of a person or object as representative of the whole (*pars pro toto*), for example a steering wheel standing for the car, a capital city for the government or the head for the entire person – also occupy an intermediate position. For instance, the body can be shown through metonymic instructions that it is capable of suppressing reflexes using the example of the eyes, and this knowledge will involuntarily be applied by the body to the suppression of hiccups (the original problem). This approach is exemplifed by the story "The Frozen Hiccup".

These different approaches can also be combined: an object, word or situation with metaphorical connotations can be used as part of a reality-based example.

### Positive models, negative models and searching models

Both metaphorical and paradigmatic stories can be divided into several categories depending on the therapeutic purpose for which they are used (Hammel 2012b: 151); Bandler and Grinder distinguished between isomorphic (structurally similar) and directive (warning) metaphors (Bandler & Grinder, 1981: 134).

Listeners respond to isomorphic metaphors by applying them to their own lives; by way of contrast, directive metaphors engender a desire to avoid experiences similar to those described in metaphorical terms. I prefer a different categorisation, based on the work of the communications theorists Watzlawick, Jackson and Beavin Bavelas (Watzlawick et al., 1976: 56), who postulate three basic human forms of response; acceptance ("yes"), rejection ("no") and disqualification ("neither yes nor no"). Three types of metaphorical or paradigmatic stories can be identified on the basis of this categorisation; those which the listener is likely to accept, those which the listener is likely to reject and those which are likely to leave the listener in a state of uncertainty. I refer to these three types respectively as positive models, negative models and searching models.

As a general rule, positive models engender an attitude of internal agreement (rapport) which can serve as a useful basis for the ongoing counselling relationship, and most metaphorical stories belong to this type. Metaphorical positive models demonstrate a productive way of behaving and experiencing in a sphere of life other than that described by the client, thus manifesting in the world of the imagination (which is free of stresses and blocks) potential solution structures that can be transferred back into a real world full of stresses. Although these models resemble dreams, the solutions they contain may have a parallel application in real life, allowing the listener's unconscious mind to examine the associated opportunities without experiencing any stress. One example of this approach is the metaphorical story "Almost Too Late and Not Too Early";

> A lifeguard once told me, "If someone who is drowning is still panicking and flailing around, it's impossible to get them to dry land. You have to wait until they've calmed down, and then you can rescue them."

The story "Love" is another example of a positive model as a paradigmatic story;

> I was travelling in the same train carriage as them. My diary was stuffed full of meetings, whereas they were two people in love who had all the time in the world. She looked into his eyes and smiled. He smiled back.
> "If you hadn't talked to me when I was sitting on the park bench that day, I'd still be sat on my own in the home with all the other old dears."

It is easy for a listener to apply stories such as these to his or her own life, since all he or she needs to do is to replace the characters before envisioning his or her own "happy ending". Individuals with a pronounced "yes, but" habit will however sometimes raise cognitive objections to these positive paradigmatic stories precisely because they are so easily transferrable, and these consciously expressed objections may develop into negative autosuggestions telling the individual that "there is no way out"; in such cases preference should be given to metaphorical stories or the negative or searching models described below. The messages in these latter stories are applied to the listener's own life through a more complex procedure, meaning that the logical (and sceptical) conscious mind is for the most part bypassed, and the story is primarily responded to by the creative and associative unconscious mind. This avoids "yes, but" discussions which stifle motivation ("that will never work for me," "I've already tried all of those things," "if you only knew...") and which impede the search for creative solutions.

In literary terms, negative models are sometimes referred to as tragedies, and the well-known stories of the German Struwwelpeter ("Shock-headed Peter") are exclusively negative models, aimed at engendering resistance to and avoidance of the described behaviour; in a worst-case scenario, however, they also provoke reactance. All aversive methods in the field of hypnotherapy are related to this type. Negative models demonstrate an outcome of a situation that must be prevented at all costs, and the actions that must accordingly be avoided. Their message resembles that of a nightmare in that they send a signal to the unconscious to avoid all associated situations, come what may. The following is a negative model in the form of an unreal paradigmatic story;

> A man was driving along the road in his car when he spotted a police car at the edge of the road. He stopped, got out and spoke to the police officers: "You're not doing roadside checks, are you? I haven't drunk anything! Not a drop!"

A further example can be found in the story "A Single Request". An example of a metaphorical negative model can be found in the story "The Potential of Weeds":

> They were silent for a long time. Then the little dandelion asked his much larger neighbour, "What are you doing?"
> "I'm growing my taproot."
> "That's what I'm doing too. But I've made no progress for days. My root has hit a stone."
> "Just do what the couch grass does and grow your root around the stone. Grow more roots if necessary," said the big dandelion.
> "I can't do that," said the small dandelion. "A taproot is a taproot."
> And he never grew any larger.

A further example can be found in the story "The Cart, The Mud and I".

Stories which are suitable for use as searching models are those to which the listener cannot spontaneously answer "yes" or "no" because of the difficulty involved in assessing the relevance of the story to his or her life. Instead, the listener's response is one of perplexity, confusion or bafflement, placing him or her in the searching and questioning state of mind that is necessary to solve the story's puzzle. Stories based on a searching model are therefore similar to mysterious dreams in that they invite the listener to embark on a search while deliberately providing no answer or solution. An example of a searching model is the metaphorical story "Children's Shoes";

> "I've only just started learning what to do," said the apprentice. "How can I pretend to know everything already?"
> "Buy children's shoes which are one size larger," replied his instructor.

The listener can also be invited to embark on a search by means of stories based on questions rather than puzzles. The following is an example of a searching model in the form of a paradigmatic story:

> Do you know the story of the woman who had a pair of surgical scissors left in her stomach by a surgeon? What happened to her in the end?

Further examples include the stories "My Aim in Life", "What Does That Make Me?" and "The Creation of the World".

Many stories cannot be clearly assigned to one of these three types; they are of a composite nature, and it is often possible to identify individual elements belonging to the first, second and third story type in them.

### Classification model for therapeutic story types

Therapeutic stories can therefore be classified into six story types, which are listed in the table below together with examples.

| Story as... | Example | Metaphor |
|---|---|---|
| Positive model (isomorphy, promoting acceptance) | Stop | Pulling the Goat Home |
| Negative model (warning, promoting resistance) | The Consultation | The Cart, The Mud and I |
| Searching model (puzzle, incongruity, promoting a searching attitude) | The Creation of the World | The Cave Dwellers |

The boundaries between the various story types are fluid, and composite types such as the following can often be found:

Example as negative model and searching model: "Theatre Trip".
Metaphor as positive model and negative model: "The Lipoma".
Example and metaphor as positive model: "The Sailor on Shore".

## Basic forms of suggestion

### Declarative suggestion

Verbal suggestions can be divided into four basic types, which I refer to as declarative, directive, implied and questioning. Implied suggestions are not expressed out loud, instead being concealed in the context of the statement, whereas directive suggestions are formulated as orders and therefore involve an (as yet) unreal element. Declarative suggestions are identical to explicit statements, while suggestions that are disguised as questions represent a special form of implication which is accepted or rejected by the client in his or her silent or voiced answer. Erickson and Rossi refer to declarations and imperatives as "direct suggestion", and to implications, ambiguities, connotations, verbal allusions and similar therapeutic methods that act suggestively by association as "indirect suggestion" (Erickson & Rossi, 1979: 18).

There are open and concealed forms of all the different types of suggestion; an example of an open declaration would be the storyteller saying to the listener after telling the story "Pirate Anaesthesia":

"Hey, you can't move your leg any more!"

An example of a hidden declaration would be as follows;

Then the pirate told himself, "Never mind, you can't move your leg anyway!"

Or

"That's the thing about being a sleeping pirate – you can no longer move your leg."

This statement is ambiguous in that it suggests that both pirates and "you" (the listener) can no longer move their leg. The following is a further example of a hidden declaration;

"I'm sure you realise how difficult it is for pirates to move their wooden leg while they're asleep. Imagine that you're a pirate yourself, confident that you'll no longer do it consciously – and just think how much less you'll do it unconsciously!"

The following declarations are integrated into these statements:

You're self-confident!
You'll no longer do it consciously!
You'll do it even less unconsciously!

If the story is told in isolation and without any context, the declarations will probably only be understood as a prompt to lose the ability to move the leg, and the association previously established between "motionless" and "numb" will probably also result in the leg feeling numb. If the story is told in the context of the problems which prompted the client to come to counselling, however, the unconscious mind will also understand the declarations to mean, "Do not consciously do the action which has previously caused problems!" and "You'll unconsciously do the action much less frequently (than before)!" The likelihood that the listener will relate the suggestions to his or her problem and implement them increases if a number of similar suggestions are incorporated into the story one after another.

Declarative instructions to the body represent one example of suggestive declarations; the client – or his or her therapist – tells the body what it already (perhaps unconsciously) knows and can do and what it will therefore (definitely) do. The target audience for instructions of this kind can be not only the body as a whole, but also a part of the body or a bodily function, as in "Mrs Brain". This constitutes a form of psychoeducation for the body, based on the idea that the mind is part of the body, and indeed such an integral part that the body naturally understands and can implement what the mind understands.

### Directive suggestion

It goes without saying that many suggestions can also be issued as orders. Although many therapists are reluctant to use this register of speech, the following suggestion by a therapist to a client can nevertheless have a very powerful effect: "Bow down to yourself in the mirror at home and say to yourself, 'I have not treated you well. Please forgive me!'" In my opinion, however, it is important to respect the client's autonomy by not insisting on compliance with therapeutic instructions.

A less direct but perhaps gentler and more elegant method is to tell a story about someone who received the above instructions from a wise old woman, and was first irritated by them, but then found himself or herself unable to fall asleep in the evening, repeatedly tried out the words that had been suggested and felt increasingly contented.

Directive suggestions can also provoke reactance, particularly if they are difficult for the client to understand on an objective or emotional level. An example of this problem can be found in the Biblical tale of Naaman, a commander who fell ill with leprosy and asked the prophet Elisha to heal him;

> [103] "So Naaman went with his horses and chariots and stopped at the entrance to Elisha's house. Elisha sent a servant out to tell him to go and wash himself seven times in the Jordan River, and he would be completely cured of his disease. But Naaman left in a rage, saying, 'I thought that he would at least come out to me, pray to the Lord his God, wave his hand over the diseased spot, and cure me! Besides, aren't the rivers Abana and Pharpar, back in Damascus, better than any river in Israel? I could have washed in them and been cured!' His servants went up to him and said, 'Sir, if the prophet had told you to do something difficult, you would have done it. Now why can't you just wash yourself, as he said, and be cured?' So Naaman went down to the Jordan, dipped himself in it seven times, as Elisha had instructed, and he was completely cured. His flesh became firm and healthy like that of a child." (2 Kings 5:9)

People who – as a result of their upbringing or professional experience – are used to following orders and demonstrating obedience often respond to directive suggestions by involuntarily but wholeheartedly executing what has been requested. It was therefore a good idea for Elisha to issue an order, but the prophet perhaps forgot the importance of establishing rapport beforehand in order to ensure that the therapist is perceived by client as a parental or superior figure. It is however more likely that he responded to the double bind, "Heal me, I am armed," with the counter double bind; "I reject you. If you accept that, I will accept you." Further examples of a counter double bind are given in the stories "How Do You Break a Spell?" and "The Man Who Wins When He Loses".

Auto-suggestions issued as orders represent a very different form of directive therapeutic suggestion. Directive instructions to the body follow the pattern "Dear body, please do this and that for me"; since we often do not know which behaviour will benefit the body most and which side effects might be associated with a changed behaviour, it is generally also useful to ask the body to carry out checks: "Dear body, please check whether..., and if it proves useful, keep on doing it" as in the stories "Keep All Cells Alive" and "The Silent Hand". The spirit, the soul, the memory, the imagination, the brain or one's own name can be addressed in a similar fashion.

Directive instructions of this kind can be issued openly by directly and clearly addressing the client or part of his or her body. They can also be issued in a concealed form if they are incorporated ambiguously into a story in which they primarily express something else (cf. the story "Placebo IV").

### Implied suggestion

Implications are the unspoken messages which the listener automatically associates (or can be expected to associate) with the messages expressed out loud, but which are not generally perceived by the conscious mind. The statement "Do not change yet" implies "Change, but do it at a later point in time". The statement "Think hard about a number" implies that other irrelevant things that come to mind more readily should be ignored. The sentence "I think you should overhaul your alarm system" in the story "Call-Out" relates primarily to a troop of firefighters, but is also an instruction to the body to overhaul its immune system.

Metaphors often contain complex and multi-layered implications. If you tell a child a story about an eagle chick, the child will probably identify with the animal, and accept the implication that chicks fly the nest, travel far away from home and later establish their own eyrie. In all likelihood, the story will help the child to become more independent of his or her parents, or at least examine the option of behaving more independently.

The effects of implications are far-reaching. In the story "Pirate Anaesthesia", the listener is invited to identify with a pirate. This is an intriguing prospect which reawakens childhood memories, and most people will engage with it and remember their boyhood or girlhood dreams. Children will see it as entirely plausible that a pirate should wear a wooden leg, and so most people will accept this. Wood feels no pain and cannot move, so imagining a wooden leg induces numbness and immobility. In the story, the pirate unstraps his wooden leg; it is plausible that a wooden leg should be unstrapped, and most people will also accept this. A body part that has been separated from the torso cannot be felt and cannot move, and imagining the unstrapped wooden leg therefore induces yet deeper anaesthesia and immobility. According to the story, the pirate goes to sleep and dreams, which is logical and will therefore generally be accepted. People do not usually feel anything when they are asleep, and also mostly move less than when they are wide awake, so this induces yet deeper anaesthesia and immobility. In the story, the pirate dreams of his wooden leg swimming on the ocean like a sailing boat; this is also readily comprehensible, and will therefore again be accepted. It is implied that during the rest of the story the wooden leg no longer belongs to the first reality which is experienced when awake, but to the second reality which is experienced when dreaming, and that an object which disappears further and further into the distance is less and less under the control of its owner, in particular when the owner is asleep. According to the story, the wooden leg disappears over the horizon; this too is plausible and will be accepted, and implies a complete loss of control over the limb.

If a storyteller takes his or her time and tells the pirate story properly, it is therefore likely that the mobility and sensitivity of the listener's leg will be greatly reduced. The pirate could be left dreaming that he is made entirely of wood, or that he himself is the sailing ship, in which case the immobility and numbness would spread out throughout the entire body.

The story therefore incorporates implicit instructions for hypnotic anaesthesia, catalepsy, dissociation and amnesia. *Anaesthesia* is achieved as follows: (1) through trance induction in general; (2) through the implication that wood does not feel anything, (3) through the analogy of the blind eye; (4) through the shifting of attention to the sense of sight and the sense of balance; (5) through the implication that a leg separated from its torso does not feel anything; (6) through the implication that we do not feel anything when we are asleep; (7) through the implication that the leg is merely a dream in the rest of the story; (8) through the fact that the leg floats away and disappears; (9) through the statement that the pirate no longer knows where the leg is. *Catalepsy* (rigidity of the body) is achieved in particular through the reference to "a wooden leg made from strong and solid old oak" and the "hard, rigid oak leg". *Dissociation* (mental separation) of the leg from the torso is achieved by imagining that the leg is made from another material, by unstrapping the leg, by imagining sleep and by dreaming that the leg is floating away. *Amnesia* (gaps in memory) is achieved by imagining sleep and by the concluding statement that the pirate no longer knows where his wooden leg is. It can be reinforced by a subsequent suggestion of a deep and dreamless sleep.

The storyteller could end the story with the invitation, "And now just try to make a single movement with your leg!" He or she would still be using implications, but at the level of "real" bodily experiences rather than at a metaphorical level. The word "try" implies that failure is pre-programmed, the word "just" implies that the listener should under no circumstances do more than try, and the word "single" implies that only one attempt should be made. Since the unconscious is always listening on several levels, these instructions will be unconsciously understood and generally also implemented.

Changes in bodily reactions – as a potential goal of therapeutic stories – can be achieved not only through declarative or imperative suggestions as discussed above, but also through metaphorical instructions (as in "The Recovery Game" and "The Villa"), metonymic instructions (as in "The Frozen Hiccup", "The Bladder Alarm Clock" and "The Silent Hand") or otherwise implicit instructions to the body (as in "Risk of Contagion"). Just like most bodily functions, most mental and social functions can also be influenced by way of implications incorporated into metaphorical instructions. (For further information on the forms and effects of suggestive implications, see Erickson & Rossi, 1979: 38.)

### Questioning suggestion

A special form of implied suggestion involves suggestion through questioning. Most of the questions asked during a therapy session – or at least those that are not anamnesis-related – contain open or hidden implications which can produce a solution to a problem. For example, a dichotomous question implies that the listener must choose between the proposed alternatives, while other suggestive questions (such as rhetorical questions, which allow only one answer or one type of answer) might advocate a point of view that was previously alien to the client but which might be useful for problem-solving purposes. Many systemic questions, such as exception questions, divert the listener's attention away from his or her paralysing problems and towards the energy-bestowing resources inherent to the situation. Many questions, in particular puzzling or unanswerable questions (as the closing question in the story "Releasing the Spring" and the questions in the story "Dot to Dot"), also serve to induce a searching attitude in the client (and in the therapist). This function of stimulating a seaching attitude can be exemplified by the questions in the story "The Creation of the World".

## Basic therapeutic storytelling interventions

### Real and unreal reframing

People invariably describe the situations in their life through the prism of a particular interpretation, and many such interpretations exist for any perceived event or action. After inviting a client to consider a situation from an alternative perspective, we can therefore propose a different retelling of his story, using identical events but reconstructing the relationship between them – the same picture, but in a different frame. In the field of systemic therapy, the term "reframing" is used to refer to the procedure of retelling a client's life stories from a solution-based perspective rather than the original problem-based perspective.

The technique of reframing can be used somewhat more elegantly if we ask the client to imagine someone else seeing the situation in an alternative way, and ask what difference that makes. We can of course also tell the client about a colleague of ours and what she would say if she heard the story; this approach will potentially result in less resistance and a more positive attitude on the part of the client.

The technique of reframing can be used yet more elegantly if the therapist explains the very different interpretations that other people have ascribed to a similar situation. The examples that can be used include case studies from the therapist's own practice, a personal experience or a scene from a TV drama or a novel, or of course an invented story, such as a short dialogue that summarises the different points of view or a fable in which animals are responsible for illustrating a different interpretation of a story similar to that told by the client.

The technique of reframing can therefore be applied to the situation described by the client (cf. the story "On the Threshold"), a comparable paradigmatic situation or an isomorphic metaphor (cf. the stories "The Pruned Tree" and "Noah's Brothers"). A distinction can be made between situational, paradigmatic and metaphorical reframing, depending on the starting point used as a basis for reinterpreting the story. In the case of paradigmatic reframing, and particularly in the case of metaphorical reframing, it is to be expected that the offered solutions will be processed to a lesser extent by the conscious mind and to a greater extent by the unconscious mind, resulting in a lower level of scepticism ("yes but" attitude) on the part of the client.

When discussing the goal of reframing (reinterpretation), a distinction should be made between two different types of stories, which I refer to as real reframing and unreal reframing. This distinction is particularly important during situational reframing, or in other words when the actual situation presented by the client is reinterpreted.

Paradigmatic and metaphorical reframing almost always involves real reframing, since the stories involved can be freely shaped and flexibly designed without recourse to unreal interpretations.

Real reframing means the introduction of a new perspective which is compatible with our usual interpretation of reality. Within the framework of a therapeutic conversation, a woman who has previously perceived her husband's jealousy as an insulting lack of trust can attempt to reach an understanding of the same behaviour as an expression of his love and passion for her, or as evidence of her own attractiveness. If the woman reinterprets her husband's behaviour, her behaviour towards him will also change, and the reverse applies to her husband; if he can reinterpret her hurt as an expression of her faithfulness, it is likely that his behaviour towards her will also change.

The above-mentioned methods of transforming problem metaphors into solution metaphors on the basis of a rules approach or an exception approach involve real reframing on the basis of metaphorical positive models (isomorphic metaphors).

Unreal reframing is characterised by the fact that an unreal interpretation is imposed on a real situation in order to make the latter more pleasant and facilitate helpful responses. The woman mentioned above could imagine her jealous husband singing a wistful serenade and say to herself, "He's searching for the words to describe my beauty." One advantage of unreal reframing is that quite literally any change whatsoever can be enacted in the form of internal images, and although this does not result in a direct change to external reality (or perhaps it does, because there is no such thing as external reality, and only internal reality?), unreal reframing may extensively remodel psychological, physical and social patterns of behaviour and also provoke entirely new responses to the social environment through a change in attitude. The above-mentioned method of transforming problem metaphors into solution metaphors using a cartoon approach involves unreal reframing on the basis of isomorphic metaphors.

Unreal reframing can be used as a healing suggestion (cf. the stories "Morbus Feivel" and "Risk of Contagion"), to lighten the mood (cf. the story "November Blues"), to overcome anxiety and shyness (cf. the story "Peer and Rasputin") or to boost work motivation in stressful situations (cf. the stories "That Day", "The Film" and "Social Noises"). Unreal reframing is an effective way of inducing a wide range of trance phenomena, such as hypnotic anaesthesia and amnesia, dissociation from body parts, catalepsy, hypermnesia and time distortion. Examples of the therapeutic use of the above-mentioned trance phenomena in this way include the stories "A Walk Along the Beach, "The Unscrewable Body", "Pirate Anaesthesia", "The Archivist" and "Time Adjustment" (listed in the same order as the trance phenomena).

Thanks to enormous scope it provides for creativity, unreal reframing also offers a treasure trove of opportunities for self-coaching. Some forms of unreal reframing have proved particularly useful for remodelling physical, psychological and social patterns of behaviour.

In cases where invisible friends are used for therapeutic purposes (for example the stories "Peer and Rasputin", "Mr Peabrain" and "Invisible Friends") resources are imagined in externalised form as helpers, following the example of children who acquire imaginary friends who support and entertain them. In hypnotherapeutic settings such figures are often referred to as "power animals", but their benefits extend far beyond their traditional use as a tool to boost self-confidence, as demonstrated by "Mr Peabrain", an imaginary companion who takes away pain. In a similar way, the character in the story "Selling Pain" hands over her physical pains to invisible customers.

Mental games are an important subgenre of unreal reframing, for example in the form of imaginary computer games or films ("The Recovery Game" and "The Film") but also in the form of a thought experiment which allows the imaginative reinterpretation of real-life experiences ("That Day", "Social Noises" and "The King Is Coming"). Mental games can be used to strengthen the immune system ("The Recovery Game"), to improve mood ("November Blues") or to boost one's ability to withstand and defend oneself against insults ("Life as a Game").

Stories which use unreal placebos – where the administration of a medication or form of treatment is only imagined, but the same therapeutic effect is achieved – have important applications in the field of medicine. The stories "Placebo I" to "Placebo IV" represent examples of the use of unreal placebos. Looking at or painting on the medication can produce similar effects on a metaphorical level ("Wart Remedy"). Instructions can also be issued to the body using a statement similar to the following; "Please behave in the way that you would normally behave when undergoing this medical treatment" (cf. "Placebo IV"). The patient will be aware that the placebo is not a pharmacologically effective medication, which is not the case for standard placebos, but it is unlikely to be difficult to prove that real placebos often produce the intended effects even if they are administered to the recipient with the comment that they are a "highly effective placebo"; studies in the field of hypnosis therapy have also shown that placebos can work effectively even if the patient knows what they are.

Other forms of unreal reframing include thought experiments which could never occur in reality (cf. the story "When You Meet Your Brother") and accounts of fictitious or real dreams which relate to events that would be impossible in our waking reality. The dreams in the stories "Pirate Anaesthesia" and "The Blade of Grass in the Crack" demonstrate this tendency.

### Destabilisation and stabilisation

Systemic and hypnotherapeutic counselling takes advantage of the fact that there are always different interpretations of reality by applying the technique of reframing, which involves looking at the patient's habitual reality from an unusual perspective and reinterpreting it in the process. More specifically, this method combines two different procedures in one, namely the deconstruction of reality and the reconstruction of reality, or alternatively the destabilisation of the construction of reality which previously prevailed and the introduction and stabilisation of a new construction. Anyone who wishes to take a slower and perhaps more thorough approach to the reinterpretation of previous beliefs about the world can therefore break the procedure down into two different stages; firstly the therapist introduces the idea that the client's previous interpretation of reality may not be entirely reliable, and then he or she works together with the client to search for possible alternative interpretations. For more information on the deconstruction of beliefs and the identities ascribed to a person (cf. Monk et al., 1996: 95).

Habitual patterns of thinking and behaving can be destabilised by asking questions based (in the broadest possible sense) on the model, "Who knows…?", or by challenging interpretations with reference to philosophical ideas. The stories "The Creation of the World", "The Cave Dwellers" and "What Does That Make Me?" can serve as examples of this approach.

The same can be achieved by counter-hypotheses; the therapist can suggest to the client that he or she can irritate those responsible for spreading gossip about him or her by spreading additional or counter-rumours (cf. the story "Good Morning Everyone!"). A woman once said that after telling her husband she wanted a divorce, her husband replied, "If you're sure that that's what you must do, then do it." His reply made her think for a while, and she ended up staying together with him. Beliefs can therefore be destabilised using statements based on the model "If you know that this is right for you, then do it (or continue doing it)". Destabilisation can also be achieved by means of warnings (as done in metaphorical terms in the stories "The Cart, the Mud and I" and "The Genie") and implicit or explicit criticism of specific patterns of thinking and behaving. For example, implicit (because it is incorporated metaphorically) criticism is contained in the statement, "It is a huge mistake to overheat a steam engine, and a mistake that will only be made by an amateur" in the story "Steam Engines".

Any type of confirmation is useful for stabilising alternative interpretations or behaviours demonstrated by the client or identified in the course of conversation. Stabilising communication may be non-verbal in the form of approving gestures, verbal and direct in the form of praise and recognition, paradigmatic in the form of case studies about clients who succeeded with a similar strategy, or metaphorical in the form of images that are compatible with the client's patterns of thinking and behaving.

Desired patterns of behaviour can also be stabilised through direct or metaphorical prefigurement of the success, which will follow the relevant behaviour, as in the stories "Bad English" and "Dung Beetle".

Suggestive questions (as the questions in the story "Dying at the Age of 26") or series of questions (a yes set, as in the story "The Legacy") can also be used to stabilise desired new perspectives and patterns of thinking or behaviour.

Stabilising desired patterns of behaviour is important not only when a therapist communicates with a client, but also when a client communicates with himself or herself. Clients can be taught not only to communicate with themselves respectfully, but also to formulate respectful instructions to their own body and mental functions and to associate them with praise. The self-communication in the story "Peace Settlement with a Tooth" can serve to illustrate this.

Within the context of systemic counselling, the expansion and optimisation of resources are a way of stabilising helpful patterns that are already present.

Resources which are less readily available (infrequent patterns of behaviour) can be tentatively established within an individual's behavioural repertoire by means of exception-based questions ("In which situations would the symptom no longer be present? What would be different, and might this have contributed to the exceptional situation?"), questions to the future ("If the problem were to stop existing at some point in the future, what would you experience and do? Once you'd overcome the problem and could look back, what steps would you have taken to get there?") and questions assuming a miracle had happened. ("Imagine a good fairy came in the night and conjured your problem away. How would you notice next morning that it had gone? What would you do differently to the day before?"). The questions alone help to stabilise the resources, since anything that is asked with interest by the therapist and acknowledged positively will generally gain in significance for the client. The therapist can then discuss which ways of behaving and thinking may result in the resource being experienced more frequently and more reliably.

A client's responses to systemic questions of this kind are based on recollected and hypothetically constructed life stories. We can stabilise the patterns of thinking and behaving which they express by telling paradigmatic stories with a similar structure from the lives of other people, thus prompting the client to come up with further ideas for solution-based structures in the relevant storytelling context.

We can also tell metaphorical stories about expanding resources which are as yet invisible, as in the fairy tale story "The Blade of Grass in the Crack", or stories that make it clear that focusing on resources instead of on problems and deficits promotes the capacity for action, as in the story "From Oasis to Oasis".

If the resources are readily available, the therapist can exchange stories with the client about the ways in which what is already good can be made better and the associated outcomes, for example in the form of anecdotes concerning the strategies applied by successful professionals, competitive sportspeople or artists: "A famous trombonist was asked for the secret of his success. He replied, 'People don't just hear the breath you use, but also the breath you don't use'" (cf. Hammel, 2012b: 27).

Another way is to supply everyday stories which support the existing resource in paradigmatic or metaphorical terms, as is done in the story "Grandma's Cooking".

### Reversing or shifting the focus of attention

Another effective technique involves reversing the focus of attention, for example by means of a metaphor, reframing or a pacing and leading strategy. In metaphorical terms, a focus on the opposite of what has previously been the case can be achieved by means of a paradoxical story, for example a story which instructs the listener to search for something that has been overlooked, as in the stories "Christmas Bell" and "Hearing Difficulty". The problem situation can also be reframed in such a way that the problem solves itself through a paradoxical effect. This is done in the stories "The Sailor on Shore" and "The Three Principles".

For example, reframing can be used to convey to the client that he or she is wrong to regard tinnitus as something that is present, when in fact it is something that is absent; rather than silence being the absence of noise, noise is the absence of silence, which means that silence is the original state, and what is important is not the volume of the noise, but the level of silence which has been achieved. From this point onwards the therapist should refer only to silence, reversing the focus of attention of the part of the mind which regularly checks to see whether the noise is still there, and interrupting the psychological mechanism that perpetuates the tinnitus. Following a similar principle, in the story "Language Rules" non-smoking is no longer viewed as the absence of smoking; instead, the opposite is true, with a smoking-free condition regarded as the positive and manifest experience and nicotine consumption defined as its non-existence and absence.

Pacing and leading can also be used to achieve refocusing of this kind if a coherent chain of thought from what is being experienced in the moment to its opposite is created and comprehended as logical by the listener. For example, a journey can be undertaken away from the suffering currently being experienced and towards its opposite, or in other words the pleasant sensations that are longed for and anticipated ever more frequently, confidently or intensively, as in the story "Go Away".

It is also possible to shift the focus of attention, for example from feeling to hearing (cf. the story "Hypnotising Dogs") or from the body to the mind (cf. the stories "Blinded by Love" und "Continent Eyes"). This results in a state of dissociation which – since it represents the absence of problems – can be deepened and stabilised or made repeatable through "anchors" (conditioned triggers).

### Separation and reconditioning

For the vast majority of the time we think, speak and behave automatically and unconsciously, and we are also unaware of what we do while we are asleep or in everyday trance states. Most of our communication during the day takes place on a non-verbal level or by means of hints and connotations of which we are never consciously aware, and all of us have conditioned reflexes and emotional responses that evade our conscious control. It is often an impossible task for people suffering from lapses in memory, post-traumatic responses or anxiety disorders to "pull themselves together", and tics and addictions are also largely impervious to conscious control. Many physical responses are equally involuntary, and can only be consciously influenced to a limited extent. Most of our opinions, associations and emotional attitudes are acquired so involuntarily that we never even consider the existence of basic alternatives, and indeed we are barely able to do so any longer. How can we change damaging behaviours and ways of seeing the world if we have so little conscious control over them?

The solution to this problem often involves separating and reconditioning trigger-response patterns, or in other words associations and ways of seeing the world and behaving which are involuntarily associated with certain triggers. This also involves interpreting our perceptions, the way we communicate with ourselves (on a physical and mental level) and our social and spiritual communications, and technically speaking this is an amplified version of the basic destabilisation and stabilisation interventions discussed above. In many cases a separate intervention for the separation of dysfunctional patterns is not required, since the old pattern is implicitly separated when the new pattern is created.

In the field of hypnotherapy, the temporary mental suspension of associations (response patterns and interdependencies) in the body is referred to as "dissociation". All physical and mental functions and areas can be dissociated, including specific body parts, memories, emotions and any sensory perceptions. Dissociations of this kind can occur involuntarily if an individual suffers a shock or trauma, sometimes resulting in serious psychological and physical problems (post-traumatic stress disorder), but the temporary separation of associations in a safe context can be beneficial. For example, techniques involving dissociation can be used to reduce pain and anxiety in acutely stressful situations; in such cases it is important to prevent the client overestimating his or her real (e.g. physical) capacities and taking on too much, however. For more dissociation techniques, see the stories "The Unscrewable Body", "Pirate Anaesthesia" and "Arm Wrestling".

The targeted conditioning of a response is identical to the technique of "anchoring", which involves practising a particular response with the aim of ensuring that it occurs involuntarily every time that a particular trigger is perceived externally or imagined.

One example of this approach is the eradication of a phobic response such as the one described in the story "Fear of Moths", where the trigger-response pattern which has been learned involuntarily is replaced with a new pattern, which may be just as nonsensical but which no longer involves suffering. Another example of an intervention involving separation can be seen in the story "A Jarful of Allergies", where the trigger-response pattern, "I have an allergic response to pollen" is mentally eliminated. A logical follow-on to this intervention is the story "The Way to the Meadow", which outlines a procedure for the reconditioning of allergy-free physical behaviours.

One simple way of separating and conditioning constructions of reality is to challenge the associations assumed by the client to exist (thus leveraging the therapist's position of authority, cf. the start of the story "Three Boxes"), or to reject these associations in an argument and put forward alternative plausible claims. Other options involve imagining metaphorical images which illustrate the separation of associations (illustrated in the story "The Filing Cabinet"), announcing that a new era has dawned in which the old associations no longer apply (as in the story "The Schoolchildren's Fairy"), or using realized metaphors, that is, actions performed by the client (rite of passage, action as a metaphor) or physical things (object as a metaphor) to illustrate the fact that a particular era has passed or is no longer necessary. This type of intervention is used in the story "Dry".

For therapeutic purposes, a distinction can be made between the conditioning of waking behaviours (cf. "Social Noises", "Fear of Moths", "Grunting" and "The Schneiders") and the conditioning of sleeping behaviours (cf. "The Bladder Alarm Clock", "Alarm Clock with a Snooze Button", "My Right Eye", "Breathless", "Stop" and "Snoring"). This should not be understood as a methodological distinction, but merely as the identification of two different areas in which the same conditioning techniques are used.

Conditioning may take place in the situation itself (*in vivo*) or by imagining the situation (*in sensu*). As a basic principle, every aspect of reconditioning is possible *in sensu*, and this form of conditioning is a much more practical option in many therapeutic situations (such as those relating to sleeping behaviours); on the other hand, *in vivo* conditioning can be assigned to the client and his or her friends and family as homework. These conditioning techniques play a significant role in relation to the systematic desensitisation ("Mrs Sing" and "Numb Feet"), of anxiety disorders such as phobias, where the therapist works together with the client to practise increasingly calm and relaxed responses to the triggers that previously gave rise to anxiety. It is equally possible to condition a behaviour that involves feeling the pleasant physical sensations and emotions associated with being in a favourite holiday destination whenever a certain trigger is experienced in future, or to reinterpret the trigger in such a way that it becomes wholly unthreatening.

There are many different examples of things that can be conditioned, ranging from involuntary physical responses (reflexes, autonomic responses, gland and cell functions ("The Way to the Meadow") and associations through to emotions and patterns of social behaviour; as a basic principle, it is possible to condition any response to any trigger. It is often useful to practise response patterns that necessitate a pattern interrupt, for example waking up at night as a response to the trigger of a full bladder or a bad dream. The conditioning of a response ritual (in the form of a symptom prescription, for example) to replace a spontaneous involuntary response (such as those caused by tic disorders) interrupts the old conditioning and allows new responses to be established. Inverse trigger-response patterns are also possible; for example, a patient with sleep apnoea can learn to perceive shallower breathing as a trigger to take a deep breath.

The therapist can teach a client techniques for self-conditioning or the conditioning of a partner's behaviour ("Stop"), by telling him or her paradigmatic stories involving other clients or stories from his or her own personal experience; alternatively, he or she can tell a metaphor-based story in which a particular word or idea is repeated so many times that the client can be expected to display the associated behaviour involuntarily in response to a particular trigger.

In some cases it may be preferable simply to avoid the trigger rather than to use reconditioning techniques, for example if the trigger occurs very infrequently or if any confrontation can easily be avoided, as illustrated in the story "Mental Block". It also makes sense to avoid triggers that are of critical importance during the client's current stage of life; for example, an addict attempting to cease consumption of a particular addictive substance should avoid the triggers associated with it (such as cigarette lighters, ashtrays, an armchair in which a smoker previously always sat and smoked or situations in which smoking took on the character of a ritual). By way of analogy, it is often a good idea for a client who has recently separated from his or her partner (a process which in biochemical and psychological terms is similar to an addict's withdrawal) not only to avoid coming into contact with the former partner, but also to avoid any triggers associated with him or her in order to avoid relapses into distressing patterns. Anyone who wishes to remain faithful to his or her partner but is tempted to play away (or use pornography) would be well advised to remove the relevant triggers from his or her field of vision and daily routine (cf. the story "Temptation").

### Reinterpreting life stories

Memories – both the client's memories and the therapist's memories – are also stories. A distinction could be made between deficit-oriented and resource-oriented memories, but what is perhaps most important when it comes to deciding whether a memory is described in negative or positive terms is not its content, but the punctuation and the meaning ascribed to it. Punctuation determines whether a story has a positive or negative ending on the basis of the particular life experience chosen as its conclusion, and this procedure is illustrated by the story "Life as a Sinus Curve":

> If we imagine that life's ups and downs resemble a sinus curve, we can draw this curve in two different ways. We can start the curve at its highest point, trace it down through its lowest point and then return to its highest point – or we can do the opposite, and draw the curve from its lowest point, through its highest point and back to its lowest point. In mathematical terms, it is exactly the same curve.

If we want our clients to repunctuate their stories and find new happiness in their lives, we can help them to change the stories they tell about their past experiences, for example by asking, "And then what happened? And after that? And what happened next?"

The same applies to clients' expectations of the future; one client may see his or her future as a series of catastrophes, while another client in exactly the same situation looks to the future with hope – not because of the objective facts, but because of their differing patterns of interpretation and punctuation.

It is a good idea for therapists to encourage their clients to develop visions of the future which start and end on a high note, with just the odd setback in between.

It was a wise man who coined the saying, "everything will be alright in the end"; if everything is not alright, the end cannot yet have been reached.

All ongoing and circular processes can be repunctuated, and the same is true for all systems involving interdependencies (static or dynamic equilibria).

Forms of punctuation include the reinterpretation (often the reversal) of cause and effect, sender and recipient (of a message) or activity and passivity (e.g. non-action as a form of action).

### Increasing and reducing complexity

In cases where a client describes his or her situation in highly complex terms, it can often be helpful to reduce the level of complexity, for example by means of stories that in just a few words get to the crux of diffuse or complex topics; the genre of aphorisms is especially suitable for focusing in on a particular topic in this way. Clients often perceive the reduction of complexity by a therapist as a provocation.

Conversely, if a client describes his or her situation in very simple terms, it is often useful to increase the level of complexity. Stories that introduce a distinction, or in other words which invite the listener to deal with different circumstances on their own merits, are a good way of encouraging differentiation.

### Utilisation

It is a paradoxical truth that a therapist who makes direct reference to a symptom (or a key element in the symptom's context) and utilises it for therapeutic purposes often has the best chance of eliminating it. There are various ways of setting about this task; for example, a basic method for utilising symptoms is the technique of symptom prescription (paradoxical prescription), which is well-known in the field of systemic therapy. The effectiveness of this procedure, which involves ordering a particular symptom to occur, derives from the fact that many symptoms can *only* occur spontaneously, and deliberately producing the symptom destroys the pattern upon which it depends. An alternative version of this method involves the use of positive triggers that prompt the client to *want* to demonstrate the symptom; the conscious effort involved in this process destroys and eliminates the pattern that formerly resulted in the spontaneous occurrence of the symptom. A somatic application of this method can be found in the story "If You Can Manage...".

Another form of utilisation involves the therapist mirroring the client's symptom-inducing patterns or outdoing the client in demonstrating the symptom. The effectiveness of this approach can be explained by the fact that the therapist positions himself or herself on the side of the symptom through the interpersonal transfer (delegation) of one aspect of the relevant ambivalence, meaning that the client is left with no choice but to position himself or herself on the symptom-free side. When using this procedure, care must naturally be taken to ensure that the client feels that the therapist is taking him or her seriously, and experiences the intervention as a useful component of the therapeutic encounter.

A third form of utilisation involves setting up situations in which the symptom is governed by the symptom itself and eradicated by the resulting paradox. One example of this procedure is the task of committing a "perfect error" by the next therapy session, frequently set as homework by therapists practising in the systemic tradition when working with perfectionists and those with compulsive personalities. Another example is the approach described above whereby the therapist promotes a sceptical attitude on the part of the client and then encourages the client to be sceptical about the scepticism.

Symptoms which are manifested through language or with the voice can naturally also be tackled using the therapist's manner of speech and story-telling techniques; an example of this procedure can be seen in the story "Mrs Sing".

Not only problems (symptoms) but also ideas for solutions can be utilised, and placebos are a classic example of this approach. Placebos are familiar to many as "pretend" medications which are taken by patients in the belief that they are pharmacologically effective drugs, and which often produce the desired effect despite the absence of any active ingredients, as in the story "The Good Gel". The effect of real placebos and "genuine medications" (which likewise attribute part of their efficacy to the placebo effect) is heightened if the method of functioning of the medication and its efficacy are verbally emphasised. Placebos can be used effectively not only for problems that can be treated with medication, but also for certain problems that cannot (homesickness tablets for children).

Placebos can also be effective if they are prescribed to patients explicitly as placebos, and the patient is given the paradoxical instruction that trials have shown placebos to be effective even if the patients knew what they were. The therapist can also point out that the placebos worked even on patients who did not believe in placebos (in order to ensure that the patient accepts on faith the idea that method may also work for sceptics like him or her). Placebos include not only medications but any simulated medical treatment, for example "pretend" acupuncture or any other treatment method that is supposedly ineffective. An example is the treatment in the story "The Lipoma" (though there may be a minor therapeutic effect in the use of spit which contains enzymes used by the body for decomposing cell material).

I refer to imaginary medications and treatment methods as mental placebos or unreal placebos; the imagined ingestion or application of these remedies causes the body to behave as though the real medication had been administered. Examples for this technique can be found in the stories "Placebo I" to "Placebo IV" and "Wart Remedy". Prescriptions of placebos (as described above) and other ritual suggestive procedures can also be understood as unreal placebos, achieving a placebo effect without administering a real placebo.

Many therapeutic effects, for example those relating to hypnosis, are based on the active use of placebo effects. "Hypnosis is based on belief, but it works even if you don't believe in it," is a paradox that can take the wind out of the sails of any sceptic; the desired effect can be produced not only if the patient believes in the placebo itself, but also if he or she professes disbelief in the placebo but believes in its effect.

Every step towards a solution and every expectation of a solution (whether rational, irrational or based on a paradox) has the potential to be utilised as a real or unreal placebo with a view to achieving the relevant solution.

Therapeutic goals can also be achieved through the utilisation of an individual's values, his or her identification with other people or aspects of interpersonal relationships. The above dialogue in which a grieving daughter is asked whether her mother forgives her for (allegedly) causing her death is one example of this approach, and similar thought experiments based on relationships with living or dead persons can also be used to prevent patients committing suicide (cf. "When You Meet Your Brother" and "A Single Request").

A further variation on this theme involves the utilisation of the communication patterns used by the client and his or her reference system, based on the technique of mirroring introduced into the field of talking therapy by Carl Rogers; counter double binds are a therapeutically important form of these mirroring techniques.

"You can't have your cake and eat it!" How does a therapist respond to double binds of this kind? One option is to use an answer along the following lines: "Of course you can, you just need the right plate," or "Chocolate cake or Victoria sponge?" As a general rule, counter double binds are the safest way of avoiding ensnarement in the double binds which are sometimes typical of therapy, and of prompting clients to process their own ambivalences independently. In order to construct a counter double bind, the therapist must identify both sides of the ambivalence which has been expressed (either intuitively or analytically), and respond positively to both, ensuring that the paradoxical communication is mirrored back to the client. Alternative forms of the counter double bind strategy include negative responses to one or both sides of the ambivalence, following the principle that the reply should be no less paradoxical that the initial message. In the example referred to above, a suitable response would be, "You can't, but I can make sure that the cake is particularly tasty. Will that be ok?"

An example of the use of counter double binds in a therapist's everyday therapeutic practice can be found in the story "The Man Who Wins When He Loses." If a client is finding it difficult to communicate with others because of the double binds they use, it may of course be useful to suggest that he or she can construct his or her own counter double binds, and then practise doing so; all of the stories in the section on double binds are suitable for this purpose.

Another method of mirroring communication patterns and utilising them for therapy is the circular argument or circular reasoning. The therapist invokes the success or failure of therapeutic communication (if necessary provoking said success or failure) as evidence that this pattern can also be expected to result in successful or unsuccessful communication in other situations, or in other words the client's everyday life ("The Converter"). For a more detailed discussion of the concept of Utilisation see Hammel, 2011, 2012a.

### Externalisation and visualisation

Problems which a patient perceives as being internal rather than external are often more difficult to overcome than those which he or she can confront and locate externally in relation to himself or herself.

Problems described as being internal can therefore often be overcome more easily if they are projected outwards by means of unreal reframing, or in other words externalised. This is as true for physical complaints as for emotional suffering, and applies as much to references to illness as to other problem constructs ("my ADS", "my inability to stop smoking").

An approach that has generally proven useful is to externalise and visualise the problem at the same time, or in other words to imagine it as a visible person, object or structure. Anyone who embellishes the form and shape of a problem that has been externalised in this way (following the cartoon approach) will generally also discover that the physical and psychological symptoms abate or are experienced as being comparatively more pleasant. The same is true if a problem is evaporated, shrunken, melted or simply transported to a remote location in the sufferer's imagination (an intervention based on phobia techniques from the field of NLP).

If a patient is unable to externalise a symptom, the problem can initially (or exclusively) be visualised within the body. The metaphorical transformation of the problem symbol into a solution symbol or the elimination of the problem symbol will then be achieved by means of a dialogue based on the rules, exception or cartoon approach. I once held the following conversation with a client suffering from generalised anxiety disorder when attempting to externalise her anxiety:

"I can't project it outwards. It's like a lump in my throat."

"A lump in your throat? Couldn't you eat it? Perhaps chop it up with a knife and fork?"

"No, it's stuck in one place."

"Is the lump hollow or full of something?"

"It's full of water."

"And there's a membrane surrounding this water?"

"Yes."

"What would happen if you poked a hole in the membrane?"

"The water would drain out." (The client began to cry.)

"And where would it go?"

"My stomach."

"And then it would flow onwards until at some point it reached a stream, and then a larger stream, and then perhaps the River Nahe and then the Rhine, is that right?"

"Yes."

"And the Rhine flows into the sea. By then your lump will be very far away! Won't you miss it?"

"No, not at all."

"And if you were standing by the sea, you wouldn't want the individual drops of water to return to you?"

"No, of course not."

"But the lump might be unhappy without you!"

"I don't care."

"But then you'll be completely rid of your lump! What will you do without any lump at all?"

"I'll be happy."

"And then you won't need me any more. Won't you miss coming to therapy?"

"I'm sure it'll be ok."

"Then we'll just have to come to terms with the fact that you don't need any more therapy sessions."

"I'll manage somehow…"

Chronic anxiety disorders, itching (for example in the case of chicken pox, skin diseases or conjunctivitis) and certain types of pain can often be reduced or cured in this way within a single therapy session (as was the case with the patient suffering from anxiety). This highlights the fact that the visualisation process can start within the body and be externalised at a later point in time, even if distancing of the symptom initially appears impossible. It also makes it clear that the therapist can control the process using a yes set (a series of statements that engender a "yes" response). The outcomes are stabilised by means of suggestive questions and paradoxical statements (which promote reactance).

Not only symptoms (in the broadest sense of the word) but also resources can be externalised and visualised; invisible internal or external resources can sometimes be made more readily available if they can be imagined in metaphorical form. Reference has already been made to the method of personalising resources as invisible friends, but symbols of this kind can also be put into tangible form as stuffed animals or other concrete symbols; this process involves using realized metaphors to turn invisible friends into visible ones. For example, after telling the story "Peer and Rasputin" a troll can be painted or shaped in playdough, or the therapist can give the child a toy troll to carry around.

Ambivalences can also be externalised and visualised. For example, a child can be encouraged to use ropes and stuffed animals to create a map on the floor with a "country of annoying animals" and a "country of kind animals". The child can then play with the animals in the relevant countries to find out which animals enjoy living there and which animals would like to live some-where else, and under which conditions they will be accepted by the animals that live in the other country or sent back to their own country, thereby creating a model of a successful social framework. Additional methods for externalising and visualising ambivalences are described in a separate section of this book.

### Interventions based on positive and negative models

A change in perspective results in a change in action over the short or long term, and what initially looks like a reframing of the way in which people see the world frequently leads to a change in the way in which they behave towards one another. We can influence people's patterns of behaving even more directly if we provide them with models and counter-models of successful behaviour, for example by means of paradigmatic stories. Suitable sources of these stories include case studies from the therapist's own practice as well as episodes from his or her life and the lives of his or her acquaintances (biographical stories). It goes without saying that fictional characters can also be used as models of successful and unsuccessful patterns of behaviour; fables represent a genre developed specifically for this purpose, for example, and fairy tales pursue the same goal in encrypted form.

Metaphors that can be used as a model of action can be found in many different areas, for example the fields of science, technology, history, politics, economics or even everyday life.

The purpose of many of our night-time dreams is to test out different behaviours in the form of examples or metaphors, and this is also true of nightmares, which realistically or allegorically highlight situations that should be avoided (through fight or flight) before it is too late.

As a basic principle, positive models of action are easier for the unconscious mind to comprehend, and negative models entail a greater risk of misunderstanding (avoidance of the learning situation as a whole instead of just the undesired option, action instead of inaction in relation to the undesired option). Although both approaches are undoubtedly effective, the sole use of negative models of action as a therapeutic measure can therefore be risky, and these models should be used as a supplement to positive models.

### Promoting expectations, searching and learning attitudes

One of the most important basic functions of therapeutic stories is to promote expectations and engender searching and learning attitudes, and many of the stories which pursue this goal follow the searching model which has already been discussed. The stories (most of which are short) leave the listener in a state of perplexity or astonishment; in order to resolve this uncertainty, the listener involuntarily embarks on a search for potential answers and explanations This technique is used in the stories "Stand Up", "Motorway Roadworks" and "Dot to Dot".

Searching and learning attitudes can also be promoted by means of stories about how people search and learn (cf. the stories "Learning to Talk" und "Learning to Walk"); in order to understand the meaning behind these stories, the client must examine his or her own experience in this area, thereby taking the first steps on the path signposted by the story. The task of changing existing learning attitudes is similar in many ways to that of promoting learning attitudes; as a general rule, paradigmatic stories can be used to illustrate alternative, supplementary or more sophisticated learning strategies.

It is often useful to use storytelling to promote positive expectations of therapeutic outcomes early on in the course of therapy, for example by means of positive case studies or recollections of previous positive experiences.

Psychoeducation techniques can also be used to promote positive expectations and searching and learning attitudes; for example, paradigmatic stories (or – less frequently – metaphorical stories) can be used to highlight problems of perception or communication. Other stories illustrate patterns of successful and unsuccessful communication between couples or demonstrate ways that people can learn to connect with others in spite of their lack of social skills. Examples are respectively the stories "The Converter" and "Of Following and Leading". Psychoeducational stories can be used to illustrate suggestive and psychosocial dynamics (as the story "A Desire for Life") and to teach strategies for attacking, defending and de-escalating a situation (as the stories "The Power of Thoughts", "Nails Make the Man" and "Gregor the Dragon"). They can be used to clarify the way in which the unconscious mind works and how it interacts with conscious experience (cf. respectively the stories "The Wrong

Audience" and "The Archivist"), and also to teach effective learning methods (cf. the stories "Exam Revision" and "A Sacred Agreement").

### Rapport-based interventions

The pack mentality, which is innate not only to certain species of animals but also to human beings, means that members of a particular group very quickly adjust their non-verbal (and often also verbal) behaviour to mirror that of the other members of the group by adopting the same postures, performing the same movements at the same time, synchronising their rate of breathing etc. The same is also true for their tone and volume of speech, the words they use and the structure of their sentences. Rapport can mean aligning one's behaviour with the average behaviour of a group, or with a person who draws particular attention to himself or herself, such as a family member, someone who is sexually attractive or an individual in a position of authority. In my experience, the transference of rapport behaviour is achieved more easily if the other individual is located at the blurred edge of the field of vision, or in other words in front of or behind the area which is in sharp focus.

Infectious yawning is a rapport phenomenon, as are the oft-reported cases of partners, twins or parents and children falling ill after learning through a telephone conversation that the other has become ill. Rapport has long-term effects; for example, people who have worked with children for many years often look younger than other people of the same age who have worked with pensioners. Individuals who identify with the suffering of those whom they are helping often bear the evidence in their habitual facial expressions, and those who work with people who move slowly, for example as a result of a stroke, can find that their own movements are affected. The idea that dogs and their owners grow to resemble each other appears less absurd in this context.

The phenomenon of rapport can be used for a variety of therapeutic purposes. It is only logical that approximating one's own bodily behaviour (speech, breathing etc.) with the client's initial (often problematic) behaviour will as a general rule lead to a higher level of identification, in most cases benefiting the therapeutic process; the term "pacing" is used to refer to this procedure. The therapist then gradually changes his or her own bodily behaviour towards a desired outcome, resulting in similar changes on the part of the client; this procedure is referred to as "leading".

The transition from pacing to leading is a basic hypnotherapeutic intervention, during which the therapist copies the client's bodily behaviour and then gradually modifies this behaviour until the desired outcome is achieved. In many cases this allows agitation, panic, hysteria, certain types of pain and mental blocks to be allayed within a very short space of time, leaving the client in a state of relaxation. For example, the story "Instead of a Lullaby" illustrates the procedure using the example of an infant. (For further information on the pacing and leading of physical behaviours, cf. also Bandler & Grinder, 1981: 64.)

Pacing (and rapport) can also be achieved by using words and topics from the client's vocabulary, identifying commonalities (biographical or otherwise), agreeing with the client's views and expressing support for his or her particular skills and interests (cf. the story "Sorting Screws"). A link therefore exists between pacing and the establishment of rapport on the one hand and utilisation on the other.

Reference was made above to the use of the "ambivalence seesaw" in the context of suicidal tendencies and mania. This technique involves the therapist demonstrating that he or she fully understands the client's perspective, but also implying an ambivalence (initially minimal) that does not exclude the opposing view. To begin with, this counter-position is put forward so tentatively that the client does not raise any objections, and a yes set is then used to put forward the counter-view (for example life instead of death) ever more positively in incremental steps, whereby the other option (for example death) is still repeatedly referred to as a comprehensible option and perhaps the right option. By constantly seesawing between both options or perspectives and gradually assigning more weight to one of them, the client's positive attention is imperceptibly shifted from one extreme to the other.

The ambivalence seesaw is a version of the ambivalence swing technique used in systemic therapy, which involves the therapist behaving in a consistently neutral manner by starting and ending in the centre and then taking the sides of each of the parties in turn and to the same degree, until the client has opted for one of the sides, for both of the sides, for neither of the sides or for an interim position. It goes without saying that there is also plenty of scope for highly beneficial therapeutic stories about seesaws, swings, slides and cable cars, which refer only briefly to the problematic experience and then focus on a playful form of problem solving…

The method of stimulating an overall psycho-autonomic state through simulation of the relevant state can be described as a type of self-pacing and self-leading. As in the case of systematic desensitisation, a patient who breathes calmly and assumes a relaxed posture will stimulate a state of low anxiety despite being in a situation that may provoke high anxiety. The story "Manta Ray" illustrates this phenomenon. It is equally possible to stimulate waking up from sleep by conditioning the performance of an aspect of waking behaviour in a particular sleeping situation until the waking condition is reached, as shown in the story "My Right Eye". Conversely, the simulation of sleeping behaviours (including the use of conditioning triggers such as a bed, a stuffed animal or a hot water battle) often induces sleep, and the simulation of trance results in a trance.

Mental gymnastics is an umbrella term for physical exercises which are performed in the imagination or "demonstrated" by the therapist and which are aimed at improving the patient's mobility. The underlying principle is that every movement which is imagined gives rise to the same processes in the brain as the movement itself, simply in diluted form. A movement or other bodily behaviour that needs to be learned or practised can be based on a memory, examples demonstrated by other people (as in "Learning to Walk"), metaphors from other spheres of life (as in "Pantomime" and "The Nail") or metonymic illustrations of similar bodily functions (as in "The Frozen Hiccup"). It should likewise be possible for patients suffering from certain neurological problems to regain feeling in numb parts of the body by repeatedly imagining sensations in the relevant part.

It goes without saying that rapport or the process of pacing and leading can also be imagined. Imagined rapport will have the same effect as if it had been experienced in real life, and many of the interventions in this book are based on this principle. The story "Manta Ray" establishes rapport with an imagined manta ray, ensuring that the heartrate and rate of breathing can be approximated with the beat of this creature's fins in a crisis (heart attack, asthma attack, hyperventilation, panic attack).

Invisible friends, which were mentioned in the context of unreal reframing and which also have repercussions on real-life behaviour and experiences, also belong under this heading, as in the story "Invisible Friends".

Other stories bring to mind memories of how a mother taught something to her daughter, and use the imagined rapport between the mother and the daughter to teach the mother or daughter something in the present day or to motivate them to learn something, as in the stories "Learning to Talk" and "Learning to Walk".

In some cases it is essential for rapport to be interrupted, for example if the therapist experiences a sensation of paralysis as a result of the problems described by the client. The interruption can be achieved through any kind of communicative non-sequitur, for example by telling a story that is deeply puzzling or wholly inappropriate and not commenting any further on it. An interruption of rapport, or in other words a deliberate failure to follow on from what has been previously communicated, is however also a form of intervention that can be taught to clients in order to overcome challenging everyday situations; for example, strategic interruptions of rapport are a good way of shutting down physical or verbal aggression, as in the stories "How to Handle Sexual Assault..." and "Thank You".

Interrupting rapport involves using an element of surprise to confound a habitual relationship with other people or a particular person, for example the therapist, thereby momentarily suspending expectations and beliefs. This can be achieved by means of a stimulus such as a metaphor that directs the listener's attention in an unfamiliar direction and leads to an internal searching attitude. Not only relationships with people, but also relationships with objects, topics or patterns of behaviour can be used as the basis for interruptions of rapport. Erickson and Rossi refer in this context to "disrupting the client's habitual frames of reference and belief systems" (Erickson & Rossi, 1979: 5).

In the field of systemic counselling, the interruption of rapport is generally viewed from the perspective of a change in well-rehearsed relationship
patterns, and referred to as a pattern interrupt or pattern change (Mücke,
2001: 19).

### Interventions based on rewards and punishment

There are various different ways in which rewards and punishment can be used
effectively in therapeutic stories. As a basic principle, every positive resolution
to a problem in a story corresponds to a prefigured reward (benefit) provided
that a similar approach is taken to a comparable problem, whereas negative
models correspond to a prefigured punishment (harm) in the event of unsuitable
behaviour. Provided that the rewards or punishments are a logical consequence
of fate or the rules of nature or culture, the client is unlikely to demonstrate
any reactance; if the protagonists in the story (including the therapist in the
indirect role of storyteller) reward and punish others, care must be taken to
ensure that the story does not provoke resistance in the client. The therapist
must give careful thought to whether a directive procedure might be suitable,
both for himself or herself and for the client; in the case of patients suffering
from addiction or depression or patients who have been raised by authoritarian
parents, greater change can sometimes be achieved by more authoritative lead-
ership, and the therapist will furthermore be in a better position to avoid sinking
into a problematic trance together with the client. A potential objection which
can however be raised to the use of rewards and punishments is that it does little
to promote the client's autonomy and creativity.

Interventions based on the use of rewards and punishments include the
ordeal technique developed by Erickson, as well as stories based on promises,
contracts or bets. The other party involved in such agreements may be the
client himself or herself (self-policing agreement), a family member, a friend
or the therapist.

An ordeal involves a binding agreement that an undesirable consequence,
for example a punishment, will take place in the event that the client performs
an undesired involuntary behaviour. If the punishment is guaranteed to be
meted out, the subconscious mind will decide to avoid the undesired behaviour, as in the story "Returning the Key".

As a general rule, care must be taken to ensure that interventions based
on the use of rewards and punishment are underpinned by the client's value
system (his or her "principles" or "honour") in such a way that the reward or
punishment is guaranteed to take place as agreed. Ambivalent or inconsistent
implementation will counteract the therapeutic goals being pursued, as in the
story "A Sacred Agreement"

Another variation on the use of reward and punishment is the implicit
or explicit use of praise and scolding, as explained in the section on
"Destabilisation and stabilisation".

## Storytelling structures

### Traditional structure

Anyone wishing to develop a story to use with clients in a counselling situation can draw upon a wide range of tried-and-tested structures as a basis for this task. The most common pattern embodied in these structures (exposition – build-up of tension and rapid elimination of escape routes – resolution) forms the basis – with minor modifications – for many fairy tales, myths, theatrical plays and novels, and can be adapted for therapeutic stories as follows:

1. Introduce the protagonist and his or her world. The protagonist may be an animal, a colleague, a previous clientor the therapist himself or herself during an earlier stage of life. If the cartoon approach is being followed, anything can become a protagonist, including a chair, the abstract concept of justice.
2. Introduce the protagonist's problem, which will have parallels with the client's problem.
3. Refer to unsuccessful attempts to find a solution. Previous experiences from the client's life or a blueprint for future failures can be used for this purpose (negative models). Antagonists and purveyors of bad advice (external or internal voices) may also appear at this point in order to complicate the situation or highlight unfeasible solutions.
4. Clearly describe the protagonist's downfall. If the story includes several attempted solutions, the sum total of all of the perplexity and sadness experienced by the protagonist should be described at the climax of his or her failure.
5. Bring an external or internal advisor into the story. This may be a different person or an idea, for example a voice who takes part in an internal dialogue.
6. Ensure that the protagonist and anyone else involved enjoys and celebrates his or her success, or leave the end of the story open to encourage further contemplation.

This procedure can be illustrated on the basis of the story "The Bulls Are Coming"; other examples of this pattern include the stories "Gregor the Dragon", "The Desert" and "Dark Room".

1. My children and I were enjoying a picnic. Sarah was eleven at the time, and Thomas had just turned four. Our little dog Woyzeck was also there, and we sat and ate in perfect harmony.
2. Yet we hadn't noticed that there was no fence between us and the herd of bulls grazing in the meadow behind the woods where we were picnicking – and suddenly the bulls started to thunder towards us.

3.  I grabbed the dog and ran until I was safely behind the fence. The children didn't make it as far as me.
4.  (The story omits the mother's horror, which will nevertheless be experienced by the listener.)
5.  "Get behind me!" yelled Sarah, positioning herself in front of Thomas. Stretching her arms out wide, she confronted the galloping bulls…
6.  …who screeched to a halt. For a while the bulls and the girl stared at each other. Then the herd turned around.

Many stories, like the tale about the bulls, represent a variation on the pattern in that they omit an element (although the listener may nevertheless fill in the missing element in his or her imagination), repeat an element or change the sequence of the elements. As a fundamental principle, all stories with a plot and a climactic turning point can be described as contracted or extended versions of this basic form. As I discuss the following approaches to the invention of therapeutic stories, I will therefore focus on the ways in which these stories differ from the basic pattern.

### Rules, exception, cartoon and paradoxical approaches

As discussed above, problem metaphors can be converted into solution metaphors not only by means of a dialogue, but also by means of a monologue told as a story. For example, a metaphor that suggests that someone has a memory "like a sieve" could be converted on the basis of the rules approach as follows:

A gold panner once lived in a hut by a river, high up in the mountains. He had lived there for many long years, and had panned many tonnes of sand. Some days he found a little gold, but rarely more than he needed to cover his daily requirements for food, clothes and tools. He had long dreamed of finding a large nugget of gold, but he now suspected that this dream would never come true. Most of the time when he looked into his pan he saw nothing but small pieces of gravel which glinted in the sun. One day he received a visit from an old schoolfriend, who worked as a jeweller in a large city and had amassed a considerable fortune for himself. He was curious to find out how the gold panner lived.

"Show me how you pan the gold," he said to his old friend.

The gold panner hesitated, but then stood up, took his pan from the wall and walked to the river with his guest. He dipped the pan into the river, shook it and let the water run through it.

"Nothing at all – it's always the same," he sighed and looked up at his friend.

His friend had gone pale, and said, "I can't believe it. Diamonds everywhere!" (Cf. Hammel, 2012b: 88.)

Anyone wishing to invent a solution-based story using the exception approach should initially introduce the concept to be reinterpreted and mention the rule that normally applies in this respect. He or she should then mention with surprise and interest a case that plausibly diverges from this rule, if necessary adding a hint that there are more such exceptions. An example of this is the following story about back alleys;

> I once knew someone who had been visited by a man who could see no way out.
> "There's nothing else I can do," he said. "I'm at a dead end."
> Then my friend remembered something, and replied, "Where I live there are sometimes little back alleys between the houses which run from one street to another. You can only walk along them by foot, and they are barely any wider than a grown man. There's a dead end where I live, and if you drive in you can't continue – like every other dead end. But this dead end is different, and I think it's probably not the only one; if you go right to the end, somewhere on one side, hidden between the houses, you'll find a back alley." (Cf. Hammel, 2012b: 92.)

The following story follows the cartoon approach since it is based on the assumption that anything is possible, but it also follows the rules approach in that it thinks the metaphor "loss of face" through to its logical conclusion in line with the principle that "everything that can be lost can be found":

> Once upon a time – and I'm not making this up – a man living in Japan woke up one morning and had lost his face. As I'm sure you can imagine, this was extremely embarrassing for him, and he could not contemplate showing himself to another person in this state. So he started looking for his face on his own; he used his fingers to search over the surface of his bed and the floor under his bed, and eventually he felt over the surface of the entire room. He tried to find his face by himself for a long time, until he finally understood; if you lose your face, it's impossible to find it again by yourself – after all, you can't see or hear anything! How did he manage to get out of this mess? With the help of his friends, who searched everywhere again for him and finally found it – in the bathroom mirror, where he had left it during a nighttime trip to the toilet. (Cf. Hammel, 2012b: 89.)

The opposite tactic can of course also be used by following a paradoxical approach (a metaphorical paradoxical intervention) which dictates that the metaphor should end in disaster.

> When I forgot to steer the cart around the mud, I said to myself, "It's too late to do anything now", and I waited to see what would happen. When

> I pushed the cart right into the mud, I said to myself, "It's too late to do anything now," and I waited to see what would happen. When the cart sank in the mud and I sank along with it, I said to myself, "It's too late to do anything now," and I waited to see what would happen. When the cart disappeared in the mud, and I disappeared along with it, I knew what I had always known.

Using Watzlawick's forms of response as a frame of reference, the first of the two solution-based stories referred to above provoke acceptance in the listener (positive model). By ignoring the world of experience familiar to the listener, the third solution-based story creates perplexity and results in a questioning and searching attitude (searching model). By way of contrast, the story which ends in disaster provokes Watzlawick's "rejection" response and is likely to encourage the client to resist the idea that his or her life could follow a similar course (negative model).

### Competence and incompetence at work

A simple way of inventing stories, in particular when working with children, is to choose a job which the client is likely to find appealing (children can be asked what they would like to do when they grow up, or what their favourite hobbies are, for example), and then to describe the problems experienced by a fictitious apprentice until he or she is able to do the relevant job competently and reliably, at which point his or her master proudly announces that the apprenticeship is over and that the apprentice has earned a special award.

There are many different variations on stories of this kind; for example, a Japanese archer who is unable to stop his arm from trembling, and who is told by his master to trace a large figure of eight with his arrow tip, to make this figure of eight ever smaller and to think only of the figure of eight instead of the target, and at some point to let the arrow go involuntarily, or a story of a perfumer who loves eating garlic and who cannot choose between his two passions – garlic and perfume – until he finds a solution that is right for him...

### Periods of success

A widespread intervention in the field of family therapy is to ask couples whose relationship is in crisis to talk about how they fell in love. When they reply, they will find themselves returning to and re-experiencing the sensations they felt at the time (in keeping with the principle of age regression). They can then think about what attracted them to the other partner back then, and how these sensations might be recreated.

Milton Erickson would remind clients facing challenging situations how difficult it was for them as children to learn to write and to tell the different letters apart, and how easy this task later became (Pelletier, 1990). He would then establish a connection between the earlier experience and the client's current – and apparently similarly challenging – situation. He would list other examples such as learning to walk and learning to talk, all of which represented a huge challenge at the time but later became automatic, and allow the clients to conclude for themselves that they would be able to overcome the present challenge with the same confidence and thoroughness as the earlier ones, and one day wonder how these things could ever have appeared difficult...

A therapist who wishes to incorporate a similar therapeutic concept into a story can either talk about the client's previous learning successes or about what he or she has successfully taught his or her children or other persons under his or her care, before concluding that the client will be able to complete a forthcoming task in the same way that he or she (or his or her children or pupils) completed the earlier task. For the purpose of reinforcement, the therapist can repeat the suggestion that the client will succeed now as he or she did before in slightly different variations, as illustrated by the story "Learning to Talk" (an account of what I told a stroke patient towards the end of her hospital stay and shortly before the start of her convalescence):

> When your daughter was very young, you helped her learn how to talk. You probably had to repeat some words to her two or three times before she could understand them and pronounce them correctly, but finally she managed it. Later she even learned English and French... as second languages, of course. German was and still is her mother tongue. And your parents also helped you learn how to talk. Like all children, you couldn't understand anything to begin with – that must have been a difficult task! And yet you finally managed it. Gradually you learned more and more words, a whole world of them. Now you are grown up. You are no less clever than you were then, and you must perform the same task. With one difference; this time you understand a lot of what you are learning, and you can draw on many valuable experiences from your past. Most importantly, you know that if you've learned it once, you can learn it again.

As an alternative to age regression, age progression can also be used to transport a client to a period of success. A well-known exercise in systematic therapy (as well as hypnotherapy and mental training) is for the client to imagine what it would be like if he or she had solved his or her problem or achieved his or her goal. As a general rule, it is preferable to use the indicative form of any verbs ("will") rather than the conjunctive form ("would"), although an exception should be made in cases where the patient is extremely ambivalent about solutions and puts up a high level of resistance (a situation frequently encountered with patients suffering from addiction, depression or suicidal tendencies). The therapist can make subversive use of the conjunctive form in order to destabilise ideas such as, "I'll never have a happy life," "If

I don't get my hopes up, I won't be disappointed," and "I don't want to win so that I don't have to risk losing."

An age progression to a period of success is demonstrated by the metaphor in the story "The Schoolchildren's Fairy":

> The kindergarten children's fairy is beautiful, but her big sister, the schoolchildren's fairy, is even more beautiful and magical. The schoolchildren's fairy makes children dream about numbers and letters, and teaches them clever thoughts and fun games to play in the playground. When the kindergarten children's fairy grows up, she wants to become a schoolchildren's fairy too, and she hopes that this will happen as soon as possible. Then a younger fairy can take over her job and become a kindergarten children's fairy.
>
> (See also the paradigmatic story "Love")

Since ideas about the future are always fictitious, unreal scenarios can be developed as well as realistic visions of the future. The above example illustrates a metaphorical and fairy tale version of the future, whereas the miracle questions developed by Steve de Shazer stay comparatively closer to real-life experiences, and involve asking something along the following line: "Imagine a fairy came at night while you were sleeping and the problem had disappeared by the morning. How exactly would you know, what would you do and experience differently to before, and who else would do and experience things differently?" These questions are based on a fairy tale situation, but they result in realistically described (non-metaphorical) scenarios.

It is important to ensure that any unreal future scenarios that are developed create resources for a real future. As a basic principle, the client should understand that there is "a grain of truth" in the story, regardless of the unusual way in which it is presented or perhaps precisely for that reason.

### Locations of success

Instead of using periods of success as a point of reference, the therapist can naturally also refer to locations and contexts in which the client experienced success, as demonstrated by the story "Renewed Life":

> A number of researchers wanted to find out why salmon die after spawning, so they fished a number of specimens out of the river, fitted them with radio transmitters and placed them back into the sea. And what do you think happened? The animals stayed alive.

Either external or internal locations can be chosen to construct resources of this kind, and reference can be made not only to experienced contexts, but also to contexts that have been heard about or invented. In the case of symptoms that occur on only one side of the body, the therapist can arrange with the client – either by means of a direct discussion or in the form of a paradigmatic or metaphorical story – that the two halves of the body should learn from each other. This is the procedure followed in "Learning to Walk":

> Imagine that your left-hand side, the one which can move, is a mother, and your right-hand side, the one which can't move quite so well, is her young daughter [...].

The same applies to the case study "Taekwondo".

Similarly, any type of imaginary location can also be used; if the listener finds the analogy expressed by a metaphor plausible, he or she will generally incorporate what is implied by the story into his or her view of the world.

As was the case for the above examples, stories based on "locations of success" generally compare one (or more) location(s) associated with a problem to a location associated with a solution. See also the stories "The Winter Rose", "The Eagle Chick" and "The Little Cat".

As ever, negative models that use the possibility of failure as a guide to success are a viable alternative to success-based stories. An example can be found in the fable "The Potential of Weeds".

### The inner parliament and the tea table

The field of communication science uses the terms "inner team" or "inner parliament" as metaphors to visualise ambivalences and polyvalences and to help a client facing a complex situation to gain an overview of his or her various "inner voices" or "personality parts", to understand better how they relate to each other and (if necessary) to reassess and reorder these relationships. The concept of the "inner team" was developed by Friedemann Schulz von Thun, cf. Schulz von Thun, 1998; Schulz von Thun and Stegemann, 2004.

The "inner parliament" can be introduced into the therapeutic conversation not only by means of the well-known dialogic structure, but also as a story in which various members of parliament (or committee members, colleagues or family members) hold a discussion and reach a conclusion. If it appears preferable to avoid any content-based suggestions, the story can be left ambiguously open and concluded with a question or an enigmatic hint.

Another variation on the inner parliament is the "body parliament" or body team, which can be useful when coaching managers or in the context of mental training for competitive sportspeople in order to prevent bodily functions being damaged through one-sided stress. An example of this approach can be found in the story "Day's March":

> "I was an officer in the army for many years," he said. "There were many times when I had to lead my soldiers on a long day's march. I always made

sure that the weakest members of my troop were well prepared but not overstretched, and that the strongest were challenged but also learned to watch out for those less strong than themselves. This approach – focusing on the troop as a whole rather than the individuals within it – was not only more humane but also produced better results."

The story serves as a metaphor for work/life balance and the balance that must be achieved between existentially important goals and ambitions, for example in relation to the patient's health. One patient suffering from Crohn's disease developed an intervention that involved her intestine and immune system sitting down at the kitchen table with a cup of tea while she did the washing up and listened to what the two of them were discussing. Other people would join in the conversation as necessary, including one called Yoho who liked to sit on her shoulder and advise her on questions concerning the relative priority she should attach to her job, her private goals and her health.

### Externalising ambivalence as a dialogue

Metaphors form the structural basis for our self-perception and our perception of the world; we use spatial metaphors when we say, "*on* the one hand… and *on* the other hand…", "*in* my dreams… and *in* reality", "*out* of my subconscious". We use social metaphors when we hold internal discourses in conversation with ourselves, give human names to areas of high or low pressure and hurricanes, speak of connections or relationships between things and ascribe human feelings to objects ("wine needs to breathe", "money talks"). We use movement-related metaphors to imply the passage of time ("it *caught* my eye", "I've left everyone else *behind*").

Whenever we are dealing with several (complementary, contradictory or ambivalent) perspectives or ways of acting, we can tell stories about different people, locations, times and forms of movement and divide the various options between them.

In its simplest form, this can happen as follows; Person A says, "On the one hand…", and Person B answers, "On the other hand…" This is the structure followed by the stories about Mr Gundolf, for example the story about cake, which can be used in relation to unfaithfulness, withdrawal from an addiction and changes in habits;

> This disturbs Mr Gundolf; "I can't look at a piece of cake without wanting to eat it." (Thesis)
> "Then don't look at the cake." (Antithesis)

The aim behind a story of this kind should not be for the client to accept the antithesis; one possible goal might instead be for the client to explain why he or she does not choose the obvious solution (not looking at the cake). Once good reasons for both of the options have been identified, the value and price of the first option (thesis) can be weighed up against those of the second (antithesis). This storytelling pattern can also be used to represent complex problems; in the fable "The New Word", the questioner receives many contradictory answers and finally decides that although there is no generally valid answer, there is an answer that is right for him.

Interactions between personified positions illustrate dilemmas and facilitate the discussion of solutions. For example, the fable "From the Crocodile's Mouth" provides a model for shedding light on the dynamic of double binds. The friendly and unfriendly messages are attributed to two individuals which can be distinguished from one another but which live in symbiosis, resulting in the following structure:

*Friendly verbal message;*
> "Good morning, my dear zebra!"

*In symbiosis with a hostile non-verbal message;*
> The small bird [...] was sitting in Ali the crocodile's wide-open jaws and picking remnants of food out of his teeth.

*Negative response to the hostile non-verbal message...*
> The zebra looked at him with a terrified expression, took a step backwards and then ran away.

*Reproach for negative response, again presented as a friendly verbal message;*
> "But zebra, you don't need to be afraid of me! We've always..."

*No answer. Friendly verbal message, again in symbiosis with the hostile non-verbal message...*
> The bird looked at the crocodile. "What's up with him? Do you know?"

*The outcome: confusion and underlying aggression;*
> Ali shook his head. "No idea. Zebras are strange animals."

The personality parts that are externalised as animals illustrate the dilemma and make it possible to separate out the contradictory messages and demonstrate how each response is inappropriate for one of the parties involved. It is relatively easy to find various solutions to the problem embodied in the model; the bird could fly after the zebra and meet him somewhere else, or perhaps the crocodile could close his mouth and dive under the water next time, or the zebra could wait at a safe distance and call the bird when he is ready to talk... Within the framework of counselling, the therapist and the client can discuss which real-life solutions correspond to the metaphorical solutions, or alternatively the therapist can refrain from commenting and leave it to the client's unconscious mind to use the metaphor as a prompt for embarking on creative changes in day-to-day life.

As well as assigning ambivalences to different people, the therapist can do the same with rooms, times, spheres of life and types of movement. The key factor is that the symptom is described in externalised form, or in other words as an external counterpart rather than as part of the client's own identity.

### Externalising ambivalence as two locations

The therapist can invent a country of cooperation and a country of competition, and discuss which laws and patterns of behaviour would apply in each of these countries. He or she could offer a true-to-life description of how an individual tried out opposite solutions to the problem in the two different countries, both of which delivered unsatisfactory results, and how the individual finally found a third location and a third solution which lived up to expectations. The story "A Lovely Christmas" uses different Christmas celebrations as examples of solutions to a relationship problem that result in failure and a solution which results in success. Things can only be truly lovely if they are up-to-date and authentic.

The therapist can refer to the soul as a house, and discuss where the room of hope and the room of despair would be situated, what furniture they would have in them and at which times the client plans to spend time in these rooms. The metaphor implies that the client can make a conscious decision over whether or not to stay in a particular mood.

### Externalising ambivalence as two types of movement

Different patterns of behaviour can be described as dancing, running or limping, and the effects of these different forms of movement can be considered. Different speeds or directions of movement can also be compared in order to raise a metaphorical question regarding the qualitative and quantitative criteria which should be applied to good work or good development;

> Once again, Ludwig, the carp, was bundled into a bucket. We carried him home through forests and across fields. Ludwig swam round and round his bucket in circles – quite small circles, because Ludwig had grown over the winter, and an old paint bucket is no mansion for a carp of his size. We also lost over half of the water from the bucket on our way. However we finally arrived, and with a flip of his tail Ludwig landed back in his pond with his old friends. What he did next astonished us; Ludwig kept on swimming in circles, as though he were still in a small bucket instead of in a pond. He swam six or seven circles with a diameter of not more than half a metre. Then the circles gradually turned into a spiral – first a narrow spiral, and then ever wider. Finally Ludwig realised where he was, and shot out of his bucket-shaped orbit on a long straight trajectory (cf. Hammel, 2012b: 70; see also the fables "Speed" and "Progress").

It is of course also possible to use a combination of externalisation types (different people, places, times and movements). The ambivalence expressed in the story about the carp Ludwig could also be represented as a discussion between two astronauts who disagree about whether they should keep their rocket in orbit or land on Earth, and who put forward arguments for going around the Earth again or landing straight away – arguments which coincidentally reflect aspects of the client's own life. Perhaps there is a third astronaut who would like to visit the moon before landing on Earth?

## Genres

### Biographical stories and anecdotes

Biographical stories are paradigmatic stories which highlight opportunities and solutions by offering alternative pathways for a particular stage of life or an entire lifetime. This principle is illustrated by the following (biographical) positive model;

> When Anton was 20, he travelled around the world, and his favourite country to visit was France. He left his wife and two daughters at home, and stayed in rooms above pubs even when he was in his home country – he was very fond of the taste of beer.
>
> When Anton was 22, he got divorced. He did not pay his ex-wife any maintenance, and instead drank away his money.
>
> When Anton was 26, he saw his daughters for the last time; his ex-wife refused to allow any further contact. When Anton was 55, he made a new friend who was supposed to be managing his money for him, but in fact kept most of it for himself. Anton was almost always drunk if he wasn't at work.
>
> When Anton was 61 he stopped drinking, and it was around this time that he met Frieda. Anton worshipped Frieda. Frieda had spent her entire life in a small house in the country, and had never been interested in drinking alcohol.
>
> By the time Anton was 70, he had taken Frieda to Paris and also to London, Brussels, Berlin and Budapest. He had introduced her to his relatives in Dessau and had hiked through the countryside surrounding their home town with her and their friends.
>
> When Anton was 71, Frieda became ill, and he took her to see many doctors. Anton said, "You're the best thing that has ever happened to me. You won't end up in a care home as long as I'm alive."
>
> When Anton was 72, he married Frieda. He ran the household, did the vacuuming and the shopping and cooked the meals.
>
> When Anton was 75, Frieda died. Anton outlived her by only 18 months, and drank a glass of sparkling wine every day during this period. "For my circulation," he would say. "Doctor's orders." (Cf. Hammel, 2012b: 84.)

This story can be used with patients who believe they are too old to embark on a major change, to endure withdrawal from an addictive substance or to find the love of their life. Depending on the specific counselling situation, Anton's age at the time when his life turned around can be changed, or the client can be told that what Anton achieved at the age of 61 can logically be achieved by the client at an earlier age. Biographical negative models can also be used as aversive suggestions, or in other words as a warning or encouragement to be mindful of a potential hazard:

> My great-grandmother often received visits from a neighbour who would pour out her heart to her. My great-grandmother was a good listener, and she had a deep Christian faith. She was good at giving advice to other people, and at helping them whenever she could. This particular neighbour used to tell my greatgrandmother about her marriage, which must have been miserable. Her husband was often drunk, and he beat and mistreated her. The woman was so desperate that she decided to get a divorce – a brave step for a lonely woman in a Bavarian village 80 or so years ago. She shared her plan with my great-grandmother, who advised her against it. "What God has joined together, let no man put asunder. Those were the words of our Saviour." And my great-grandmother advised her neighbour to try this or that to improve the situation with her husband. Things went on like this for a while, with crisis after crisis, but one day the word went around the village that the neighbour was dead. She had hanged herself. (Cf. Hammel, 2012b: 63.)

Negative models often function as provocations. The listener may be deceived into believing that they will have a happy ending until almost the very last moment – and the more unpleasant the surprise, the more vehement the resistance provoked. A story of this kind should however be told in such a way that there is a clear implication that the calamity could have been averted, for example by means of a divorce in the story above. Reference can also be made to several alternatives in order to highlight the fact that different options are available (a temporary separation or a separation without divorce in the story in question), or a general statement can be made to the effect that those providing advice identified several solutions, which were however rejected by the therapist or both parties in the conversation, avoiding a content-related suggestion ("Get a divorce!") in favour of a structural suggestion ("Look for alternatives and act accordingly!"). The villagers' thoughts about the disaster and the ways in which it could have been avoided could also be added at the end of the story, triggering a long-lasting searching attitude in the listener and encouraging him or her to search for as many different alternatives as possible.

Anecdotes function in a similar way to biographical stories, although in the narrower sense of the term they tend to be less vivid than stories, which still retain some characteristics of real-life experience. They therefore engender a lesser degree of identification in the listener as a general rule, and function instead (like aphorisms) as an illustrative example or a prompt for conversation.

### Case studies

Every therapist makes tacit use of lessons learned from previous courses of therapy when working with his or her current clients, and it is often useful to make explicit reference to experiences of and with other clients (while maintaining their anonymity). Case studies in the form of positive and negative models can be used to illustrate options for successful and unsuccessful behaviour, and new strategies for communicating with oneself or others can be thought through and examined in terms of their relevance to the current situation. It is almost impossible for a therapeutic conversation about case studies of this kind to take place without it giving rise to change, and clients regularly remodel their previous patterns of behaviour and communication strategies within a matter of days. Stories about previous clients' experiences may appear to be neutral information, but they provide clients with ideas for new ways of thinking and behaving and represent a very powerful therapeutic intervention.

The effectiveness of case studies of this kind is increased if several similar or complementary stories are told. The technique of stringing together and interweaving paradigmatic stories is illustrated in the story "Pest". Stories of this kind can be used in supervision to train perception and illustrate therapeutic techniques.

### Fables, fairy tales, farces and legends

The transitions between biography and legend are blurred, and this applies as a general rule to the boundaries between fiction and non-fiction. In the same way that biography and legend often blend into each other, biography, science and fable are interfused in the story "The Route Through the Mountain", in which a real fact (swallows flew through the St Gotthard Tunnel on their annual migration) is used as the basis for a modern fable with elements of an inventor biography. Fables are ideally suited for use in a counselling context, and even though the genre is somewhat less popular than it once was, any therapist who uses it as a source of stories will find that it has lost nothing of its fascination, even for modern-day listeners. Examples of fables which can be used for the purpose of coaching and therapy include "The Potential of Weeds", "From the Crocodile's Mouth" and "The New Word".

Stories that resemble fairy tales likewise fascinate both children and adults (although often not adolescents), and it is interesting from a therapeutic perspective to note that listening to a fairy tale involves an age regression into childhood, or in other words a period generally associated with a learning attitude characterised by curiosity and a willingness to obey those in positions of "parental" authority. (Contemporary features and fairy-tale elements are combined in the story "Heaven on Earth".) This attitude is reactivated during listening and can be utilised to encourage the listener to embark on the task of self-motivated learning.

The same applies to myths (as in the story "Noah's Brothers"), legends, pranks and farces (as in the story "Morbus Feivel") as well as any similar genres which clients can be expected to have encountered in their childhood.

### Novellas and adventure genres

Most modern storytelling genres are too broad in scope to be used within the confines of a single therapy session, although it is conceivable that a soap opera or adventure novel could be told in episodes over a series of meetings with the client, like a thread that is spun endlessly further. New events that occur in the client's life can then be flexibly integrated into the therapeutic "family saga" (or crime series, medical drama etc.). In most cases, longer genres can be integrated into the therapeutic context more easily in the form of allusions or heavily abridged versions; depending on the preferences of the therapist and the client, therapeutic messages can for example be disguised as novellas, as in the story "The Desert", or pirate stories, as in the story "Pirate Anaesthesia".

### Nature studies and research outcomes

Nature studies and reports from the field of technology or the social sciences can also serve as a starting point for therapeutic stories. For example, real examples of communication between animals or plants or between animals and humans can be used as a model for successful and unsuccessful life choices, in an alternative form of the traditional fable. (Compare the stories "Renewed Life" and "The Eagle and The Falconer".)

Historical accounts, travelogues (compare respectively the stories "The Spanish Conquistadors" and "From Oasis to Oasis") and various data formats from the field of mathematics (compare the story "Life as a Sinus Curve") can be used in realistic or abstract form as metaphorical instructions for mind- or action-based solutions to problems, and the outcomes of biological, medical and psychological research (compare the story "Renewed Life") can be cited with a view to prompting clients to develop their own solution models. It is irrelevant whether a study cited in this way meets the standards of the scientific community or is merely a traveller's tale; what matters is that it facilitates the search for potential solutions and provides inspiration for new ways of thinking and behaving.

## Lists and descriptions

Repetition is a particularly useful technique for integrating a suggestive message in such a way as to ensure that it is implemented by the unconscious mind, as illustrated by the story "Selling Pain". Descriptions and lists – examining a metaphor from many perspectives without an underlying storyline – are a simple way of repeating suggestions often enough that they are highly likely to be implemented:

> Some engineers specialise in designing valves. They do nothing but design valves, all day long. You might think that spending so much time thinking about valves would be boring, but in fact it is an extremely interesting topic. There are many different types of valve; air valves and steam valves, water valves and oil valves, pressure valves and thermostatic valves. There are mixer valves which can be used to set the temperature of a liquid, for example in a shower. There are valves which operate automatically and those which can only be operated manually, and there are also valves which operate both automatically and manually.
>
> A huge range of different valves can also be found in nature. Natural valves can be found at the entrance to the oesophagus and the trachea, at the exit of the stomach and the bladder and at the end of the intestine. Many glands also have a kind of valve. The heart has valves, and the veins contain valves to ensure that the blood flows in the right direction.
>
> One might even say that the mind has valves, since it regulates everything we think and feel on the basis of what it believes to be important. If it turns out that something has not proved useful, it can change the focus of its experience and try something new... (cf. Hammel, 2012b: 49).

A listener who hears so much about valves and learns everything that they can do, including in his or her own body and mind, will understand that he or she can in many ways adjust the "settings" of the body or mind which are perpetuating his or her problems. A monologue of this kind will encourage him or her to carry out checks (both conscious and unconscious) to identify whether a new approach could be taken to his or her current challenges.

The metaphor of the valve is a figurative suggestion with the underlying message, "you can handle it." A systemic question can also be used to express the weighing up of priorities as a metaphor;

"Imagine that the two options you are struggling to decide between were the two end positions of a slider switch, and that one end was marked "zero", and the other end "ten", with "five" being right in the centre – where would the switch be right now? Where would you like it to be? Push the switch to that position, and see how that feels. What has changed? What is better now, and what is worse? If you wanted to choose 70 per cent of one option and 30 per cent of the other, what should the 30 per cent include if at all possible? Of course, you can always push the switch to a different position if something changes in future and you need to make an adjustment..."

Every basic human experience can be described in similar ways; learning, searching and finding. Waiting, maturing and defending oneself. The underlying message is: "You can do it. Make the most of the opportunities available to you!"

It goes without saying that the various examples can also be assigned to different people, rooms or times, as illustrated by the following description in relation to the topic of "searching":

> What is the best way to search for Easter eggs? Why do some people search and search without finding any? If you happen to be one of these people, let me give you a few tips.
>
> Possibility one; very small children are unable to find Easter eggs because they don't know what they are.
>
> If they get sent off to search without being given any instructions, they may well return with twigs or daisies.
>
> Possibility two; slightly older children know what Easter eggs look like, but do not understand what "searching" really means, and that there are many different ways of searching. Just in case you're an Easter egg yourself, it's important to know that a good way of finding something is to let yourself be found.
>
> Possibility three; even older children know what Easter eggs look like and how to search for them, but might look for them at the wrong time and in the wrong place. Have you ever searched for Easter eggs and not found them anywhere? If so, you'll understand what I mean.
>
> Possibility four; the Easter eggs are there, but they don't look quite the same as they did last year. Perhaps they have always been red and blue in the past, and now they are camouflage green – your internal image of an Easter egg doesn't correspond to the external reality. People often can't find what they're searching for because it doesn't look like they expect it to look.
>
> Possibility five; the Easter eggs are there, and they look like they did last year, but they are hidden by something – grass, a piece of bark or an old gutter. The things in life that are truly valuable are often hidden and need to be searched out.
>
> If you follow all this advice and still can't find any Easter eggs, there's only one thing for it – take out a paintbrush and some pots of paint, paint some Easter eggs yourself in red, yellow and blue and hide them everywhere, preferably so that there is always a little splash of colour visible among the green grass! (Cf. Hammel, 2012b: 60.)

## Quotes and aphorisms

Quotes can also be used as stories, and this includes both fictitious quotes (such as those in the stories involving Fedor the magician, that is, "Finding Treasure", "How Do You Tame a Dragon?" and "How Do You Break a Spell?") and statements which have really been spoken and written down. Questions and explanations narrated in the third person can also be used to break up a long monologue, as illustrated by the following story:

> We were talking about music.
> "The ear is merciful," she said. "It hears what is meant rather than what is actually played."
> The woman who said that to me was a piano teacher who had been teaching pupils for decades, all the while thinking about how music is processed by the ear and the brain.
> "The ear is merciful," I repeated. "What do you mean?"
> She replied, "When we sit in the audience and listen to music, we generally ignore any mistakes and hear what we are meant to hear – what arrives in the conscious mind is a perfect melody. The musicians and their teachers hear the mistakes, but the audience hears the music." (Cf. Hammel, 2012b: 71.)

The purpose of a quote of this kind may be the paradigmatic representation of an internal ambivalence or the simple illustration of a metaphor, as in this case where it symbolises a possible approach to the need for logical, aesthetic or moral completeness. When using monologues of this kind, it is important to remember that they should not merely represent the opposite of the client's beliefs, but use these beliefs as a starting point for moving in new directions. This corresponds to the principle of pacing and leading, which is well known in the field of hypnotherapy; if we wish to change something about the client's experiences and behaviour, it is a good idea to start by following in the client's footsteps and only afterwards lead the way.

Aphorisms are short mottoes that get to the crux of complex or ambivalent aspects of human existence in just a few words, and in such a way as to prompt the listener to consider the matter further. Many aphorisms have a metaphorical/descriptive and narrative quality, and deliver useful therapeutic effects when used wisely. Their effectiveness derives from the fact that they stand alone and are not debated ad nauseam during the subsequent conversation; although this is a general rule which applies to all stories, it is particularly true of aphorisms.

The following sentences are examples of aphorisms which can be used for therapeutic purposes;

> "Finished!" said the egg after it had been laid. ("Finished")

"The job of parents is to make sure that their children can manage without them." (Cf. the story "Managing Without Them".)

"Well done," said the tree when the snails overtook him. (Cf. the story "Speed".)

### Poetry

Poetical texts and literary prose can also be used as suggestive prompts for further consideration; for example, in tinnitus therapy I use the lyrics of the Simon and Garfunkel song "The Sound of Silence" to encourage the patient to refocus his or her attention from the intensity and quality of the noise to the intensity and quality of the silence. An example of a poetical story is "The Cave Dwellers", which can be used to challenge the listener's belief in the supposedly unalterable nature of reality.

# Chapter 10

# Telling therapeutic stories

## Before storytelling

Many of the interventions presented in this book will seem unfamiliar to clients, and perhaps also to therapists; some violate the normal rules of logic, while others are framed as pranks. These interventions are most likely to succeed in situations where the counsellor can tell the story with an ironic twinkle in the eye.

Interventions of this kind may need to be announced in advance to clients who believe that a therapist should take himself or herself seriously; in such cases the therapist can use a few preliminary remarks to integrate the stories into the relevant context, for example by pointing out that a number of friends think that he or she is crazy for coming up with such strange ideas, and that perhaps they are right, but since the ideas are often helpful to clients it seems a shame to stop talking about them.

Almost any ideas that the therapist believes to be useful can be expressed in a story after an introduction of this kind; self-proclaimed madness and ignorance are familiar territory for therapists, and the fool always held a privileged position at the king's court. For example, a therapist could say, "When I work with children, I often use these Lego blocks to help explain a conflict of this kind, and afterwards the children see the situation quite differently. Some of them completely alter their view of events – it's really quite fascinating. Now obviously as a Chairman of the Board you're too important for things like that..." The therapist might repeat this statement and then, when the Chairman suggests trying it out anyway, ask, "Are you really sure?" and "I don't know whether that would be appropriate for a man in your position..." The client might then remind him that he has children of his own with whom he plays, and the two of them can then get down on their knees and play with the Lego.

Almost any method can be used for almost any client if it is introduced correctly.

## Starting storytelling

There are lots of different ways in which a therapist can train himself or herself to find appropriate stories and to tell them during counselling sessions, and a number of pointers are given in the section above on "Using intuition". Yet many therapists set the bar so high when it comes to the quality of their storytelling that they never get started, which is both a shame and entirely preventable...

Therapeutic storytelling and aesthetic storytelling are two different arts, each of which can only be learned with practice; what is artistically valuable is not always therapeutically valuable, and vice versa. I believe that it is important to be clear about the distinction between literary and therapeutic quality before starting to tell stories, and that anyone who wishes to learn to tell stories for the purpose of counselling should temporarily set aside his or her desire for aesthetic perfection, particularly if there is a risk that the pleasure of experimenting with a new therapeutic technique might be overshadowed by the search for beauty and refinement.

There are many questions that are more important for therapeutic work than linguistic panache, such as the following; what are the implications of my story which the client – if he or she accepts the story – will apply by analogy to the search for solutions to his or her own problems? Which isomorphic (i.e. with a similar structure to the content of the story) ways of seeing the world and behaving is the story intended to promote in the client?

Alternatively, which searching and learning processes is it intended to trigger? If a therapist tells a particular story to several different clients, its aesthetic appeal can gradually be refined.

It goes without saying that anyone keen to use stories which are particularly well-crafted in linguistic terms can write them down before or after a counselling session and then read them aloud at the next available opportunity; by doing so, the therapist will also gain clearer insight into the implications, potential applications and effects of his or her stories, as well as accumulating a growing collection of stories at his or her fingertips. The story "Bad English" illustrates how storytelling can be learned:

> When I was growing up, my parents took us to America to visit relatives. My elder sister wanted to speak English correctly, and so didn't say anything. I just wanted people to understand me, and so I gestured with my hands and feet and made countless mistakes. My relatives were impressed, my parents were proud and I suspect my sister was envious. I learned English by speaking bad English.

We tell each other stories all day long, and many of these stories are suitable for purposeful use in a counselling context. A therapeutic effect can often be achieved if we simply tell these everyday stories as we would tell them when sitting around the kitchen table or chatting with friends, with the only difference being that we should remain silent after the climactic turning point in order to give the listener time to think. There are three factors that turn an everyday story into a therapeutically effective story; the counselling situation itself implies and suggests that the story is aimed at producing a therapeutic effect, the story is told in a situation that has parallels with its content, or the story is told in such a way that the client searches for parallels with its content. The client's unconscious mind will ultimately decide whether the story is relevant to his or her problem and whether the message it contains should be implemented.

Some therapists claim that they are unable to tell stories; it is helpful to ask whether they are also unable to tell stories when sitting in a pub garden or coffee shop, or whether they mistakenly believe that a story told in a counselling room should sound different to one told around a table with friends. Most therapists are in fact already accomplished at the art of storytelling – they are simply not used to thinking about it as such.

A therapist who wishes to start telling stories should do so by building on the aspects of his or her therapy work that are already more personal and narrative in nature, such as the small talk at the start of a therapy session or the stories that naturally crop up when trying to set a date for the next session; all will easily accommodate metaphors and statements that promote searching attitudes and a focus on solutions.

## Trusting the power of stories

### Reduction to what is essential

The delivery of a story can be either powerful or weak; a story is delivered powerfully if it is reduced to what is essential and vivid, and if questions are asked and a questioning and searching attitude is triggered in the listener. The power of a story can be intensified by using surprise, ritualistic repetition and a choice of words which allows the kind of rhythmical emphasis we normally expect to find in poems.

A good rule of thumb is that every superfluous word weakens the story, and it is easy to test this out by deleting any unnecessary words from a sentence, reading both versions aloud to yourself and comparing their effect. Anyone writing down a story should therefore take care to ensure that every single word is necessary. It is often a good idea to remove auxiliary verbs such as "can" and "should", and certain relativising words such as "perhaps" and "sometimes"; entreating or placating phrases such as "surely" and "in fact..." are also dispensable in most cases.

What the resulting story loses in its differentiation of reality, it will gain in aesthetic and therapeutic effect. Any relativising or specifying statements which are genuinely indispensable should be presented in a subsequent sentence instead of a subordinate clause.

The last recommendation is based on the second rule of thumb, namely that subordinate clauses weaken the power of the main clause, and parenthetical statements weaken the power of the main statement. A *single* example often results in a more powerful story than two or three; for example, instead of the phrase "cares and concerns" it would be preferable simply to use the noun "cares".

All grammarians know that every rule has its exception, and this also applies to the grammar of a powerful story. There are sometimes good reasons for including apparently superfluous elements in a story, and these reasons are discussed in the following sections.

### Reduction to what is vivid

The goal of human communication is often (but by no means always) to speak in a way that does not overtax the listener's comprehension and concentration, so that he or she can easily follow the speaker's train of thought and listen consciously for long periods.

The use of vivid language also benefits the unconscious mind; as a general rule, the unconscious mind is more receptive to positive statements than to sentences which include the word "not" or other negative phrases.

It is therefore a good idea to revise sentence structures which use the words "but", "instead" and "not...but rather", since it is likely that the story will be more powerful without them; they can either be omitted in keeping with the above principle of reduction to what is essential, or replaced ("but" can often be replaced by "and" or "therefore", for example).

It is furthermore often useful to replace the word "or" with the word "and"; in order to understand a sentence structured around the word "or", the first part of the sentence must be imagined and then forgotten so that the second part can be imagined, since the ultimate aim of a sentence structure of this kind is to juxtapose two ideas which exclude each other. Paradoxically, however, none of the individual sentence elements may be completely forgotten, since it would otherwise be impossible to compare the two options. The listener must therefore expend a great deal of concentration on decoding "or"-based sentences, and part of the information is therefore not processed (at least consciously). Preference should be given to the use of "and"-based sentences wherever possible, since the unconscious mind imagines the two elements alongside each other and metaphorically compares them.

The content of abstract statements (including nominalisations, i.e. verbs, adjectives and other word types which have been turned into nouns) is difficult to imagine in vivid terms. Nouns such as those ending in —ness (happiness, from happy), —ation (hibernation, from hibernate) or —ship (ownership, from own) are difficult to represent in metaphorical terms and therefore hard for the unconscious mind to comprehend. The word "nominalisation" itself provides a good example of this phenomenon; although its meaning is cognitively clear, it does not create any kind of internal image which would be accessible by the unconscious mind. Politicians' speeches which sound meaningful but contain little of any real demonstrable meaning contain a high concentration of abstract nouns of this kind; a therapist who wishes to use vivid language should therefore turn nouns back into the verbs and adjectives on which they were originally based.

## Trances and trance phenomena

### Using trances

A therapist wishing to intensify the therapeutic effect of a story can use trance-inducing words and sentence structures, trance-inducing non-verbal elements and implicit trance suggestions. Each of these options will be examined in detail below.

According to the Italian psychotherapist Camillo Loriedo (Loriedo, seminar presentation, 2003), the advantages of using trances in family therapy conversations include the following:

- The level of aggression of the participants is reduced significantly; the conversation can be held in a more relaxed atmosphere, and emotionally charged situations remain under control.
- A good rapport is established not only with the therapist but also with the other parties in the conversation, meaning that mutually agreeable solutions are easier to find.
- Interactions take place at a slower rate, leaving the counsellor more time to think and intervene.
- The participants are simultaneously more independent in their behaviour and more attuned to each other, which is otherwise almost impossible to achieve in a waking condition.
- The participants are more receptive and willing to learn.
- Blocks and barriers which exist in the waking state are often reduced or eliminated.
- Participants are more open to different interpretations and perspectives.

In my experience, many symptoms of physical and psychological stress (in particular anxiety, aggression, nervousness, pain, breathing problems, muscular tension, allergic reactions and withdrawal symptoms in addicts) are greatly reduced or eliminated during trances induced involuntarily by storytelling; anchoring techniques and concluding interventions (post-hypnotic suggestions) can be used to perpetuate this stress-free state and to ensure that it can be recreated in the future.

## Trance-inducing content

One way in which a therapist can prepare a client for a trance or induce a trance in the client is to describe a trance situation, or in other words an experience associated with a trance. He or she might talk about a visit to the cinema, the intense concentration displayed by an archer during an archery tournament or the boredom of a school pupil towards the end of a double period on a rainy Friday afternoon. (For further details on trance induction through trance memories, compare Bandler & Grinder, 1981: 72.) The therapist can likewise induce a trance in the client by asking him or her to describe an experience associated with a trance. Finally, the same goal can be achieved by naming or describing trance phenomena and other aspects of a trance. For example, the therapist can illustrate everyday phenomena such as dissociation, hypnotic anaesthesia, positive and negative hallucinations and catalepsy by means of the stories "Pirate Anaesthesia" or "The Unscrewable Body". For further details of drawing on the therapist's experiences to describe trance situations and trance phenomena in order to induce a trance in the client, compare Bandler and Grinder, 1981: 50.

## Trance-inducing patterns of speech

A standard format for trance-inducing stories is to start with a question, and preferably a whole series of questions, as in the stories "The Creation of the World" and "When You Meet Your Brother". Or questions which incorporate additional methods of trance induction. For example, it might be useful to ask a series of questions about the client's childhood or situations that already involve a trance; the therapist could ask the client to describe the plot of a thrilling novel based on the client's problem, and then discuss how (after a number of false starts) a successful combination of different solutions is found and the novel concludes with a happy ending.

Stories can be used to induce a trance by generating confusion, for example by means of perplexing and paradoxical statements or ambiguous wordings, or by diverting part of the listener's attention with incomplete or grammatically incorrect sentences, logical incongruities and factually incorrect statements. A trance can be induced by making the familiar unfamiliar, by forcing the conscious mind to "switch off" by overtaxing its attention with a sequence of complex statements, or by deliberately promoting boredom. Sentences that might be profound or might just be profoundly stupid can be interspersed in a story, and unreal statements can be used ("assuming... imagine... what if...").

## Trance-inducing ways of speaking and moving

A therapist wishing to deepen a trance in his or her listener can tell stories using a different pitch and a slower pace of speech, and with a quieter and softer voice which perhaps sounds more mysterious and meaningful. He or she can reinforce the trance yet further by using a slurred and mumbling way of talking, breathing more slowly, incorporating long pauses into the story and synchronising the pace of the story with the rhythm of the listener's breathing (breath pacing).

A therapist can promote a trance in his or her client by going into a trance himself or herself and displaying the physical behaviours which are typical of a trance; movements which are less frequent, less distinct and somewhat jerky, and which occur with a delay after the verbal or non-verbal impulses which trigger them.

### Using trance phenomena

All traditional trance phenomena (even in their somewhat unassuming everyday forms) can be used to induce a trance or to deepen an incipient trance, stimulated either non-verbally on the basis of rapport or verbally on the basis of spoken suggestions. These phenomena can furthermore be used for therapeutic purposes.

For example, a therapist can induce a trance in a client through dissociation, or in other words by distinguishing between different parts of the client's personality, as in the story "Dinner for One", or different body parts and giving them different instructions. If the therapist then suggests that they should embark on different and mutually incompatible experiences, they will become alienated from one another while these experiences are being imagined in order to comply with the therapist's instructions.

This technique can be used to induce anaesthesia (see the last section of this sub-chapter) or to use a region of the brain which is working properly as a model for an area which is not working properly (subjectively experienced as encouraging a sick part of the body to learn from a healthy part). Examples of stories where one part of the body functions as "teacher" or "parent" and another as the "pupil" or "child" are "Taekwondo" and "Learning to Walk". Mental functions and parts of the personality can also be dissociated; the separation of associations or functional areas of the mind (as in the story "Dinner for One") can eliminate harmful trigger/response patterns and embed new response patterns. New messages and relationship patterns can also be practised between parts of the personality which are in conflict with each other. (Compare the story "The Three Principles".)

In cases where this creates a state which is free of symptoms, the client can be informed while he or she is still in the trance (following the principle of psychoeducation) that he or she should unconsciously evaluate this state and then display it ever more frequently while in a waking condition. A structural (i.e. not content-related) suggestion can also be directed to the client asking him or her to tell his or her unconscious that it should check how the dissociation currently being experienced can be used in modified form to solve his or her problem.

Another way in which trances can be induced is to tell stories which trigger memories. When the therapist talks about his or her childhood (as in the story "Dot to Dot") or someone else's childhood, the listener will automatically think of his or her own childhood, inducing a trance through age regression. The same will happen if the therapist uses a genre of stories which are typically told to children, for example fairy tales or stories about animals. Simply starting a story with the words, "Once upon a time…" or "A long time ago, in a land far far away…" promotes a trance by triggering age regression.

The client can be told that past, present and future are experienced concurrently in the human brain as memories, momentary experiences and expectations, and that the resources of the experienced "present" and "future" can be used to heal the experienced "past", that earlier memories can be used to heal later memories and vice versa and that these experiences do not relate to different (sequenced) times but to different (unsequenced) locations in our body.

Using this framework suggestion and psychoeducational information as a basis, positive life experiences and the associated bodily experiences and emotions can be recollected in great detail and metaphorically taken (using a basket, a lorry or a pipeline) to a time where they are needed or were once needed. (Compare the story "Peace Settlement with a Tooth".)

The client can imagine people from a later stage of his or her life visiting an earlier stage (or vice versa) to provide assistance. The person of today can enter into a conversation with the child of long ago in the role of "big brother" or "big sister", or the client as he or she was before a trauma can visit the person after the trauma in order to provide assistance. Age regression can also be used as a form of beauty treatment; the client imagines himself or herself at a younger (wrinkle-free, happy) age and anchors the psycho-autonomic responses to this imagined experience in order to make them accessible again in the present as well as in stressful situations in the future. (Compare the story "The Difference".)

It goes without saying that the technique of age progression can also be used to induce trances.

When undertaking journeys of this kind into a fictitious future, it can sometimes be important to introduce the story with framework suggestions in order to promote positive expectations on the part of the client.

The client can be taken forward in time to a period, "when you have left your problem behind", using all of his or her senses to imagine this period and looking back to see what helped him or her to solve the problem. He or she can gaze with pride and thankfulness at what has been achieved, and return to the present with the same sense of pride and look forward to achieving the goal. The phenomenon of age progression can likewise be used by telling positive stories about older people; the lessons from these stories can then be applied to the patient's own life, promoting positive expectations about the future, as in the story "Love". Age progression can also be used for the purpose of thought experiments; when working with suicidal patients, a fictitious journey beyond death itself can be undertaken in order to engage in dialogue with the introjects of previously deceased family members, as in the story "When You Meet Your Brother".

In the case of therapy involving children, progression to the age of an older child or adult can motivate the patient to act as though he or she were older (or simply the appropriate age), as in the stories "The Little Cat" and "The Schoolchildren's Fairy". It is also possible for a child, by imagining that he or she is older than his or her real age, to stimulate unconscious behaviour, which means that he or she is treated as older or as a grown-up by others. An example for this is the attempt by the fourteen-year-old girl to imagine herself as a seventeen-year-old in the story "Pest".

The phenomena of amnesia and hypermnesia can be promoted by describing situations which imply a deterioration or improvement in memory in paradigmatic or metaphorical terms.

"I don't know", "you can forget about that", "none of that matters" – the increased use of expressions like these promotes amnesia in respect of what happens in the story or aspects of the problem that caused the client to seek help from the therapist.

In the interests of psychoeducation, the client can be told that people unconsciously decide what they should remember and forget, and that they can always unconsciously change these decisions later if it would be useful to do so. The terms "remember" and "forget" merely indicate whether our unconscious mind makes a memory accessible to our conscious mind or not. A structural suggestion, for example a paradigmatic story about another client who experienced something similar, can therefore be used to suggest to a client that he or she should reexamine what he or she remembers and forgets in the midst of experience. The therapist can tell a story about how the other client remembered new things, at first in his nighttime dreams and then increasingly during the day, but how a friend pointed out that he seemed to have forgotten other things.

The phenomenon of catalepsy is used if a client is asked to imagine a bandage or plaster around a body part that needs to be kept immobile (for example a sprained ankle); the potential medical risks must be kept in mind if catalepsy is used as a technique to improve sporting performance, as in the story "Arm Wrestling". The phenomenon can also be used in its everyday form to silence bullies – the client does something that results in seconds (or minutes) of surprise or shock associated with immobility and speechlessness (compare the story "Thank You", which can usefully be combined with the story "How to Handle Sexual Assault…"), after which the other party lacks a point of reference to continue with his or her previous behaviour (and often lacks the associated memories as a result of amnesia).

Stories and storytelling interventions can induce hypnotic anaesthesia in many different ways. Methods of doing so without using formal hypnotic techniques are illustrated in the section on "Bodily sensations and the perception of pain", but it is also possible to intersperse details with anaesthetic implications throughout a story or to describe images which imply the absence of pain or bodily sensations; this includes techniques for the dissociation of bodily parts (compare the stories "The Unscrewable Body" and "Pirate Anaesthesia"). Physical discomfort can also be externalised, visualised and transformed on a metaphorical level. Age regressions can be used to prompt clients to return pain to its time of origin, as in "Peace Settlement with a Tooth" or even to a time before the pain started, as in "A Walk Along the Beach".

## Therapeutic interventions in detail

### Clarification of goals and orders

Stories can be used in a counselling context to clarify goals and orders. For example, the story "My Aim in Life" can be used to raise the issue of the patient's fundamental goals directly, but the therapist can also use stories to draw the patient's attention indirectly to problems which require an appropriate response and which prevent the victim from searching for solutions. A good example of a story that can be used in this way is "The Cave Dwellers".

### Anamnesis questions

Questions can be used for suggestive or informative purposes. It goes without saying that anamnesis questions should be formulated as neutrally as possible, and as a general rule open questions starting with "who", "how", "when" etc. are often preferable to dichotomous questions which may restrict the patient's interpretations of reality rather than expanding them.

Anamnesis questions may be aimed at determining how long a problem has been present, the contexts in which it occurs, the triggers for and typical progression of the symptomatic behaviour and any points at which a pattern interrupt may be possible. See for example the questions in the story "The Bladder Alarm Clock".

One technique for asking anamnesis questions is to observe any changes in the client's voice which reveal increased stress when using certain words or discussing certain topics; if the client's voice sounds sad, shaky or hesitant, or if his or her speech is loaded with Freudian slips or meaningless slips of the tongue. Associated questions can then be asked on these topics as a form of brainstorming; if this procedure is repeated several times, the questions often lead rapidly to the crux of the problem, as in the story "A Girl Like Robin Hood".

Words that are "misheard" by the therapist can also be used in this way; the brain often mishears things when it unconsciously notices infinitesimal triggers such as a change in pronunciation indicating that the speaker was thinking of another word at the same time, or when connotations are communicated non-verbally. Asking clients to repeat the word that was "misheard" often reveals the underlying problem and uncovers a deeper meaning behind what was apparently meant.

### Preparation and follow-up

I use the term "framework suggestion" to refer to the process of laying the groundwork for therapeutic suggestion by means of preferments, verbal hints, the explanation of a treatment method or symptom or implications associated with the treatment situation. Practitioners of traditional hypno-therapy refer to such forms of targeted influence by the therapist as "pre-hypnotic suggestion"; therapists following the teachings of Milton Erickson and carrying out hypnosystemic work, which rarely uses formal trance induc-tion, prefer the term "seeding", while others use the term "priming". Manfred Prior has carried out a detailed investigation into the use of such interventions during a telephone conversation before the first therapy session, in the form of stories, questions and observation exercises (Prior, 2007: 42).

The underlying aim of suggestions of this kind – which are extremely effective and often operate at an unconscious level, even for the therapist – is to establish an optimal framework within which the central suggestions can be accepted and implemented. The mere fact that the client is attending a course of therapy is a powerful framework suggestion, and he or she will consciously and unconsciously investigate everything that is communicated in this context to identify helpful or healing impulses. Anything the client has heard about the therapist and his or her work from a referring doctor and any experiences during the initial telephone call and the first therapy session also constitute framework suggestions. If the client achieves significant results after his or her first meeting with the therapist, progress will continue to be rapid because this is what the client now expects and therefore unconsciously facilitates. Anything that the therapist announces to the client at the start of the course of therapy or an individual therapy session also represents a framework suggestion, and – provided a good level of rapport has been established – will influence the client's behaviour.

Key framework suggestions include comments by the therapist in relation to the positive experiences of other clients, the innate human traits of curi-osity and imagination, the ability of children to learn or the satisfaction of achieving a long-held goal. As a general rule the listener will be induced to implement what has been discussed, thus ensuring that the foundations are laid for the appropriate changes.

Preventive suggestions that are aimed at preventing a foreseeable but undesirable behaviour represent a special subcategory of pre-hypnotic suggestion. In the context of trauma therapy, it is often useful to make it clear at the start that the client can actively regulate the way in which he or she experiences earlier events and the associated emotions. Before tackling the problematic events, the client can be asked to imagine a remote control which can be used to adjust every aspect of the brightness, contrast, colour, volume and emotional intensity of the experience. Preventive suggestions can also be used to minimise the impact of impending injury, as in the story "Keep All Cells Alive", and to equip the immune system to fight off infectious pathogens, as in the story "Risk of Contagion".

Concluding interventions or post-hypnotic suggestions, which can also be effective when used in an everyday trance situation without induced hypnosis, represent the counterpart to seeding or pre-hypnotic suggestion.

One form of post-hypnotic suggestion is the use of statements such as "Every time when you…, you will…", linking an unavoidable occurrence (such as seeing the colour red or opening and closing a door) with a desirable mental change such as reinforcement of the decision to remain a non-smoker. For further information on post-hypnotic suggestions (cf. Erickson & Rossi, 1979: 85).

In addition to post-hypnotic suggestions in the narrower sense of the term, homework (compare the case study "Pest") and rituals, as used in systemic counselling, can also be employed as an effective follow-up to therapy sessions.

### Personalising the content of stories

It goes without saying that in certain cases it can be a good idea to adapt invented stories to the client's situation, for example by giving the protagonist a similar age and a similar job and placing them in a somewhat similar situation. It is, however, rarely advisable for the protagonists of stories or the situations in which they find themselves to be more or less identical to real people and circumstances; certain differences must remain in order to encourage the listener's mind to apply the story to his or her own life. A lack of dissimilarity between fictitious events and real experiences sometimes also provokes resistance on the part of the client.

Certain differences can be introduced on purpose; for example, the protagonists in paradigmatic stories for children can be one year younger than the "real" child. In the same vein, if the child attending counselling is a boy, the child in the story can be a girl, and vice versa, because as any seven-year-old boy knows, "If a six-year-old girl can do it, then I certainly can!"

Similarly, solutions are generally found more readily if the exemplary protagonists of stories have a job that enjoys somewhat more or somewhat less social prestige than the client's profession, building on the idea that "you can do that too!" in order to develop new ways of seeing the world and behaving.

### Prioritising the content of stories

How can we ensure that a story is heeded by the unconscious mind and that its implications are implemented? Most of the other stories people hear as they go about their day-to-day lives are regarded as being of no great relevance and have no major impact. Whether or not a story prompts further thought by the unconscious mind depends on whether it is given greater priority than these other stories as a result of its context and the way in which it is told.

The implications of the setting in which the story is told are of decisive significance in this respect. A story told in the context of a therapy session will be examined by the unconscious mind for its therapeutic benefits, whereas the same story told during an evening at the pub will probably have no therapeutic effect. A catchy advertising slogan which is quoted during a counselling session may lead to a decisive turning point in a patient's life, but the same slogan on a billboard which is read by the patient in passing will probably not have the same effect, or at least not until it has been reinterpreted within the framework of counselling.

The second key criterion is that the client believes that the story contains a solution and relates to his or her problem. In this respect it is important that the situation described by the story should be structurally similar to the patient's own life, ensuring that the outcome of the story has plausible parallels with a possible outcome of the patient's own problem. The third decisive factor is whether the story (or parts of the story) are emphasised by the storyteller as being significant.

There are a variety of different ways of ensuring that a story or an element of storytelling is ascribed particular importance by the unconscious mind. For example, anyone who tells several stories which are structurally similar highlights the significance of the elements shared by these stories, and implies that they should be accorded particular attention by the unconscious mind. A sentence which is repeated several times in a story is prioritised, and anyone who uses a word or refers to a topic repeatedly shifts the listener's focus of attention to this word or topic.

A word, a group of words, a topic or a sentence can be prioritised by emphasising the relevant elements nonverbally, for example if the therapist turns his face in a different direction every time he says the relevant words, pauses briefly beforehand, raises his or her voice, speaks more loudly or quietly, rubs his or her nose or otherwise changes the presentation of the words. This method was developed by Milton Erickson and is described in NLP as "analogous marking". For further information on analogous marking, compare Bandler and Grinder, 1981: 63.

The same naturally also applies to stories as a whole, and merely the act of switching to the genre of storytelling (which is somewhat unusual in a counselling context) serves as a first indication that the content of the story is significant. In order to make it even clearer that the unconscious mind should treat a story as a priority, the therapist can alter the volume and sound of his or her voice and the speed at which he or she speaks, at the same time inducing a trance in the listener which promotes unconscious (i.e. multi-faceted) processing of the material covered in the story.

### Interspersal of topics

A deliberate increase in the use of indirect methods such as ambiguity, connotation and metaphorical and logical implication is referred to under the term of "interspersal technique", and is used either to prepare for interventions (in which case it is referred to as "seeding") or as the intervention proper. The technique involves using storytelling elements to weave words or topics with solution-based implications and connotations into a story or a dialogue until the suggested solution is accepted by the client's unconscious mind.

In addition to the story "Snail Race", in which the focus is on the use of ambiguity and connotations, the story "Selling Pain" can also be used as an example of the interspersal technique (a method developed by Milton Erickson) where the focus is more on metaphorical implications.

### Using ambiguity and connotations

It should be clear from the above that ambiguity can be used to convey messages to the unconscious mind. Everything that is ambiguous is also suggestive. The listener can only consciously respond on *one* level at a time; if he or she wishes to respond to all the messages, it is necessary to examine the significance of the various levels one after another, meaning that his or her attention will be fixed for a while on this single sentence and he or she will be unable to listen consciously to the meaning of the following statements. As a general rule, therefore, a listener only consciously responds on one level; if he or she accepts the message as plausible, the other levels of meaning will also be accepted. For example, if the listener accepts the sentence, "Imagine that you're a pirate yourself, confident that you'll no longer do it consciously", he or she will also accept the declaration "you're self-confident" without undertaking the complex task of distinguishing between the different levels of interpretation.

A declaration or implication is more likely to be accepted if the listener's conscious attention is held by distinctive storytelling aspects in the vicinity of the statement which mean that it would take even longer to distinguish the various levels of meaning. These may include sentence elements that must be processed cognitively or which are disturbing or emotionally loaded.

In the story "From Oasis to Oasis" we hear the following about the Bedouins:

> He [...] admired the Bedouins for their sense of calm they exuded. They rode from oasis to oasis, constantly reassured by thoughts of the next oasis as they journeyed through the desert.

This passage includes the following hidden declarations targeted at the listener; "You exude a sense of calm. You are constantly reassured by thoughts of the future..."

It is unlikely that statements of this kind could be made directly to a patient suffering from anxiety, grief or depression without provoking a protest and becoming ensnared in discussions that would remove much of the power of the positive declaration. Yet if the storyteller makes exactly the same statements about Bedouins, his or her statements will be accepted, and it will be difficult for the listener to differentiate between the accepted meaning of the sentence in the immediate context of the story (Bedouins) and the rejected potential meaning in the wider storytelling context (client).

A woman who says that she acts like a headless chicken when it comes to choosing a romantic partner could be told a story which starts as follows:

> Way down south below the equator, in the heart of the African bush, there once lived a brave chicken who was afraid of nothing. She was unafraid of cats, squirrels and weasels, and she was only perhaps a little bit afraid of the great shaggy lion.

A distinction can be made between the use of ambiguity in the normal sense of the word (for example "shaggy"/"shag") and the use of connotations which reveal a further meaning behind the actual text.

The example referred to above includes therapeutically relevant connotations for the expressions "down below" (in an anatomical sense and in the sense of somewhere deep), "down south" (down, internally), "African" (curly-haired, dark, mysterious, hidden) and in the bush (in the pubic area).

The story "Snail Race" also talks about animals...

> ...the length of time taken by these moist creatures to make progress, and how slowly they expel slime as they moisten the ground over which they glide [...] how the snails strain forward to make progress! How they straighten their smooth, solid feelers, and stretch them out towards their goal! How the sides of their body move with a wave-like motion in order to push them onwards!

Although none of the individual words are ambiguous, the high density of words with sexual connotations creates a context in which everything is imbued by the listener with a second, sexual meaning.

### Using assonance

Assonance – that is, words that invoke associations because they sound similar to other words – can be used in a similar way to ambiguity. The following sentence could be added to the example above:

> "She was not afraid of men...ding anything in her house."

The suggestion to the unconscious mind (that the listener should not be afraid of men) is not contradicted by the conscious mind because it is forced to interpret the word as "mending". The unconscious mind however understands the significance of the pause and the relevance to the problem being discussed, and continues to think about the possibility of being unafraid of men.

Similarly, the following sentence could be included in a story about someone who suffers from vertigo:

> When she started to learn more about architecture, she discovered that verti...cal lines and height are just as important – if not more so! – than horizontal lines.

The conscious mind will accept the suggestion that vertical lines and height are positive things in the context of architecture, while the unconscious mind will understand the hidden reference to vertigo and interpret the statement as suggesting that heights in general are nothing to be feared.

### Avoiding resistance

If the storyteller wishes to take additional steps to ensure that this second level of meaning is accepted, there are various ways of avoiding resistance on the part of the listener; for example, the listener's conscious attention can be diverted by means of cognitive information, as in the following example:

> "Did you know that elephants can weigh up to four tonnes and live to the age of 60? Elephants are useful.
> They are strong. They can carry the heaviest of loads with majestic power."

Attention can also be diverted through a disruptive element such as a grammatical error:

> "Elephants *is* useful. They are strong. They can carry the heaviest of loads with majestic power."

Emotionally meaningful elements can also be used to divert attention;

> "Elephants are useful. Oh, there they are! Just look at them! Look at how beautiful they are! The true kings of the jungle! Elephants! How strong they are. They can carry the heaviest of loads with majestic power."

Once again, the story "Pirate Anaesthesia" serves as a good example of various ways of bypassing or eliminating possible resistance against anaesthetic, cataleptic and dissociative suggestions by diverting the listener's attention:

1. The introduction "Imagine that you're a pirate…" suggests through ambiguity that anything contradictory that might be imagined is ruled out.
2. A false alternative is offered; would you rather be a pirate with or without an eye patch? This eliminates the alternative of not being a pirate at all; in the event that the listener nevertheless chooses not to be a pirate, he or she can be someone thinking about a pirate; soon the storyteller and the listener will be on the same page, and attention will be diverted from the wooden leg (which is important in conceptual terms) to the eye patch (which plays no role in the rest of the story).
3. Use of the words "Either way" create a sense of indifference.
4. References to the pirate's work and the swaying of the ship encourage the listener to focus on other senses, in particular the sense of sight and balance.
5. Use of the phrase "of course" suggests that the following statement is indisputable.
6. The irrevocability of the previous suggestions is implied by the floating away of the wooden leg.
7. Sleep implies unconsciousness and defencelessness on the part of the listener.
8. If the storyteller claims not to know something, this induces a phase of "not knowing" in the listener. The technique of talking about "not knowing" or "not doing" in order to promote a trance in connection with a positive attitude to learning was introduced and described by Milton Erickson (Erickson & Rossi, 1979: 24).

## Stringing together and interweaving stories

The stringing together of a sequence of any metaphorical stories that may occur to the storyteller, without analysis of the individual stories, has proved to be an extremely useful technique. In his later years, Milton Erickson often told a series of anecdotes during teaching seminars as though he had forgotten where he was. This approach can be extremely refreshing for client and therapist alike, because the problem is no longer apparently the focus of attention, and the unconscious mind can search for solutions without being disturbed by symptoms of stress.

If several stories with a similar purpose are told one after another, their suggestive effect is increased. This is firstly because repeated suggestions are prioritised by the unconscious mind, even if it is merely the structure or purpose of the stories that is repeated rather than specific wordings. Secondly, the choice of several stories highlights to the unconscious mind the common denominator (or in other words common purpose) and complementary solutions offered by the individual stories, intensifying the effect of the common factors and at the same time offering a wider range of solutions (or interpretations of the key message).

A therapist who wishes to tell several stories with contradictory solutions must take care to ensure that the power of the individual stories is not weakened as a result. He or she can do so by asking the client to search for anything useful in the stories, and to reject anything that is unsuitable; as Gunther Schmidt once said, "To my clients I'm a waiter serving up different versions of reality" (Schmidt, seminar discussion, 2001). This attitude can also be conveyed to clients through stories, for example by asking, "Do you prefer to be on the defensive or on the attack? Do you behave like the protagonist in the story 'The Bulls Are Coming', or the protagonist in the story 'The Power of Thoughts', or perhaps quite differently? I'll have to tell you these two stories some time – I'd be interested to find out which one fits your situation best, or whether you can think of a third story which captures the essence of your situation even better." There is no need to worry that the client will be overtaxed by such complex instructions, since anything which exceeds the capacities of the conscious mind will be processed by the unconscious mind and will nevertheless produce an outcome. Cognitive overtaxing as a result of complex tasks leads to a deeper state of trance, which can be very much an advantage in a counselling context.

Instead of telling stories one after another, it is also possible to interweave a series of stories in the form of a frame story or embedded narrative, following the pattern: "Someone once told me that someone had told him…" Variants on this theme might involve seeing what someone sees, reading what someone reads, imagining what someone imagines and combinations of these forms of experience, all of which are based on the perception of someone perceiving something, the imagination of someone imagining something, the construction of machines that construct things, the reflection of a mirror that reflects things etc. The method of sequencing stories is frequently combined with that of interweaving frame narratives. The story "Pest" is based on the sequencing and interweaving of related stories. Complex encapsulation of therapeutic stories can be found in Hammel, 2006, and in Trenkle, 1998. Intricately encapsulated stories occur frequently in the storytelling tradition of the Ancient Orient, for example in *The Tale of Four Dervishes* (Mir Amman, 1803), in the fairy tales from *The Thousand and One Nights* and in the book of Job in the Bible.

## After storytelling

What should follow a story? How should the counselling session continue? An explanation by the therapist of the story's meaning is a bad idea, since explanations rob a story of much of its power and restrict the listener's freedom to find his or her own interpretation of what has been told. Explanations also have a slightly defensive feel, as though some kind of justification were required for the incorporation of a story into the counselling session. Since explanations often provide answers, they prematurely curtail the journey on which the listener had just embarked.

The best way to continue the counselling session is to be silent after the story until the client speaks and ends the silence.

Alternatively, the therapist can tell further stories which vary, interpret or complement the first story.

The therapist can of course also ask the client to explain what he or she is thinking or imagining after hearing the story, and then start a discussion on this basis. Equally, the therapist can simply ask, "Does that mean anything to you?" Clients generally respond to this question in the affirmative, but another abstruse prompt for discussion can be offered in addition to the story if they do not. If the listener asks the therapist, "What was that supposed to mean?" the therapist can answer cryptically, "It just came into my head, and I had a feeling that it might be useful for you." The therapist does not in fact need to be able to identify a specific purpose for a story, provided that he or she has a feeling that it is appropriate – the less clear the reasons why the story has been told, the more intently the client will search for the solutions it contains.

It is not necessary to explain metaphorical stories. If the story holds meaning for the client, he or she will intuitively understand this meaning and respond to it. If the story is irrelevant, it will not become meaningful simply by being explained.

It is interesting to note that clients generally discover some benefit in a story told by a therapist, but often for reasons that are completely different to those which motivated the therapist to tell the story, suggesting that even stories that do not appear to the therapist to be of any concrete benefit might help clients in their search for solutions. Some of the main effects achieved by storytelling include a state of relaxation, a sense of hopeful expectation and a searching attitude on the part of the client, in turn making it more likely that solutions will be found. In the absence of any explanation of the story, there is a chance that the listener will search for its meaning until he or she has discovered something of use, even if it is not what the storyteller intended.

# Chapter 11

# Experiencing therapeutic stories without words

## Painted and sculpted stories

Most of the metaphors presented and discussed in this book are of a verbal nature, but paintings, drawings and sculptures can also serve as effective therapeutic metaphors. It can be useful to encourage a client to position in a central location in his or her home a picture that symbolically represents the relevant conflict or part of the personality (e.g. a wolf if the client is dealing with aggression problems). If the client is confronted with the symbol on a daily basis, he or she is likely to find solutions for dealing with the relevant situation.

One example of how stories can be incorporated into a therapeutic conversation in pictorial form is the therapeutic map "The Island of Love" (see below), which can be used in couples therapy to clarify goals, conflicts, commonalities and differences between the partners.

The therapist first asks the partners to locate themselves or (hypothetically) each other on the island, and to think about the routes they follow together and alone. He or she asks each of the partners to explain their wants and wishes for the relationship or a particular situation and to locate these on the map, or to indicate their present location on the basis of current circumstances. The map can also be altered if necessary to better represent the couple's situation.

The therapeutic conversation can focus on how near or far the partners' current goals are to each other, whether both of the partners' goals are valuable and justified (which is of course the case) and how both of the partners' wishes and wants can be achieved. Should this be done individually or together? Should they take turns? Who should go first, and who should get a go more often, or for longer, or if there is any doubt?

The therapist can ask about the boulders which must be cleared out of the way and the swampy patches, and any roads or telephone lines that will need to be built.

The therapist can also use circular questions, that is, ask the man in the presence of his wife, "Imagine I asked your wife where she was located on the map in the situation you've described, what do you think she would say?" The wife can be asked the same in reverse, and the therapist can then encourage the partners to reveal what they really think, revealing how much (or how little) the partners' self-assessments correspond to their assessments of each other.

The therapist can ask the partners to describe their arguments by rating the violence of volcanic eruptions, wind strength or wave height, and then discuss why a volcanic eruption rated as a ten by one partner was only rated as a two by the other.

The different areas on the island can be discussed to make it clear that "love" can take many different shapes, that the behaviour of both partners can still be "love" even if it looks completely different, and that all forms of expressing love are valuable.

The therapist and clients can talk about why it is impossible to be on the Peak of Excitement (or the Coast of Falling in Love) at the same time as being amongst the Gentle Slopes of the Familiar at the foot of the Hill of Home, and discuss how all these different types of "love" can be incorporated into life without incurring too many other losses. They can discuss the possibility of round trips, departures, shipwrecks etc. in metaphorical terms, avoiding concrete references to these options that might otherwise be perceived as huge threats, stirring up conflict or paralysing the conversation; the use of metaphors to express opportunities and risks will thus ensure that the dialogue is more open.

The therapist can of course also set the couple the task of producing their own "Island of Love" as homework. It is best if this task if completed separately at first, without discussing it with the other partner, and only then should the maps be compared, for example at the next therapy session. The partners can ultimately negotiate and produce a joint map of their very own "Island of Love". (See Figure 11.1: the map of the island was first published in Hammel, 2006: 156.) The story "The Island of Love" can also be told when introducing the map:

> Far out in the sea, off the coast and behind the Cape of Storms, is a small island. It is so small that it only appears on the most detailed of maps, and yet it enjoys a certain level of notoriety among experts in the field. Sailors refer to it as the "island of love". Many people take a trip there once in their lifetime, or perhaps even more than once. They undertake a thorough exploration of the island, and they make some amazing discoveries. Some of them – before they get to know the island better – think that they can travel straight from the Coast of Falling in Love to the Hill of Home, and are surprised at the round-about route they have to take through the Valley of Mystery at the centre of the island. Others are amazed that it is impossible for them to visit the gentle Slopes of the Familiar while remaining on the Peak of Excitement. Yet others look forward to visiting the Cauldron of Passion (the large volcanic crater on the island), and are puzzled when they discover that the ascent is extremely

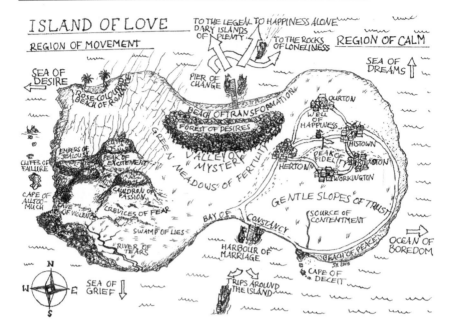

*Figure 11.1* Therapeutic map: The Island of Love.

challenging, and the path leads by the bubbling Crevice of Fear and the smoking Chimney of Rage. Thrill-seekers bathe off the Cliffs of Failure near the Cape of Alltoomuch, but even the easterly Ocean of Boredom has claimed victims among practised swimmers who have got into trouble there or even drowned. The reason I'm saying this is because people often forget that the only visitors who discover the full beauty of the island are those who explore all of it, notwithstanding all its difficulties and dangers. Some people build houses on the island or put up tents there, and I've noticed that these old-timers look with a wry grin at the eager newcomers who still hope to explore the island in just one day or one week." (Cf. Hammel, 2012b: 62.)

The map of the island can be obtained in A2 (coloured, hard plastic) or A3 format (black and white, laminated paper) from the publisher. A more detailed description is found at www.stefanhammel.de.

Following the same principle as the "Island of Love", teams or individual team members can draw a map of an island representing their workplace or team as part of supervision.

The procedure can be varied by drawing and discussing the floor plan or cross section of a house (the House of the Mind, the House of Relationships, the Team House) instead of an island.

## Pantomime stories

In cases where two people cannot make themselves understood verbally, pantomime can be used as a form of communication in addition to painting pictures and showing photographs and videos. This may prove necessary if the two parties do not share a common language or if one of them suffers from a mental impairment or a neurological disorder that has affected his or her ability to speak.

When considering the use of pantomime-type stories, we should remember that even animals communicate using symbolic rituals, and our dreams tell us stories both night and day without using verbal language.

These prelinguistic stories form the basis for our thoughts; they are examples and metaphors that provide us with inspiration for new ways of seeing the world and behaving. The story "Pantomime" provides an example of how a therapist can use pantomime-type paradigmatic and metaphorical stories to shape the therapeutic process.

## Concrete stories and lived stories

The intervention type I refer to under the term "realized metaphor" is extremely useful in a therapeutic context, and can in fact be divided into two different types of intervention. In the first, the client (or more rarely the therapist) performs an action as a symbolic metaphor expressing or triggering past or future changes in the life of the client or others; this was the procedure followed by Milton Erickson when he sent clients to walk up the nearby "Squaw Peak" and watch the sunrise (O'Hanlon & Hexum, 1991: 29, 256). Those who undertook this task found that it became a symbol of a positive change in their lives, and allowed them to gain a fresh perspective. Their unconscious mind took the metaphor experienced in such an immediate way as a prompt to implement something similar in the analogous spheres where the patients were facing problems. Compare for example the painting of the body in the story "Crossed Out".

The second of these intervention types involves presenting an object as a metaphor, or in other words showing or giving the client an object which acts as a metaphorical instruction to carry out a particular change. Compare the plant in the story "Dry" and the story "The Bin Monster".

The technique of giving homework is well known in the field of systemic therapy (compare the case study "Pest"). The tasks assigned for this purpose generally involve experiments which heighten the client's perception of their situation (increasing complexity), promote new interpretations (real reframing) and change their interactions with the rest of the world (pattern interrupt). Similarly, rituals in therapy (like the pilgrimage in the story "Dry") make it possible to mark the end of one chapter of life with a sense of gratitude, and to celebrate the start of a new one (punctuation of life events).

Rituals can also be used to prioritise a healing suggestion (by way of analogy to marking). Nursery rhymes such as "Rain, rain, go away..." are well known, and medieval folk medicine is a rich source of magic spells and actions which (if we disregard the assumed presence of some higher spiritual power) use the placebo effect to activate the body's own self-healing powers. An example is the spell and ritual in the story "The Lipoma".

One's entire life can be regarded as a story which is written or painted as the years roll by.

I remember the colouring books we were given as children, with outlines of figures which we coloured in with brightly coloured crayons. We tried hard not to go over the lines, and we put a great deal of care, love and passion into these pictures, spending hours at a time on them. When we had finished we would show our work to our parents, who would praise our efforts and stick them up on the wall. I learned a great deal from my elder siblings – I learned to believe that I could colour in. Sometimes I tried to colour like them, but then I learned to colour the pictures in my own unique style. Every individual is a work of art. Every picture is an original. And every copy is also an original – the original of the copy.

# Chapter 12

# Appendix

## List of stories

A Desire for Life 169
A Girl Like Robin Hood 166
A Glance into the Garden 99
A Good Reason to Stop Therapy 93
A Jarful of Allergies 40
A Lovely Christmas 150
A Sacred Agreement 181
A Single Request 139
A Walk Along the Beach 59
Africa 72
After the Storm 71
Alarm Clock with a Snooze Button 82
Almost Too Late and not Too Early 142
Anna's Submarine 131
Arm Wrestling 50
At the First Fart 148
Bad English 191
Balance 190
Behind the Wardrobe! 170
Blinded by Love 60
Blocked-Up Ears 163
Boat Ride by Night 86
Breathless 84
Call-Out 44
Catching Up 184
Celibacy 136
Children's Shoes 177
Christmas Bell 61
Compass and Magnet 94
Continent Eyes 79
Cow Bells 86

Crooked and Straight 61
Crossed Out 55
Dark Room 114
Day's March 189
Different 175
Dinner for One 101
Dirty Children 189
Dot to Dot 27
Dry 96
Dung Beetle 184
Dying at the Age of 26 121
Exam Revision 180
Exemplary 191
Expanding Time, Contracting Time 59
Fact 148
Fear of Moths 117
Finding Treasure 103
Finished 176
From Oasis to Oasis 100
From the Crocodile's Mouth 111
Glasses 27
Go Away 53
Gockle's Good Luck 24
Good Morning Everyone! 30
Gramophone 126
Grandma's Cooking 199
Gregor The Dragon 172
Grunting 120
Hearing Difficulty 63
Heaven on Earth 185
How Do You Break a Spell? 111
How Do You Tame a Dragon? 115
How to Handle Sexual Assault... 90
Hypnotising Dogs 65
I'll Come Again 144
If You Can Manage... 51
Illness on Order 40
Instead of a Lullaby 88
Invisible Friends 177
Jellyfish I 152
Jellyfish II 153
Keep All Cells Alive 48
King of the Wood 119
Language Rules 95

Learning to Talk 74
Learning to Walk 75
Life as a Game 105
Life as a Sinus Curve 100
Love 154
Love of Cats 162
Managing Without Them 168
Manta Ray 34
Marks Out of Ten 187
Me Too 137
Memory 73
Mental Block 182
Morbus Feivel 38
Motorway Roadworks 143
Mr Peabrain 53
Mrs Brain 133
Mrs Flow 67
Mrs Sing 68
My Aim in Life 23
My Right Eye 83
Nails Make the Man 104
Noah's Brothers 98
Nosebleed 32
November Blues 102
Numb Feet 126
Of Artists and Strategists 188
Of Cars and Men 99
Of Following and Leading 179
Of Pain and Lice 52
On the Riverbed 142
On the Threshold 168
Outbreaks 94
Pantomime 70
Past the Expiry Date 154
Peace Settlement with a Tooth 57
Peer and Rasputin 106
Pest 159
Pirate Anaesthesia 56
Placebo I 35
Placebo II 35
Placebo III 43
Placebo IV 43
Playing I 195
Playing II 195

Playing III 195
Playing IV 196
Progress 193
Pulling the Goat Home 163
Releasing the Spring 87
Renewed Life 23
Returning the Key 200
Revenge 107
Risk of Contagion 39
Sacrilege 24
Selling Pain 54
Shifting Interests 76
Shiny or Matt 150
Slides 124
Snail Race 89
Snoring 85
Social Noises 109
Soiled Underwear Again 80
Sorting Screws 76
Speed 192
Stand Up 142
Start of Term in the Staffroom 118
Steam Engines 35
Stop 85
Surfing the Waves 143
Table Tennis 112
Taekwondo 63
Target Practice 190
Temptation 151
Thank You 106
That Day 109
The Archivist 73
The Bin Monster 199
The Bladder Alarm Clock 81
The Blade of Grass in the Crack 125
The Bulls Are Coming 103
The Camel 196
The Cardboard Box Dressing 173
The Cart, The Mud and I 96
The Cave Dwellers 26
The Cellar Spider I 112
The Cellar Spider II 113
The Consultation 187
The Converter 31

The Creation of the World 25
The Dance of the Thorns and the Knives 140
The Desert 129
The Difference 170
The Disconnectable Body 55
The Door 192
The Eagle and The Falconer 149
The Eagle Chick 156
The Eagle's Journey 36
The Emergency Alarm Button 153
The Fat Woman and the Thin Woman 91
The Filing Cabinet 124
The Film 109
The Frozen Hiccup 51
The Gang of Pigs 116
The Genie 178
The Goal Behind the Goal 194
The Good Gel 58
The Hindenburg Path 62
The Keys 72
The King Is Coming 198
The Left-Handed Person 78
The Legacy 146
The Lipoma 47
The Little Cat 164
The Man Who Wins When He Loses 127
The Nail 77
The New Word 197
The People of Lensland 92
The Persecuted I 134
The Persecuted II 135
The Potential of Weeds 188
The Power of Thoughts 104
The Price of Success 182
The Pruned Tree 66
The Recovery Game 42
The Replanted Tree 161
The Route Through the Mountain 183
The Sailor on Shore 65
The Schneiders 155
The Schoolchildren's Fairy 165
The Secret Name 110
The Shoelace Debate 164
The Silent Hand 48

The Spanish Conquistadors 107
The Three Principles 176
The Villa 45
The Way to the Meadow 41
The Winter Rose 160
The Worry Catapult 49
The Wrong Audience 122
Theatre Trip 30
Three Boxes 123
Time Adjustment 169
Tourette's 119
Trying It Out 144
Ugly and Beautiful 151
Wart Remedy 47
Wasted Time 123
What Does That Make Me? 28
What Use Are Friends? 173
When Someone Says 'Stefan Hammel' 159
When You Meet Your Brother... 139
Without Words 29
You'll Manage It 176
Zero-Problem Therapy 158

# Literature

Abraham, H. (1990). Suggestion for Prevention of Seasonal Allergies. In: D. Hammond (ed.), *Handbook of Hypnotic Suggestions and Metaphors* (pp. 265–266). New York: Norton.

Bach, R. (1991). *Jonathan Livingston Seagull: A Story*. London: Thorsons.

Bambaren, S. (1994). *The Dolphin: Story of a Dreamer*. Punta Sal (Peru): Bambaren.

Bandler, R., & Grinder, J. (1981). *Trance-formations: Neurolinguistic Programming and the Structure of Hypnosis*. Boulder (CO): Real People.

Bonder, N. (1999). *Yiddishe Kop: Creative Problem Solving in Jewish Learning, Lore, and Humor: The Way of Creative Problem Solving in Jewish Learning, Lore and Humor*. Boston: Shambhala.

Crasilneck, H., & Hall, J. (1985). Hypnotic Technique for Treating Warts. In: D. Hammond (ed.), *Handbook of Hypnotic Suggestions and Metaphors* (pp. 223–224). New York: Norton, 1990.

Edel, J. (1959). Nosebleed controlled by hypnosis. *American Journal of Clinical Hypnosis,* 2: 89–90.

Erickson, M., & Rossi, E. (1979). *Hypnotherapy: An Exploratory Casebook.* New York: Irvington.

Erickson, M., & Rossi, E. (1981). *Experiencing Hypnosis: Therapeutic Approaches to Altered States by Milton H. Erickson*. New York: Irvington.

Erickson, M., Rossi, E., & Rossi, S. (1976). *Hypnotic Realities. The Introduction of Clinical Hypnosis and Forms of Indirect Suggestion*. New York: Irvington.

Gibbons, D. (1979). Suggestions for Warts (modeled after Hartland). In: D. Hammond (ed.), *Handbook of Hypnotic Suggestions and Metaphors* (pp. 224–225). New York: Norton, 1990.

Hammel, S. (2006). *Der Grashalm in der Wüste: 100 Geschichten aus Beratung, Therapie und Seelsorge*. Mainz: Verlag, Nierstein.

Hammel, S. (2007). Ist mein Kind reif für die Schule? *KidsLife*, 1/07: 50–51.

Hammel, S. (2008). Meine Tochter kann sich nicht durchsetzen! *KidsLife,* 1/08: 12.

Hammel, S. (2009). Tinnitustherapie durch Hypnose: Der Heidelberger Pilotversuch. *Musica Sacra*, 4/09: 223–224.

Hammel, S. (2010). Von Möwenfelsen und Felsenbirnen: Aufbruchsgeschichten für Kinder und Jugendliche. In: Familiendynamik. *Systemische Praxis und Forschung*, 2/10: 136–143.

Hammel, S. (2011). *Handbuch der therapeutischen Utilisation: Vom Nutzen des Unnützen in Psychotherapie, Kinder- und Familientherapie, Heilkunde und Beratung.* Stuttgart: Klett-Cotta.

Hammel, S. (2012a). Utilisation. In: H. Kleve, & J. Wirth (eds), *Lexikon des systemischen Arbeitens: Grundbegriffe der Systemischen Praxis, Methodik und Theorie* (pp. 441–444). Heidelberg: Carl Auer.

Hammel, S. (2012b). *The Blade of Grass in the Desert: Storytelling, Forgotten Medicine for Healing the Soul: A Story of 100 Stories for Counseling and Therapy.* Mainz: Kidslife Medienverlag.

Hammel, S. (2014). *Therapie zwischen den Zeilen: Das ungesagt Gesagte in Beratung, Therapie und Heilkunde.* Stuttgart: Klett-Cotta.

Hammel, S. (2015). *Das Stühlespiel: Eine neue, radikal wirksame Therapiemethode.* Freiburg (Germany): Kreuz.

Hammel, S. (2016). *Alles neu gerahmt!: Psychische Symptome in ungewöhnlicher Perspektive.* Munich: Reinhardt.

Hammel, S. (2017). *Grüßen Sie Ihre Seele!: Therapeutische Interventionen in drei Sätzen.* Stuttgart: Klett-Cotta.

Kohen, D. (1990). A Hypnotherapeutic Approach to Enuresis. In: D. Hammond (ed.), *Handbook of Hypnotic Suggestions and Metaphors* (pp. 489–493). New York: Norton, 1990.

Kohen, D., & Olness, K. (2011): *Hypnosis and Hypnotherapy with Children.* New York: Routledge.

Kopp, S. (1971). *Guru: Metaphors from a Psychotherapist.* Palo Alto (CA): Science & Behavior

Lamprecht, K., Hürzeler, A., Hammel, S., & Niedermann, M. (2016). *Wie das Krokodil zum Fliegen kam: 120 Geschichten, die das Leben verändern.* Munich: Reinhardt.

Lamprecht, K., Hürzeler, A., Hammel, S., & Niedermann, M. (2018). *Wie der Bär zum Tanzen kam: 120 Geschichten für Kopf und Bauch.* Munich: Reinhardt.

Mir Amman (1803). *A Tale of Four Dervishes.* London: Penguin. (Urdu translation of Amir Khusrau's 13th century tale, retranslated and reedited 1994.)

Monk, G (1996). *Narrative Therapy in Practice. The Archeology of Hope.* San Francisco: Jossey-Bass.

Mozdzierz, G. (1990). Suggestion for Alleviating Hickups. In: D. Hammond, *Handbook of Hypnotic Suggestions and Metaphors* (p. 267). New York: Norton, 1990.

Mrochen, S. (2002). Das RMI-Konzept (Relaxation Mental Imagery). Hypnosetherapie bei der Behandlung kindlicher Verhaltensstörungen – dargestellt am Beispiel Enuresis. In: S. Mrochen, K.-L. Holtz, & B. Trenkle (eds), *Die Pupille des Bettnässers. Hypnotherapeutische Arbeit mit Kindern und Jugendlichen* (pp. 117–123). Heidelberg: Carl Auer.

Mücke, K. (2001). *Probleme sind Lösungen: Systemische Beratung und Psychotherapie: Ein pragmatischer Ansatz.* Potsdam: Mücke.

O'Hanlon, W., & Hexum, A. (1991): *An Uncommon Casebook: The Complete Clinical Work of Milton H. Erickson: Complete Clinical Work of Milton H. Erickson, M.D.* New York: Norton.

Pelletier, A. (1990). Suggestions for Concentration, Studying, and Overcoming Test Anxiety. In: D. Hammond, *Handbook of Hypnotic Suggestions and Metaphors* (pp. 460–462). New York: Norton.

Prior, M. (2007). *Beratung und Therapie optimal vorbereiten: Informationen und Interventionen vor dem ersten Gespräch.* Heidelberg: Carl Auer.

Prior, M. (2017). *MiniMax Interventions: 15 Simple Therapeutic Interventions That Have Maximum Impact.* Carmarthen: Crown House.

Rosen, S. (ed.) (1982). *My Voice Will Go with You: Teaching Tales of Milton H. Erickson: Teaching Tales of Milton H. Erickson.* New York: Norton.

Schmidt, G. (2004). *Liebesaffären zwischen Problem und Lösung: Hypnosystemisches Arbeiten in schwierigen Kontexten.* Heidelberg: Carl Auer.

Schulz von Thun, F. (1998). *Miteinander reden 3: Das innere Team und situationsgerechte Kommunikation:* Reinbek (Germany): Rowohlt.

Schneider, P. (2009). Musik, von Engeln vorgesungen: Entstehung und Ursachen von Tinnitus und Geräuschempfindlichkeit bie Kirchenmusikern, Chorleitern, Bläsern und Sängern. *Musica Sacra,* 4/09: 220–222.

Schneider, P., Andermann, M., Wengenroth, M., Goebel, R., Flor, H., Rupp, A., & Diesch, E. (2009). Reduced volume of Heschl's gyrus in tinnitus. *Neuroimage* 45: 927–939.

Schulz von Thun, F., & Stegemann, W. (eds) (2004). *Das innere Team in Aktion: Praktische Arbeit mit dem Modell.* Reinbek (Germany): Rowohlt.

Short, D., & Weinspach, C. (2007). *Hoffnung und Resilenz: Therapeutische Strategien von Milton Erickson.* Heidelberg: Carl Auer.

Singer, I. B. (1968). *When Shlemiel Went to Warsaw and Other Stories.* New York: Farrar, Straus & Garoux.

Thurber, J. (1983). *Fables for Our Time and Famous Poems Illustrated.* New York: Harper & Row.

Trenkle, B. (1998). *Die Löwengeschichte: Hypnotisch-metaphorische Kommunikation und Selbsthypnosetraining.* Heidelberg: Carl Auer.

Trenkle, B. (2002). Ericksonsche Hypno- und Psychotherapie bei Bettnässen. In: S. Mrochen, K.-L. Holtz, & B. Trenkle (eds), *Die Pupille des Bettnässers. Hypnotherapeutische Arbeit mit Kindern und Jugendlichen* (pp. 124–153). Heidelberg: Carl Auer, 2002.

Watzlawick, P., Jackson, D., & Beavin Bavelas, J. (1976). *Pragmatics of Human Communication: A Study of Interactional Patterns, Pathologies and Paradoxes.* New York: Norton.

Watzlawick, P. (1976). *How Real Is Real?: Confusion, Disinformation, Communication.* New York: Random House.

Weber, G. (ed.) (1997). *Zweierlei Glück. Die Systemische Psychotherapie Bert Hellingers.* Heidelberg: Carl Auer.

Williams, D., & Singh, M. (1976). Hypnosis as a facilitating therapeutic adjunct in child psychiatry. *Journal of the American Academy of Child Psychiatry* 15: 326–342.

Zeig, J. (2014). *A Teaching Seminar With Milton H. Erickson.* London: Routledge.

Zelling, D. (1986). Snoring: A disease of the listener. *Journal of the American Academy of Medical Hypnoanalysis* I/(2): 99–101.

# Index

abortion 139
acne 46, 49
acute coronary syndrome 34, 36
addiction 90–91, 94–96, 113, 126, 137,
     143, 151, 173, 181, 193, 232, 246,
     251, 254
adolescence *see* growing up
adoption 156, 160–161
age progression 10, 139, 144, 155, 159,
     165, 171, 210, 251–252, 272
age regression 10, 27, 57, 59, 75, 114,
     116, 127, 171, 210, 250, 251, 260,
     272, 274
ageing 144, 155, 161, 170–171, 192
aggression 35, 50, 54, 152–153, 57, 90,
     103–113, 116, 125, 152–153, 156,
     158–159, 170, 172–173, 192, 195, 245,
     255, 269, 284
alcohol 94, 96, 151, 257
allergy 41, 44, 46
Alzheimer's disease *see* dementia
ambiguity 36, 57, 72, 86, 88–9, 91, 141,
     278–9, 281
ambivalence 23, 91, 94–95, 99, 104,
     111, 149–150, 152, 154, 164–165,
     175, 177, 188–189, 191–193, 237–239,
     241, 244, 253–254, 256–257, 263;
     *see also* ambiguity; externalization;
     prioritisation
amnesia (hypnotic amnesia) 11, 57, 225,
     228, 273; *see also* memory
amputation 57, 59, 66
anaesthesia (hypnotic anaesthesia)
     10–11, 51, 53–60, 225, 271, 273;
     *see also* narcosis
anamnesis: through bodily signals 166;
     through changes to the voice 166;
     questions 61, 81, 166, 182, 274

anchoring 41, 109, 117, 120, 127, 156,
     171, 233, 269; *see also* conditioning
angina pectoris 33–34, 36
anorexia 91–92
anxiety 34, 40, 50, 57, 59, 94, 103–104,
     106, 111, 113–119, 124–125, 136, 143,
     176, 183, 189, 228, 232–234, 240, 244,
     269, 279; with children *see* monsters
aphasia 66, 68, 70, 75
appendix 44
arachnophobia 117
Asperger syndrome/autism 29, 92, 125,
     131, 133, 175–176, 179, 193
asthma 34–36, 88, 127, 245
attention 47, 53, 61, 63–65, 68, 76, 80,
     87, 91–92, 94–95, 131, 133, 151, 153,
     159, 172, 175–179, 183, 193, 209–210,
     225–226, 231–232, 243–245, 264, 270,
     274, 277–278, 280–281
attention deficit disorder (ADD / ADHD)
     61, 87, 159, 172, 175–176, 178–179, 193
attention focus: reversal 37, 47, 53,
     61–65, 91–92, 95, 177, 183, 181–182;
     shift from body to mind 61, 80, 232;
     shift from deficit to resource 68, 153,
     231; shift from feeling to hearing 65,
     232; shift from feeling to seeing 225;
     shift from inside to outside 131
attractiveness 160–161, 168, 227
avoidance 128, 219, 248

bedwetting 81
belief 24, 27, 137–138, 145, 177,
     185–187, 189, 192, 211, 229, 230,
     237–238, 245, 263–264
Bell's palsy 50
biography 100, 146
bipolar disorder 129

bleeding 32–34
blended family 156, 160–161
blood flow 32–35, 261
blood pressure *see* hypertonia; hypotonia
body dysmorphic defect (BDD) 91–92
body language 29, 50, 70, 88, 145, 166
bone fractures 46
borderline personality disorder 35, 93, 111–112, 190
breath pacing 65, 88, 271
breathing 34, 84, 94, 234, 243, 245, 269, 271
bulimia 49, 93–94, 151, 194
bullying 40, 100, 104–110, 112–113, 116, 134–136, 153–154, 172
burning 48
burnout syndrome 8, 50, 100, 107, 129, 190–191, 193

cancer 66, 80, 96, 100, 144, 160, 193; *see also* chemotherapy
caretaking 142, 173
catalepsy 10, 51, 57, 90, 107, 225, 228, 270, 273
chemotherapy 65, 144, 160, 193
children's home 160–161, 172
chronic disease 77, 144, 160, 193
chronic obstructive pulmonary disease (COPD) 35
circular reasoning 31, 239
civil disobedience 190–191
clicking jaw 86
cold 38–39, 42–43, 49
cold sores 39
colitis 44–46, 94
coma 65, 145
complexity 236; increase 29, 110, 119, 123, 138, 141, 148–149, 151, 169, 196, 287; reduction 152, 163, 168, 185, 189, 190, 192, 195, 197, 287
compulsion (OCD) 27, 38, 40, 62, 94, 104, 119–21, 125, 137, 154, 173, 176, 178–179, 181, 189, 192–193; hoarding 154, 178, 193; washing 38, 189
conditioning: sleeping behaviours 81, 83–86, 234; waking behaviours 87, 109, 117, 120, 133, 156, 234
connotation 33, 44, 47, 57, 66, 68, 86, 89, 98, 141, 146, 153, 166, 168, 177, 213, 218, 221, 232, 275, 278–279
conscience 30, 40, 122, 139–140, 189
consultancy within an organisation 111, 190

control 35, 83, 119, 153, 225, 232–233, 276
convalescence 46, 66, 72–76, 126, 142
conversion disorder 61, 80
copycat death 139
coronary heart disease (CHD) 33–34, 36
cosmetic concerns 47, 49–50, 88, 171
counter double bind 112, 127, 152–153, 224, 238–239
crisis 98, 100, 129, 142–144, 206, 245, 250
criticism 99, 230
Crohn's disease 44–46, 254
crying *see* eye liquid; tears
cults *see* sects
culture *see* intercultural conflict
cutting 104, 111, 141, 190
cyclic illness 100, 144

dandruff 49, 94
death 145, 169, 210, 238, 244
debt 193
de-escalation 109, 156, 158–159, 170, 172, 192
delirium 145
delusion 27, 130; persecutory 134–137; poisoning 189, 215; poverty 166
dementia 27, 65, 76, 170
dental treatment 36, 57
depression 26, 77, 94, 96–102, 104, 114–116, 122–127, 169, 177, 187, 207, 246, 251, 279
desensitisation (systematic) 41, 68, 126, 145, 234, 244
destabilisation 164, 229, 233; of beliefs 177; through antitheses 176; through counter-rumours 30; through countertheses 26; through irritation 90, 107; through multi-partiality 91; through the prefiguration of negative consequences 93, 96, 108, 178; through unanswerable questions 26–28
developmental delay 131–133, 192
disability 65, 76, 133, 175, 192–193
dissociation 8, 11; of body halves 64; of body parts 56–57; of connotated notions 66, 110, 123–124, 127, 141, 199; of mental functions 101; of parts of the personality 110; of the two sides of the body 75
divorce *see* separation

double bind 93, 111–112, 127, 141, 152, 154, 187, 190, 224, 238–239, 255
dream 11–14, 84, 129–130, 178, 185, 187, 199, 204, 206, 210–212, 219–220, 225, 229, 234, 241, 248, 252, 273
dying 121, 144

eating disorder 151, 189, 193
economy 144, 154, 180, 183, 188–189, 192, 196
emetophobia 49
emigration 150, 166
encopresis 80, 86
enuresis 83–84
erectile dysfunction 89, 119
erotomania 134–136
erythrophobia 33, 44
exam nerves 34, 36, 44
exam revision 73–74, 180–182
excretion 79, 94
exhibitionism 90
externalisation: of ambivalence as a dialogue 23, 95, 99, 111, 149, 152, 154, 164, 175, 177, 188–189; of ambivalence as two categories of objects 94; of ambivalence as two locations 149–150, 165; of ambivalence as two patterns of movement 192–193; of ambivalence as two persons 91, 104, 191; of the problem as a game 105; of a problem as an object 41, 54; of a problem as a person 103, 116; of a problem as writing 121
eye liquid 49
eyes 61, 80, 218

facial wrinkles 50
faith 98
faithfulness 148–149, 151, 154, 228
falling asleep 87–88, 114, 119
falling out of bed 84
family 104, 108, 110, 127, 139–140, 146, 150, 153, 155–156, 159–160, 163, 166, 169–170, 185, 187, 190, 250
fear of exams 182–183
fertility 66
fever 94
flu 38–39, 42
forgiveness 62–63, 122
foster care 161
freedom 125, 149, 163
freezing 48
friends 111, 163, 171–173, 176, 215

gastroenteritis 38–39, 94, 194
giftedness 29, 159, 175, 179
goals 23–24, 27, 95, 107, 129, 168–169, 175, 178, 185–187, 190, 197, 209, 274, 284
gossip 30
grandparents 127
Graves' disease 44
grief 60, 72, 94, 100, 114, 126–127, 139, 142–144, 146, 156, 160–161, 173
growing up 24, 27, 77, 110, 120, 141, 144, 150, 152, 156–151, 163–168, 176, 184–187, 189, 192, 198

habit 61, 96, 149
haematoma 33
hair loss 77
hallucination 130, 138
Hashimoto's disease 44
hay fever see allergy
health 23, 32, 99, 142, 169, 190
hearing impairment 63
heart attack 34–36
hebephrenia see schizophrenia
hiccups 51–52
homework 29, 80, 96, 120, 133, 159, 166, 276
homosexuality 175
hope 100–102, 236
human resource management 108, 154, 164, 183, 190
hyperactivity see attention deficit syndrome (ADD / ADHD)
hyperhidrosis 49, 94
hypermnesia 10, 74, 228
hypersensitivity 10, 57
hypertonia 33, 35–36
hyperventilation 34, 36, 245
hypnotic amnesia see amnesia
hypnotic anaesthesia see anaesthesia
hypochondria 92, 189
hypotonia 35
hysterectomy 66

identity 24, 28, 100, 110, 129, 143, 146, 149–150, 175, 185–187, 189, 256
immune disease 44–46, 104
immune system 38–40, 42–46, 160, 189, 224, 229
impulse control 35, 153
incontinence 80, 86
infants 65, 88, 243
infection 37–39

inflammation 44–46
inner team 30, 56, 91, 101, 104, 111, 122,
    127, 139, 177, 190, 253
intelligence *see* giftedness
intercultural conflict 127, 150, 153, 166
interspersal technique 54, 89, 91, 127,
    145, 164, 278
invisible friends 54, 106, 133, 178, 228,
    241, 245
irradiation 48, 96, 100
itching 55, 240

jealousy 149, 152–153, 227

kindergarten 165, 172, 252

labour pains 60
language and speech 70, 75
larynx 66
learning 70–76, 176–178, 180–183, 189,
    191–195, 199, 242, 246, 251, 260
learning attitude 64, 67–68, 73, 75–76,
    165, 176–178, 180–181, 183–184, 191,
    199, 242, 260
left-handedness 78
life expectancy 23
lipoma 47, 238
loneliness 129, 160, 169, 172–173, 179,
    185–187
love *see* family; friends; parents;
    relationship; sexuality
love triangle 111
lupus erythematosus 44

magic spell 47, 288
mania 113, 128–130, 178, 192, 244
mastectomy 76
meaning 23–25, 146, 235, 283
medication 237–239; *see also* placebo
memory 15, 17, 69–78, 100–102, 170,
    200, 235, 273; *see also* amnesia;
    hypermnesia
mental game 102, 105, 108–110, 116,
    199, 229
mental gymnastics 52, 67, 70, 75, 77
metaphor 54, 70, 115–116, 203–210,
    211–215, 217–221, 227–231, 248–249,
    252–257, 260–263, 283, 284–287;
    action as 55, 96; object as 110; *see also*
    reframing
metonymy 49, 52, 81
migraine 34

mirroring 31, 112, 120, 127, 140, 210,
    237–239
misunderstanding 29–31, 37, 63, 111,
    138, 168, 242
mitral valve prolapse 86
mobilisation 126, 142
monsters 106, 114, 116, 136
motivation 118, 126, 133, 142, 163,
    177–178, 180–184, 190–198, 219, 228
moving house 77, 141, 150, 160–161,
    166, 185
multiple sclerosis 77
Munchhausen's syndrome /
    Munchhausen's syndrome by proxy
    141, 190
murder 139
muscular tension 10, 49–50, 86, 114, 269
mutism 70, 131

nail biting 131
names 110
narcosis 57, 83, 126, 155
nausea 65
neglect 94, 96, 154, 175, 178, 189, 193
nervous muscle twitching 52
neurodermatitis 104
night terrors 84
nightmare 11, 83–85, 220, 241
noise 86–87, 109

obesity 151, 193
obsession *see* compulsion (OCD)
oophorectomy 66
openness 118, 173
operation 57, 59, 66, 126, 142, 169
orchiectomy 66
ordeal 158, 200, 246
order (tidiness) 178, 188, 193, 198
overprotectiveness 164–165

pacing and leading 20, 36, 53, 67–68,
    83, 98, 127, 131, 134, 138, 179, 209,
    231–236, 263
pain 10, 15, 34, 48, 50, 52–60, 77, 114,
    119, 126, 69, 225, 233, 269, 274;
    *see also* phantom pain
painting 229, 284, 284–288
panic disorder 36, 143, 179, 192, 219,
    243, 245
pantomime 70, 215, 287
paradox: "Don't perceive what you
    are perceiving!" 63; "Don't think

about hot chocolate!" 117; "Failure is success!" 191; "I am not here!" 177; "Imagine a flat staircase!" 67; "Perceive what you are not perceiving!" 61; "What is wrong is right!" 127; "You'll wake up asleep!" 131
paradoxical intervention 51, 80–81, 96, 117, 120, 123, 141, 249
paralysis 75–76
paranoia *see* compulsion (OCD); phobia; schizophrenia
paranoid personality disorder 134–136
parenting 77, 119, 150, 162–169
parents 8, 24, 71, 75, 79, 104, 110, 111, 114, 127, 150, 155–156, 158, 161–163, 168, 288
pattern interrupt 234, 246, 274, 287; by the client 24, 90, 93, 105, 107, 112, 150, 158, 179; by the therapist 93, 173, 192
penitentiary system 125
perfectionism 62–63, 127, 176, 185–191
peripheral artery disease (PAD) 33
personality disorder *see* anxiety; borderline personality disorder; compulsion; symbiosis
phantom pain 127
phlebitis 44
phobia 15, 32–33, 36–37, 41, 44, 48–49, 57, 117, 233–234, 239
pilgrimage 96, 287
placebo 9, 79, 237–238, 288; real 47, 58, 229, 237–238; unreal 35, 41, 43–4, 47, 229, 238
political resistance *see* civil disobedience
positive connotation 47, 57, 66, 98, 117, 141, 166, 168, 177, 213
positive expectations 23, 71, 74–75, 77, 101, 114, 125–126, 145, 156, 160–161, 163–164, 168, 172, 176–178, 183, 185, 187, 196, 203, 242, 272
post-traumatic stress disorder (PTSD) *see* trauma
poverty 160, 163, 166
prejudice 28
premature ejaculation 89
premature labour 24, 36
premenstrual syndrome 152
pretended achievement ("act as if" intervention) 177
prioritisation 44, 94, 109, 145, 190
process structuring 180, 142–144, 180, 194

prolonged reversible ischemic neurological deficit (PRIND) 33
prostate 66, 80
provocation 127, 148–149, 169, 178, 191, 236, 258
psychoeducation 29, 31, 53, 73–75, 80–83, 85, 105, 119, 122, 148–149, 154, 163–164, 169, 172, 179, 181, 183, 196, 223, 242, 271–273
psychosis 130–136
psychosomatic disorder 32, 61, 80, 123–124, 173
punctuation 99–100, 176, 235–237

quality 185–191, 195–196, 199, 263
question 26–28, 30, 33, 88–89, 103, 139, 146, 206, 209–210, 212, 216, 230–231, 252–3, 261, 263, 270, 284; anamnesis 61, 81, 166, 182, 274–275; rhetorical 27, 121, 133, 142–143, 220, 230; suggestive 31, 62, 133, 142, 163, 221, 226, 230, 241

rape *see* sexual abuse; trauma; violence
rapport 8–10, 71, 76, 88, 120, 179, 206, 224, 243–245, 269, 271, 275; disruption 90, 107, 245–246; imagined 34, 36, 64, 67–68, 75, 138–140, 177–178, 245
reality 17–19, 26–28, 30–31, 38, 61–62, 177, 187, 192, 195, 197, 207–208, 211, 225, 228–229
reframing: metaphorical 27, 36, 44–46, 66, 72–74, 98–99, 110, 129, 137, 141–142, 151–153, 156, 160–161, 164, 192; real 28, 118, 146, 159, 166, 170, 226–227; unreal 39, 41–42, 50, 54, 56, 59, 87, 102, 105–6, 109, 116, 121, 133, 144, 178, 194, 199, 226
relationship 18, 31, 85, 96, 99, 107–108, 111, 137, 142, 144, 148–155, 163, 169, 173, 176, 179, 183, 185, 187, 190, 218, 238, 245, 250, 256, 284
resistance (avoiding) 57, 112, 246, 280
resources 13, 19, 98, 226, 230–231, 241, 252; expanding 107, 112, 125, 230–231; finding 24–28, 98–99, 164; optimising 20, 199, 230; protecting 190–191, 195–196
responsibility 107–108, 118, 129, 178, 183, 185–187, 195
reward and punishment 51, 158, 181, 200, 246

rhagades 49
ritual 47, 96, 141, 145, 150, 276, 288
romantic relationship 148
rumour 30, 230

sarcoidosis 44–46
scatological language 120
schizophrenia 133; catatonic 112, 131;
    hebephrenic 113, 177; paranoid-
    hallucinatory 131, 134–136, 138
school 104–106, 163, 165, 172, 176, 216
searching attitude 4, 23–24, 26–27, 30,
    61–63, 72–74, 76, 88, 92, 94, 103,
    112–113, 125, 142, 153, 155, 163,
    165, 171–173, 176, 177, 183, 185–187,
    195, 197, 213, 226, 245, 250, 258,
    267, 283
sects 110, 134–137, 173
sedation 145
seeding 57, 164, 275–276, 278
self-communication 95, 98, 104
self-confidence 24, 27, 30, 50, 92,
    105–106, 116, 127, 160–161, 165, 168,
    177–178, 222, 228, 278
self-harming behaviour 93, 104, 141, 190
self-perception 61, 91–92, 137, 254
sending symptoms back into the past 57,
    126–127
sense of balance 64–65, 225
separation 108, 137, 142–143, 149, 152,
    154, 156, 173, 183, 232–234, 258
sexual abuse 110–111, 152, 173
sexual harassment 90
sexuality 66, 80, 88–89, 119,
    151–153, 179
shock 126, 233, 273
shyness 92, 228
siblings 104, 156, 159, 288
simulants 190
skin (oily, dry) 46, 49
sleep 36, 57, 81–85, 87–88, 114, 119, 145,
    225, 244, 281
sleep apnoea 84, 86, 234
sleepwalking 84
slowness 170, 192, 196
smoking 95, 232, 235
snoring 85–87
somatoform disorder see conversion
    disorder
somnolence 145
specific learning disability 133, 192–193
sport (competitive) 50, 56, 194, 198

stabilisation: through praise 43, 57;
    through the prefigurement of success
    176, 185, 191; through a suggestive
    question 121
stage fright 34, 36, 44
stalking 134–136
stammering 6, 67–68
sterilisation 66
stimulation through simulation 34,
    84, 102
story series 57, 136, 159, 282
stress 7–9, 11, 15–16, 35–36, 129, 219,
    228, 253, 269, 281
stroke 68, 70–77, 243, 251
structuring of processes 142–144,
    180, 194
success 3, 24, 50, 100, 103, 107, 142,
    176–178, 180–184, 188–196, 198–199,
    231, 239, 247, 250–253
suggestion 4, 8–10, 221–226, 253,
    280–281; aversive 40, 77, 93, 96, 108,
    112, 123, 141, 152, 178, 196, 258;
    framework 95, 156, 164, 168, 272,
    275; post-hypnotic 41, 269, 276;
    pre-hypnotic 164, 275–276;
    preventive 39, 42, 48, 139–140,
    146, 275–276; test 44, 78
suicidal tendencies 138–140, 143, 173,
    190, 244, 251
survival 98, 129, 142
sweating 49, 94, 212
symbiosis 111, 255
symptom prescription 51, 80, 120, 141,
    234, 236
systematic desensitisation 41, 68, 126,
    145, 234, 244

tachycardia 34
team coaching 111
team work 108–109, 118, 153, 183, 190
tears 49, 80
teeth grinding 50, 85–86, 88
tension 49–50, 86, 88, 269
theft 166
thought experiment 139, 146, 210, 229,
    238, 273
throat clearing 94
tics 6, 94, 120, 232
time distortion 10, 60, 170, 194, 228
time management 142–144, 180–181,
    184, 192, 194, 196, 198
tinnitus 6, 15, 63–64

Tourette's syndrome 120
trance exduction 131
trance induction: through age
    progression 139; through age
    regression 27; through alienation of
    the familiar 139; through alternation
    of the familiar 74; through confusion
    54, 88, 90–91, 107, 112, 139, 175,
    177, 210; through description of a
    trance situation 57, 143; through
    dissociation 177, 271; through eye
    fixation 33, 52; through questions
    26–27, 33, 88, 133, 139, 146, 210;
    through stereotype 26, 91, 139, 146,
    210; through suggestion of trance
    characteristics 57, 143, 177
transient ischaemic attacks (TIA) 33
transsexuality 175
trauma 27, 34, 57, 72, 94, 104, 107, 110,
    117, 125, 126–127, 140, 142, 152, 176,
    199, 233, 272, 275
travel sickness 65
treatment phobia 36, 57
trichotillomania 120, 131

undercover investigators 110, 134,
    136–137
upbringing 24, 223
utilisation 236–239; of ambiguity 86,
    278; of bodily functions 52, 94;
    of connotations 68, 153, 278; of
    professional experience 46; of rapport
    71, 120, 179; of side effects and
    consequencs of treatment 66; of social
    structures 139–140; of symptoms 68,
    80, 94, 120–121, 134–136, 141, 159,
    177; of values 139–140, 145, 177

vaginismus 89
violence 104, 107–108, 110, 112, 125,
    153, 158–159, 172–173, 192
vision 100–101, 183–184, 187, 194
visual impairment 61
visualisation 41, 54, 103–105, 116, 121,
    149–150, 189, 239–240
vomiting 65, 93–94, 194

waking up 83, 244
war 12, 127, 139, 190, 211
wart 6, 47
washing see compulsion (OCD)
weight reduction see obesity
withdrawal 95, 126, 193
witness protection 110
work 190, 250
work organisation 178, 180–182, 189,
    192–193, 195–196, 198; see also time
    management
work/life balance 50, 107, 113, 129, 190,
    193, 254
workaholism 113
wound healing 46
wrinkles see cosmetic concerns; facial
    wrinkles

yes set 133–136, 146, 209, 240, 244

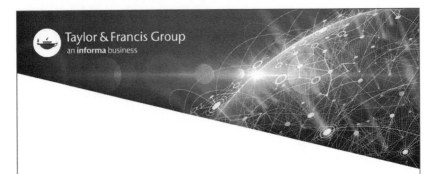